AF506307

Ganciclovir Therapy for Cytomegalovirus Infection

Ganciclovir Therapy for Cytomegalovirus Infection

edited by

Stephen A. Spector

University of California at San Diego
San Diego, California

Marcel Dekker, Inc.　　　New York • Basel • Hong Kong

ISBN 0-8247-8572-X

This book is printed on acid-free paper.

Copyright © 1991 by MARCEL DEKKER, INC.   All Rights Reserved

Neither this book nor any part may be reproduced or transmitted in any form or by any means, electronic or mechanical, including photocopying, microfilming, and recording, or by any information storage and retrieval system, without permission in writing from the publisher.

MARCEL DEKKER, INC.
270 Madison Avenue, New York, New York, 10016

Current printing (last digit):
10 9 8 7 6 5 4 3 2 1

PRINTED IN THE UNITED STATES OF AMERICA

Preface

Cytomegalovirus (CMV) is a frequent cause of congenital infection and can result in serious disease of immunocompromised persons, including organ transplant recipients and individuals with AIDS. Until recently, no drug has improved the outcome of individuals with CMV disease; CMV pneumonia was fatal in over 90% of bone marrow transplant recipients who developed the disease and CMV retinitis in patients with AIDS frequently rapidly progressed to blindness. Ganciclovir (GCV; previously DHPG) is the first drug that has demonstrated efficacy for the treatment of many of the diseases associated with CMV in immunocompromised persons.

In this book, an outstanding group of investigators and clinicians review the preclinical and clinical studies that have demonstrated the pharmacokinetics, tolerance, and efficacy of ganciclovir. Other chapters review methods for diagnosis of CMV disease, indications for initiation of ganciclovir therapy, and the potential for development of and methods of testing for ganciclovir resistance. Much of the information presented is an update and an expansion of work previously published in peer-reviewed journals. Some of the work presented represents clinical research in progress that indicates areas for which ganciclovir use may be expanded. Overall, this is a concise, up-to-date summary of the status of ganciclovir. However, even as this book goes to press, new advances are being made in the use of ganciclovir. In particular, phase I-II studies of orally administered ganciclovir have been completed and suggest that the oral formulation may be useful for maintenance and prophylaxis of CMV disease. New clinical studies are beginning, or are in development, which will address these important clinical questions.

Cytomegalovirus infections are treated by a broad range of clinical specialists, including internists, surgeons, ophthalmologists, and pediatricians. Multiple subspecialists are also involved in the care of patients with CMV disease, including those specializing in infectious diseases, gastroenterology, pulmonary, neurology, hematology, oncology, nephrology, cardiology, etc. This book will help these specialists care for patients with serious CMV disease and will be of considerable assistance in decisions regarding the institution, maintenance, and monitoring of ganciclovir treatment. Additionally, clinicians will learn what can be expected from ganciclovir therapy so as to better educate their patients regarding the benefits and risks associated with treatment.

Stephen A. Spector

Contents

Preface   iii
Contributors   vii

**1. In Vitro Inhibition of Cytomegalovirus
    by Ganciclovir**   1
Wayne M. Dankner and Stephen A. Spector

**2. Animal Models for Evaluating Ganciclovir Activity
    Against Cytomegalovirus**   15
John D. Shanley

3. Clinical Safety of Intravenous Ganciclovir   31
William C. Buhles, Jr.

4. Ganciclovir Pharmacokinetics   71
*Edmund V. Capparelli, James R. Lane, Robert L. Sonke,
    and James D. Connor*

5. Ganciclovir Treatment of Cytomegalovirus Retinitis in
   Patients with AIDS: Infectious Disease Perspective   83
   Mark A. Jacobson

6. Ganciclovir Treatment of Cytomegalovirus Retinitis in
   Patients with AIDS   91
   Douglas A. Jabs

7. Intravitreal Ganciclovir Therapy for
   Cytomegalovirus Retinopathy   105
   M.-H. Heinemann

8. Monitoring AIDS-Related Cytomegalovirus Retinitis   115
   Paul R. Montague and Thomas A. Weingeist

9. Ganciclovir Treatment of Cytomegalovirus Gastrointestinal
   Disease in Patients with AIDS   129
   Douglas T. Dieterich

10. Ganciclovir Treatment of Solid-Organ Transplant
    Recipients with Cytomegalovirus Disease   145
    David R. Snydman

11. Ganciclovir Treatment of Bone Marrow Transplant
    Recipients with Cytomegalovirus Disease   155
    John A. Zaia and Gerhard M. Schmidt

12. Cytomegalovirus Resistance to Ganciclovir   185
    M. Colin Jordan and Karen K. Biron

13. Combined Ganciclovir and Granulocyte-Macrophage
    Colony-Stimulating Factor in the Treatment of
    Cytomegalovirus Retinitis in AIDS Patients:
    Rationale for and Preliminary Results from a
    Phase II Randomized Trial   197
    W. David Hardy and ACTG 073 Treatment Group

14. Diagnosis of Cytomegalovirus Infection and
    Virologic Monitoring of Ganciclovir Therapy   215
    Stephen A. Spector

Index   235

Contributors

Karen K. Biron, Ph.D.   Division of Virology, The Wellcome Research Laboratories, Burroughs Wellcome Company, Research Triangle Park, North Carolina

William C. Buhles, Jr., D.V.M., Ph.D.   Syntex Research, Palo Alto, California

Edmund V. Capparelli, Pharm.D.   Pharmacy Department, University of California, San Diego, San Diego, California

James D. Connor, M.D.   Division of Infectious Diseases, Department of Pediatrics, University of California, San Diego, San Diego, California

Wayne M. Dankner, M.D.   Department of Pediatrics, University of California, San Diego, and University of California, San Diego Medical Center, San Diego, California

Douglas T. Dieterich, M.D.   Department of Medicine, New York School of Medicine, New York, New York

W. David Hardy, M.D.   AIDS Clinical Research Center, UCLA School of Medicine, Los Angeles, California

M.-H. Heinemann, M.D.   Cornell University Medical College and Memorial Sloan-Kettering Cancer Center, New York, New York

Douglas A. Jabs, M.D.   Departments of Ophthalmology and Medicine, Wilmer Opthalmological Institute, The Johns Hopkins University School of Medicine, Baltimore, Maryland

Mark A. Jacobson, M.D.   University of California and San Francisco General Hospital, San Francisco, California

M. Colin Jordan, M.D.   Departments of Medicine and Microbiology, University of Minnesota Medical School, Minneapolis, Minnesota

James R. Lane, Pharm.D.   Pharmacy Department, University of California, San Diego, San Diego, California

Paul R. Montague, C.R.A., F.O.P.S.   Department of Ophthalmology, University of Iowa, Iowa City, Iowa

Gerhard M. Schmidt, M.D., F.A.C.P.   Department of Hematology and Bone Marrow Transplantation, City of Hope National Medical Center, Duarte, California

John D. Shanley, M.D.   Department of Medicine, University of Connecticut and Veterans Administration Medical Center, Newington, Connecticut

David R. Snydman, M.D.   Departments of Medicine and Pathology, New England Medical Center, Boston, Massachusetts

Robert L. Sonke   Department of Pediatrics, University of California, San Diego, San Diego, California

Stephen A. Spector, M.D.   Division of Infectious Diseases, Department of Pediatrics, University of California, San Diego, and University of California, San Diego Medical Center, San Diego, California

Thomas A. Weingeist, M.D., Ph.D.   Department of Ophthalmology, University of Iowa, Iowa City, Iowa

John A. Zaia, M.D.   Division of Pediatrics, City of Hope National Medical Center, Duarte, California

1

In Vitro Inhibition of Cytomegalovirus by Ganciclovir

Wayne M. Dankner and Stephen A. Spector

*University of California, San Diego
and University of California, San Diego Medical Center
San Diego, California*

I. INTRODUCTION AND HISTORICAL PERSPECTIVE

The synthesis of ganciclovir [9-(1,3-dihydroxy-2-propoxymethyl)-guanine (DHPG) by several independent laboratories proved to be an important milestone in the development of antiviral agents with significant activity against human cytomegalovirus (CMV) (1-3). Prior to the synthesis of ganciclovir, few compounds had been identified as active against CMV, and none, including IUDR, interferons, acyclovir, cytosine arabinsoide, vidarabine, acyclovir, and trifluorothymidine, had demonstrated efficacy for the treatment of CMV disease (4). In fact, of all the other compounds evaluated, only phosphonoformic acid (PFA; foscarnet) has shown promise in clinical trials as a potential alternative to ganciclovir in certain CMV infections, particularly in patients who have failed ganciclovir therapy (4,5). Studies to compare ganciclovir and foscarnet for the treatment of CMV retinitis or colitis are ongoing. For a more complete discussion regarding the historical significance of these various agents, the reader is referred to a recent review by Verheyden (4).

II. MECHANISM OF ACTION

Despite the accumulation of both in vitro and in vivo information regarding ganciclovir, its mechanisms of antiviral action have not been fully elucidated. However, considerable research has clarified much of the drug's molecular biochemistry and its interaction with HSV- or CMV-infected cell lines.

Ganciclovir is a nucleoside analog of 2'deoxyguanosine with a structure similar to acyclovir, another nucleoside analog (Figure 1). Despite their structural similarities, ganciclovir has 10- to 100-fold greater activity against CMV than does acyclovir (6,7,17). This is best illustrated from the results of clinical trials in which acyclovir has had little therapeutic benefit in treating documented CMV disease (8,9). The lack of therapeutic efficacy demonstrated by acyclovir is probably due to its requirement for a virally specified thymidine kinase (TK), which CMV is lacking, to convert the drug to its monophosphate form (10). Interestingly, however, acyclovir has demonstrated efficacy when used as a prophylactic agent to reduce the incidence of symptomatic CMV infection in both bone marrow and renal transplant patients (11,12). The mechanism of acyclovir phosphorylation to account for its antiviral activity in CMV-infected cells has not been determined. Similarly, for ganciclovir, there is no direct evidence that the drug is phosphorylated to its monophosphate form by either a virally encoded or virally induced cellular enzyme; however, in ganciclovir, as with acyclovir, the active form is a triphosphate. Thus, some viral or possibly cellular kinase(s) phosphorylate the drug intracellularly (13,14).

Initial studies with one of the first ganciclovir compounds synthesized, BIOLF-62, revealed that HSV mutant strains lacking thymidine kinase demonstrated resistance to the drug, but DNA polymerase mutants that were foscarnet-resistant were still sensitive to ganciclovir (15). Of interest (as will be discussed in a later section) in these initial studies, the AD169 strain of CMV was found to be resistant to BIOLF-62 (15). However, subsequent

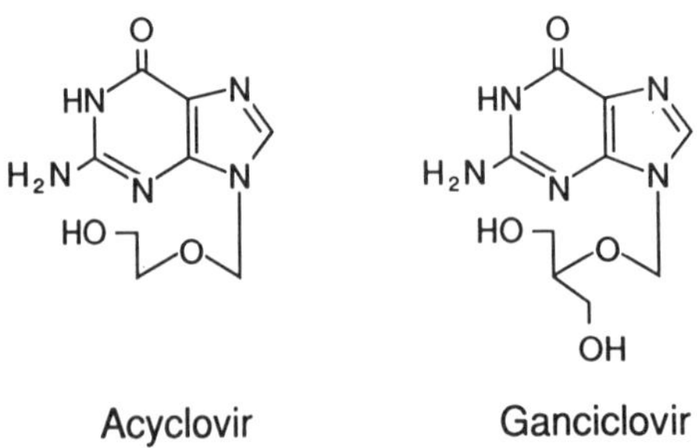

Figure 1   Biochemical structures of acyclovir and ganciclovir.

studies demonstrated that ganciclovir is more active than acyclovir against most herpesviruses, including all CMV strains (16-18).

For herpes simplex virus, TK-positive viruses, as expected, phosphorylate ganciclovir without difficulty; however, in contrast to acyclovir, TK-altered strains identified as resistant to acyclovir are as sensitive to ganciclovir as the unaltered parent strains (15,16). Additionally, DNA polymerase-altered HSV strains, resistant to either PFA or acyclovir, also maintain their sensitivity to ganciclovir (15,16). In relation to the HSV-I-encoded thymidine kinase, ganciclovir serves as a more efficient substrate than acyclovir and its monophosphate form is more efficiently phosphorylated by GMP kinase, a cellular kinase, than acyclovir-monophosphate (18). Thus, in the absence of a virally specified thymidine kinase, ganciclovir is phosphorylated to its triphosphate form much more efficiently than acyclovir (18).

As alluded to earlier, except for one report, all subsequent in vitro studies performed by a number of independent investigators have demonstrated that ganciclovir is more active against CMV than is acyclovir. The best data available, performed in CMV-infected cells, indicate that ganciclovir's major mechanism of action is the prevention of DNA elongation. In contrast to acyclovir, which acts as an immediate chain terminator, once ganciclovir is incorporated into DNA it allows the addition of usually a single nucleotide before elongation is disrupted (19). Following treatment of CMV-infected cells with ganciclovir, viral DNA synthesis can be demonstrated to be dramatically reduced. Inhibition of DNA synthesis is associated with a concomitant inhibition in the production of virus-specific late polypeptides and the apparent interruption of cell-to-cell spread associated with further virally induced cytopathic effect (20). However, the inhibition of viral DNA synthesis can be reversed when ganciclovir is removed from the tissue culture media (19,20). This failure of ganciclovir to eradicate CMV from infected cells is not surprising and has been observed with the treatment of HSV-infected cells with acyclovir (21).

Investigations into the cellular metabolism of ganciclovir have revealed that the drug is preferentially activated to its triphosphate form in CMV-infected cells. Additionally, the triphosphate form of ganciclovir is more stable than acyclovir-triphosphate (13). Combined, these differences may be responsible for much of the enhanced anti-CMV activity of ganciclovir when compared with acyclovir. In this regard, it is interesting to note that ganciclovir-triphosphate is a slightly less efficient inhibitor of the CMV DNA polymerase than is the acyclovir-triphosphate (13).

Further information regarding the mechanism(s) of action of ganciclovir against CMV has been generated by examining the mechanisms of drug resistance. In this regard, although initially a laboratory-resistant virus was thought to demonstrate resistance based on impaired intracellular phosphorylation of ganciclovir rather than an altered viral DNA polymerase, subsequent studies—described in Chapter 12—indicate that the resistance is based at least in part on an altered polymerase (14). The best apparent explanation for these reduced levels of phosphorylated ganciclovir is that CMV encodes for an as-yet unidentified nucleoside kinase that is responsible for the phosphorylation of ganciclovir. Similar mechanisms of resistance have been demonstrated for CMV-resistant viruses isolated from patients treated with ganciclovir for serious CMV infections (see Chapter 12 for details).

III. IN VITRO AND IN VIVO ACTIVITY

As discussed previously, some early in vitro studies of ganciclovir suggested that the drug was inactive against the AD169 strain of CMV (15). These erroneous findings point out some of the difficulties in establishing the sensitivity of CMV to antiviral drugs, including ganciclovir. The investigators, by using a fluorescent antibody technique to detect the presence of viral proteins, probably detected immediate early protein production that would be unaffected by ganciclovir (22). Subsequent antiviral assays, usually employing a plaque-reduction assay or a modification of plaque reduction, have found ganciclovir to have excellent activity against CMV laboratory strains and those obtained from patients who have never received ganciclovir therapy (Table 1). The ID_{50}s reported are well within concentrations of the drug achievable in patients (34). However, as reviewed in Chapter 12, patients treated with ganciclovir for prolonged periods may develop strains that are not inhibited by drug levels clinically achievable. Despite the development of resistant isolates, ganciclovir has normally demonstrated a wide therapeutic index, indicating that the drug concentrations necessary to inhibit CMV exhibited little cell toxicity. In retrospect, the initial cell cytoxicity studies performed with ganciclovir were done using human fibroblastic cell lines (13,17,22). Subsequent studies using bone marrow precursor cells have demonstrated cell toxicity at lower concentrations and help to explain the neutropenia and occasional thrombocytopenia associated with ganciclovir use in people (35).

In an attempt to improve antiviral activity against CMV, several investigators have examined drug combinations. In one such study, ganciclovir combined with recombinant beta-cysteine interferon was found to be synergistic over a narrow range of dose combinations (36). A clinical trial involving the use of both these agents was initiated, but difficulty with their concomitant administration made accrual into the study difficult. The combination of ganciclovir and foscarnet has also been examined. Although in one study this combination demonstrated synergism against HSV-II, only an additive effect was observed against CMV (37). Still other investigators have been

Table 1 Sensitivity of HCMV Strains to Ganciclovir

Name or number of strains tested	ID_{50} range (mean) μM	Reference
Laboratory-adapted strains[a]		
AD169	1.0-7.0 (3.3)	13,14,17,22,24,29
Towne	1.0-2.0 (1.5)	16,20,22
Davis	0.8-6.0 (2.9)	22,24
2	1.5-4.8 (3.2)	20
3	0.14-1.0 (0.6)	23
Clinical strains[b]		
21	0.1-10.0 (2.0)	13,16,20,22,23,25,26
54	0.4-11.0 (4.1)	27
10	1.2-11.3 (3.1)	28
25	0.9-6.3 (2.7)	29
21	1.0-5.0 (NA[c])	31
22	(3.0)[d]	32
10	0.7-4.8 (2.6)	33

[a] > 20 passages.
[b] < 10 passages.
[c] Not available.
[d] Mean only.

able to demonstrate a moderate synergistic interaction between ganciclovir and foscarnet (38). In studies performed in our laboratory, we have also examined the interaction of ganciclovir with other antivirals. We have specifically focused on determining if any antiretroviral agents used for the treatment of patients infected with HIV might alter, positively or negatively, the anti-CMV effect of ganciclovir. In these studies, we observed no antagonistic effects when ganciclovir was combined with zidovudine, dideoxycytidine, or ribavirin. We, too, noted an additive effect of foscarnet when combined with ganciclovir. Interestingly, we were able to demonstrate a synergistic effect on the CMV strains tested when ganciclovir was combined with high levels (12-15 μM) of zidovudine (39). However, the levels of zidovudine necessary to demonstrate synergism are associated with unacceptably high hematological toxicity (40). It is possible, however, that tissue levels achieved of both drugs may be sufficiently high in some patients to achieve improved anti-CMV activity.

Animal models have been used extensively to evaluate the activity of ganciclovir and other antiviral agents against herpesviruses (see Chapter 12 for details). Generally, ganciclovir has demonstrated better efficacy than acyclovir in reducing morbidity and mortality in these models.

IV. ANTIVIRAL SENSITIVITY TESTING

Antiviral sensitivity testing has become of increased importance because:
1) the increase of CMV disease in immunocompromised patients has accelerated the search for agents with anti-CMV activity and 2) the increased use of ganciclovir and the recognition that some patients treated with the drug develop significant resistance. How important the problem of resistance will become remains to be seen, but with the licensure of ganciclovir for the prolonged treatment of CMV retinitis in patients with AIDS and the use of cytokines such as GM-CSF to reduce the hematological toxicity, resistance may become an important and common clinical problem. In this regard, a recent prospective study predicted that approximately 7-8% of patients with AIDS treated with ganciclovir for CMV retinitis would develop resistant isolates (32). Thus, the need for sensitivity testing to detect these isolates and to help evaluate new drugs has become of critical importance.

Traditionally antiviral sensitivity testing has been performed using plaque-reduction assays (41,42). Although the technique may vary somewhat among laboratories, the results have usually been quite reproducible, as demonstrated by the similar ID_{50} values for ganciclovir reported by different investigators (Table 1). Thus, plaque-reduction assays are reliable, albeit work-intensive and tedious to read. In particular, they do not lend themselves well to screening large numbers of antiviral agents or to testing multiple combinations of drugs.

In view of the fact that the mode of action of antiviral compounds against CMV is usually to interrupt the synthesis of viral DNA, some investigators have utilized DNA-DNA hybridization assays to perform sensitivity testing. Through the use of viral-specific DNA probes, the percent inhibition of viral DNA synthesis produced by the antiviral agent can be quantified. The early techniques made use of ^{32}P-labeled probes and either filtered the sample DNA onto nitrocellulose filters or extracted the sample DNA before immobilization onto nitrocellulose (36,43,44). The obvious disadvantage of these techniques is the use of ^{32}P-labeled nucleotides which have a short shelf life and must be replenished for each assay. In addition, hybridization assays themselves could be cumbersome and require considerable time for completion. Recently, our laboratory has evaluated a more rapid hybridization assay that utilizes an ^{125}I-labeled, single-stranded CMV DNA probe and a novel wicking procedure to immobilize the sample DNA onto a nylon membrane (33). Once the antiviral sensitivity test has reached an endpoint, this rapid DNA hybridization assay can be performed and completed in less than one day. We have demonstrated that this assay is comparable to the traditional plaque-reduction assay in determining the ID_{50}s of several different clinical CMV strains, including resistant isolates (33) (Figure 2). A similar assay has also

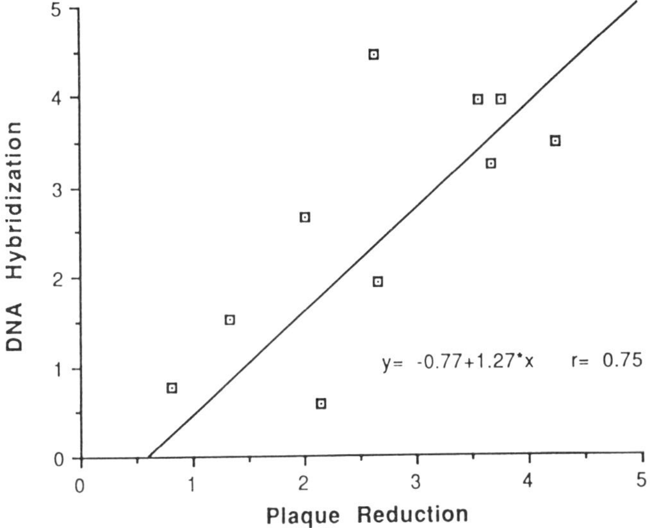

Figure 2 Linear-regression graph demonstrating comparison between plaque reduction assay and DNA-DNA hybridization assay.

been successfully used to perform sensitivity testing against HSV-I and -II strains (45).

The virus yield reduction assay, which measures the production of new viral progeny (rather than viral DNA) in the presence of antiviral compounds, has received renewed attention by formatting the technique for microtiter plates (46). However, it still requires counting plaques and at least 14 days to complete. Therefore, we do not see any advantage over the DNA-hybridization procedures other than the avoidance of radioactive probes. Additionally, because clinical strains of HCMV are highly cell-associated, the virus yield assay is frequently not useful to evaluate antiviral resistance in patient samples.

Recently another group of investigators has used a rapid culture technique, the shell vial assay, to screen CMV isolates for sensitivity to ganciclovir (47). Although this assay does not determine precisely the ID_{50} of the isolate in question, it appears to be able to detect potentially resistant isolates and allow for more detailed testing by one of the techniques described above.

Unfortunately for the detection of resistant viruses, all the above techniques require large amounts of virus to perform the assays. Because clinical isolates of CMV grow slowly, it may take several passages and possibly several weeks before sufficient virus is available to adequately evaluate the sensitivity of the isolate. Frequently, by the time antiviral resistance is determined, clinical decisions have already been made without the necessary information being available. Therefore, more rapid assays need to be developed to make the screening of potentially resistant isolates more clinically meaningful. In this regard, several laboratories are attempting to identify the genomic changes that correlate with HCMV resistance to ganciclovir. Once these areas are localized, genotypic identification of resistant viruses may provide a more rapid tool for identification of at least some HCMV strains resistant to ganciclovir.

V. SUMMARY

In conclusion, ganciclovir has excellent in vitro activity against CMV and other herpesviruses, and has demonstrated clinical efficacy. Although the molecular mechanisms of action of this drug are not completely known, there is much evidence that its major mode of action is the prevention of DNA elongation. The limited clinical success of ganciclovir has emphasized the need to develop more efficient means to evaluate antiviral activity against CMV and has stimulated the search for the identification of agents with even better activity against CMV.

ACKNOWLEDGMENTS

This work was supported in part by Public Health Service grants AI-27563, AI-27670, and AI-28270 from the National Institutes of Health.

APPENDIX: ANTIVIRAL ASSAY PROCEDURES

In this section two procedures for performing antiviral assays are described: the standard plaque-reduction assay and a rapid DNA-DNA hybridization assay.

The procedure for performing plaque-reduction assays for human CMV was described in the 1960s, first by Plummer and Benyesh-Melnick (41) and then improved by Wentworth and French (42). These early procedures used either a methylcellulose or agarose overlay and were designed for neutralization studies. Converting this assay to accommodate antiviral compounds requires only varying the drug concentrations rather than using serum dilutions. Also, most laboratories do not routinely use an agarose overlay because clinical isolates are highly cell-associated. In the case of laboratory-adapted strains that are capable of producing high-titer supernatant virus, an overlay may be indicated to prevent viral infection beyond the original plaque formation. However, we have never found this necessary using low-passage clinical isolates.

Our laboratory's antiviral assay procedure consists of growing a suitable human fibroblast cell line to confluence in either 6- or 24-well tissue culture plates. The viral isolate to be tested is passaged in this same cell line until it demonstrates 100% cytopathic effect in a 25- or 75-cm^2 tissue culture flask. Infected cells are harvested by trypsinization and added to serum-supplemented media. The cells are washed twice in phosphate-buffered saline, resuspended in serum-supplemented media, and counted, using a hemacytometer, to achieve 50-100 infectious centers per tissue culture plate well. The virus-infected cells are then adsorbed for 1 hour at 37°C before adding the antiviral compound. The antiviral compound is prepared from an appropriate stock solution that has been previously filter-sterilized. The antiviral stock solution can be made fresh or stored frozen and then thawed, if stability can be guaranteed. The working dilutions are prepared in the media being used to carry out the assay. Either the virus-containing media can be aspirated or the drug-containing media can be added directly to the wells containing the virus (in this case the drug concentration should be doubled to achieve the originally intended concentrations). The tissue culture plates are then incubated for 7-14 days (we have found that most assays require an average of 10 days) and the monolayer formalin fixed and stained with crystal violet or methylene blue. Discrete foci of virus are counted using an inverted microscope and the 50% inhibitory dose (ID_{50}) determined by using the median effect plot as described by Chou and Talalay (48). The y-axis of the graph is described by the equation $y = \log(fa/fu)$, where fa is the fraction of plaques inhibited by the antiviral agent (as compared to the infected control) and fu represents the uninhibited fraction. The x-axis is described by the equation $x = \log(D)$, where D is the concentration(s) of the drug studied. The advantage of this method is that when a combination of antiviral compounds, in fixed ratios, is used, the equations can be extended to determine the synergistic, additive, or antagonistic relationship of the compounds tested. Furthermore, these equations are now available in computer software format, further simplifying the calculations required to determine the ID_{50}s and drug-drug interactions.

For those investigators who prefer a more rapid antiviral procedure, the DNA-DNA hybridization assay may meet their needs, which has been described previously (33). The procedure is summarized below.

The assay is performed in 24-well tissue culture plates with the fibroblasts grown to confluence. Harvesting of the clinical isolate and adsorption of the virus is identical to that in the method described above, but the number of infectious centers used for the assay is increased to 3500-5000 per well in order to achieve the desired 3-4 + cytopathic effect in the non-drug-containing control wells. The desired cytopathic effect should be attained in 3-5 days (if not, then the assay may not reflect the most accurate ID_{50} for that isolate, in which case one should increase the input virus; however, input virus counts above 5000 per well usually result in higher-than-expected $ID_{50}s$ when compared to those of plaque-reduction assays). Once the desired cytopathic effect is achieved, the medium is carefully aspirated from the wells (so as not to disrupt the monolayer) and 40 μl of lysing agent (obtained in kit form from Diagnostic Hybrids, Athens, Ohio) added to each well. The resultant fluid, now containing single-stranded DNA, is wicked up onto negatively charged nylon filters by capillary action. These filters are cut into combs that bridge two wells simultaneously. When the fluid is fully wicked up, the filters are allowed to dry before the vertical portions are cut off. Once dried, the nylon filters can be stored indefinitely. The tissue culture plates may also be stored at $-70°C$ after aspiration of media from the wells. This step is convenient if one wishes to store plates for several days or weeks before performing the wicking step. Either storage method allows batching and more efficient use of the radioactive probe used in this assay. When the filters are dried, the vertical portions are placed into a vial containing the single-stranded ^{125}I-labeled HCMV probe in hybridization solution. Hybridization is carried out for 120 minutes at 60°C. The probe solution is then aspirated and the filters subsequently washed for 30 minutes at 72°C. After drying, the filters are counted in a gamma counter for 2 minutes per filter. We have found that the infected control wells should ideally yield at least 8000 counts, with the uninfected control wells usually yielding 350-500 counts. When the filters have been counted, the ID_{50} can be calculated by the method described above, where *fa* and *fu* now represent the fractions of viral DNA inhibited and uninhibited by the antiviral agent(s) tested.

REFERENCES

1. Ashton WT, Karkas JD, Field AK, Tolman RL. Activation by thymidine kinase and potent antiherpetic activity of 2′-nor-2′-deoxyguanosine (2′NDG). Biochem Biophys Res Comm 1982; 108;1716-1721.
2. Ogilvie KK, Cheriyan UO, Radatus BK, Smith KO, Gallaway KS, Kennell WL. Biologically active acyclonucleoside analogues. II. The synthesis of 9-[[2-hydroxy-1-(hydroxymethyl)ethoxy]methyl] guanine (BIOLF-62). Canadian J Chem 1982; 60:3005-3010.
3. Martin JC, Dvorak CA, Smee DF, Matthews TR, Verheyden JPH. 9-[1,3-dihydroxy-(2-propoxy)methyl] guanine: a new potent and selective anti-herpes agent. J Med Chem 1983; 26:759-761.
4. Verheyden JPH. Evolution of therapy for cytomegalovirus infection. Rev Infect Dis 1988; 10:S477-S489.
5. Walmsley SL, Chew E, Read SE, et al. Treatment of cytomegalovirus retinitis with trisodium phosphonoformate hexahydrate (foscarnet). J Infect Dis 1988; 157:569-572.

6. Plotkin SA, Starr SE, Bryan CK. In vitro and in vivo responses of cytomegalovirus to acyclovir. Am J Med 1982; 73(1A):257-261.

7. Tyms AS, Scamans EM, Naim HM. The in vitro activity of acyclovir and related compounds against cytomegalovirus infections. J Antimicrob Chemother 1981; 8:65-72.

8. Wade JC, Hintz M, McGuffin RW, Springmeyer SC, Connor JD, Meyers JD. Treatment of cytomegalovirus pneumonia with high-dose acyclovir. Am J Med 1982; 73(suppl 1A):249-256.

9. Shepp DH, Newton BA, Meyers JD. Intravenous lymphoblastoid interferon and acyclovir for treatment of cytomegaloviral pneumonia. J Infect Dis 1984; 150:776-777.

10. Elion GB. Mechanism of action and selectivity of acyclovir. Am J Med 1982; 73(suppl 1A):7-13.

11. Meyers JD, Reed EC, Shepp DH, et al. Acyclovir for prevention of cytomegalovirus infection and disease after allogeneic marrow transplantation. N Engl J Med 1988; 318:70-75.

12. Balfour HH, Chace BA, Stapleton JT, Simmons RL, Fryd DS. A randomized, placebo-controlled trial of oral acyclovir for the prevention of cytomegalovirus disease in recipients of renal allografts. N Engl J Med 1989; 320:1381-1387.

13. Biron KK, Stanat SC, Sorrell JB, et al. Metabolic activation of the nucleoside analog 9-[[2-hydroxy-1-(hydroxymethyl)ethoxy]methyl] guanine in human diploid fibroblasts infected with human cytomegalovirus. Proc Natl Acad Sci USA 1985; 82:2473-2477.

14. Biron KK, Fyfe JA, Stanat SC, et al. A human cytomegalovirus mutant resistant to the nucleoside analog 9[(2-hydroxy-1-(hydroxymethyl)ethoxy)methyl] guanine (BW 759U) induces reduced levels of BW 759U triphosphate. Proc Natl Acad Sci USA 1986; 83:8769-8773.

15. Smith KO, Galloway KS, Kennel WL, Ogilvie KK, Radatus TK. A new nucleoside analog, 9-[(2-hydroxy-1-(hydroxymethyl)ethoxy)methyl] guanine, highly active in vitro against herpes simplex virus types 1 and 2. Antimicrob Agents Chemother 1982; 22:55-61.

16. Cheng YC, Huang ES, Lin JC, et al. Unique spectrum of activity of 9-[(1,3-dehydroxy-2-propoxy)methyl]-guanine against herpes virus in vitro and its mode of action against herpes simplex virus type 1. Proc Natl Acad Sci USA 1983; 80:2767-2770.

17. Smee DF, Martin JC, Verheyden JPH, Matthews TR. Anti-herpes virus activity of the acyclic nucleoside 9-(1,3-dihydroxy-2-propoxymethyl) guanine. Antimicrob Agents Chemother 1983; 23:676-682.

18. Field AK, Daview ME, Dewitt C, et al. 9-[(2-hydroxy-1-(hydroxymethyl)ethoxy)-methyl] guanine: A selective inhibitor of herpes group virus replication. Proc Natl Acad Sci USA 1983; 80:4139-4143.

19. Mar EC, Chiou JF, Cheng YC, Huang ES. Inhibition of cellular DNA polymerase α and human cytomegalovirus-induced DNA polymerase by the triphosphates of 9-(2-hydroxyethoxymethyl) guanine and 9-(1,3-dihydroxy-2-propoxymethyl) guanine. J Virol 1985; 53:776-780.

20. Mar EC, Cheng YC, Huang ES. Effect of 9-(1,3-dihydroxy-2-propoxymethyl) guanine on human cytomegalovirus replication in vitro. Antimicrob Agents Chemother 1983; 24:518-521.

21. Klein RJ, DeStefano E, Friedman-Kien AE, Brady E. Effect of acyclovir on latent herpes simplex virus infections in trigeminal ganglia of mice. Antimicrob Agents Chemother 1981; 19:937-939.

22. Tocci MJ, Livelli TJ, Perry HC, Crumpacker CS, Field AK. Effects of the nucleoside analog 2'-nor-2'-deoxyguanosine on human cytomegalovirus replication. Antimicrob Agents Chemother 1984; 25:247-252.

23. Tyms AS, Davis JM, Jeffries DJ, Meyers JD. BWB759U, an analog of acyclovir, inhibits human cytomegalovirus in vitro [letter]. Lancet 1984; 2:924-925.

24. Frietas VR, Smee DF, Chernow M, Boehme R, Matthews TR. Activity of 9-(1,3-dihydroxy-2-propoxymethyl) guanine compared with that of acyclovir against human, monkey, and rodent cytomegaloviruses. Antimicrob Agents Chemother 1985; 28:240-245.

25. Felsenstein D, D'Amico DJ, Hirsch MS, et al. Treatment of cytomegalovirus retinitis with 9-[2-hydroxy-1-(hydroxymethyl)ethoxymethyl] guanine. Ann Intern Med 1985; 103:377-380.

26. Spector SA, Connor JD, McCutchan JA, Young W. 9-[2-hydroxy-1-(hydroxymethyl)ethoxymethyl] guanine (DHPG, BW759U) treatment of AIDS patients with serious cytomegalovirus infections. In 25th Interscience Conference on Antimicrobial Agents and Chemotherapy, Minneapolis, Minnesota, September 29-October 2, 1985.

27. Plotkin SA, Drew WL, Felsenstein D, Hirsch M. Sensitivity of clinical isolates of human cytomegalovirus to 9-(1,3-dihydroxy-2-propoxymethyl) guanine. J Infect Dis 1985; 152:833-834.

28. Shepp DH, Dandliker PS, deMiranda P, et al. Activity of 9-[2-hydroxy-1-(hydroxymethyl)ethoxymethyl] guanine in the treatment of cytomegalovirus pneumonia. Ann Intern Med 1985; 103:368-373.

29. Cole NL, Balfour HA. In vitro susceptibility of cytomegalovirus isolates from immunocompromised patients to acyclovir and ganciclovir. Diagn Microbiol Infect Dis 1987; 6:255-261.

30. Snoeck R, Sakuma T, DeClercq E, Rosenberg I, Holy A. (S)-1-(3-Hydroxy-2-phosphonyl methoxypropyl) cytosine, a potent and selective inhibitor of human cytomegalovirus replication. Antimicrob Agents Chemother 1988; 32: 1839-1844.

31. Mazeron MC, St-Jean LA, Defer MC, Gluckman E, Nebout T, Perol Y. Antiviral drug susceptibility of human cytomegalovirus (HCMV) from bone marrow recipients before and after treatment with ganciclovir. In Second International Cytomegalovirus Workshop, San Diego, California, March 27-30, 1989.

32. Drew WL, Miner RC, Mahalko S, Gullett J. CMV resistance in patients receiving ganciclovir. In 29th Interscience Conference on Antimicrobial Agents and Chemotherapy, Houston, Texas, September 17-20, 1989.

33. Dankner WM, Martin M, Scholl D, Stanat SC, Sonke RL, Spector SA. Rapid antiviral DNA-DNA hybridization assay for human cytomegalovirus. J Virol Methods 1990; 28:293-298.

34. Fletcher C, Sawchuk R, Chinnock B, deMiranda P, Balfour HH. Human pharmacokinetics of the antiviral drug DHPG. Clin Pharmacol Ther 1986; 40:281-286.
35. Sommadossi JP, Carlisle R. Toxicity of 3'azido-3'-deoxythmidine and 9-(1,3,-dihydroxy-2-propoxymethyl) guanine for normal human hematopoietic progenitor cells in vitro. Antimicrob Agents Chemother 1987; 31:452-454.
36. Rasmussen L, Chen PT, Mullenax JG, Merigan TC. Inhibition of human cytomegalovirus replication by 9-(1,3-dihydroxy-2-propoxymethyl) guanine alone and in combiantion with human interferons. Antimicrob Agents Chemother 1984; 26:441-444.
37. Freitas VR, Fraser-Smith EB, Matthew TR. Increased efficacy of ganciclovir in combination with foscarnet against cytomegalovirus and herpes simplex virus type 2 in vitro and in vivo. Antiviral Res 1989; 12:205-212.
38. Manischewitz JF, Quinnan GV, Lane HC, Wittek AE. Synergistic effect of ganciclovir and foscarnet on cytomegalovirus replication in vitro. Antimicrob Agents Chemother 1990; 34:373-375.
39. Dankner WM, Martin M, Spector SA. Inhibition of human cytomegalovirus by ganciclovir or foscarnet combined with different antiretroviral agents. In Second International Cytomegalovirus Workshop, San Diego, California, March 27-30, 1989.
40. Volberding PA, Lagakos SW, Koch MA, et al. Zidovudine in asymptomatic human immunodeficiency virus infection. N Engl J Med 1990; 322:941-949.
41. Plummer G, Benyesh-Melnick M. A plaque reduction neutralization test for cytomegalovirus. Proc Soc Exp Biol Med 1964; 117:145-150.
42. Wentworth BB, French L. Plaque assay of cytomegalovirus strains of human origin. Proc Soc Exp Biol Med 1970; 135:253-258.
43. Gadler H. Nucleic acid hybridization for measurement of effects of antiviral compounds on human cytomegalovirus DNA replication. Antimicrob Agents Chemother 1983; 24:370-374.
44. Spector SA, Spector DH. The use of DNA probes in studies of human cytomegalovirus. Clin Chem 1985; 31:1514-1519.
45. Swierkosz EM, Scholl DR, Brown JL, Jollick JD, Gleaves CA. Improved DNA hybridization method for detection of acyclovir-resistant herpes simplex virus. Antimicrob Agents Chemother 1987; 31:1465-1469.
46. Pritchard MN, Turk SR, Coleman LA, Engelhardt SL, Shipman C, Drach JC. A microtiter virus yield reduction assay for the evaluation of antiviral compounds against human cytomegalovirus and herpes simplex virus. J Virol Methods 1990; 28:101-106.
47. Telenti A, Smith TF. Screening with a shell vial assay for antiviral activity against cytomegalovirus. Diagn Microbiol Infect Dis 1989; 12:5-8.
48. Chou TC, Talalay P. Quantitative analysis of dose-effect relationships: the combined effects of multiple drugs or enzyme inhibitors. Adv Enzyme Reg 1984; 22:27-55.

2

Animal Models for Evaluating Ganciclovir Activity Against Cytomegalovirus

John D. Shanley
*University of Connecticut
and Veterans Administration Medical Center
Newington, Connecticut*

I. INTRODUCTION

In the past 25 years, the role of human cytomegalovirus (HCMV) as an important human pathogen has expanded dramatically (1,2). HCMV has replaced rubella as the leading infectious cause of congenital abnormalities, with congenital infection occurring in 1 to 2% of live births in the United States (3). HCMV is also a major source of disease for individuals whose immune system has been compromised by disease or medical therapy (4) and a major impediment to success in both solid-organ and bone marrow transplant patients (5,6). In individuals with the acquired immunodeficiency syndrome (AIDS), HCMV has recently emerged as a common and serious pathogen (7). Because of the growing importance of HCMV as a source of human disease, the development of antiviral agents with activity against this virus has become a priority. Recently, ganciclovir (Cytovene® , Syntex Research, Palo Alto, California) was licensed for the treatment of retinitis due to HCMV infection in individuals with AIDS. Animal models of CMV infection played an important role in the preclinical testing of this antiviral agent.

II. ANIMAL MODELS OF HCMV INFECTION

HCMV presents some important problems in the development and preclinical testing of new antiviral agents (8). It has been possible to identify candidate antiviral agents for HCMV in vitro, using human cell culture systems (9). However, once these agents are identified, it has been difficult to assess their effects on HCMV infections in vivo. Unlike herpes simplex virus, both human and animal cytomegaloviruses have rigorous host restrictions (10). HCMV does not replicate in any animal other than humans, making the direct testing of antiviral agents against HCMV in vivo in animal systems impossible. There are, however, a number of animal cytomegaloviruses that share strong biological and pathogenetic similarities with HCMV (11). These viruses have been well studied and developed as reliable model systems mimicking the infection and disease processes seen with HCMV. These model systems have proven useful in evaluating antiviral agents in vivo. We have come to rely on these systems to assess the potential effects of candidate antiviral agents on CMV infection and subsequent disease production. A number of animal model systems of HCMV infection were important in the development of ganciclovir.

For an animal model to be useful in the assessment of an agent for potential antiviral activity, a number of important characteristics of the model must be considered. It is important that the animal CMV be similar to HCMV in its degree of susceptibility to the candidate antiviral agent. Moreover, the mechanisms of activation, metabolism, and inhibition of virus processes should be similar. For example, ganciclovir was found to have similar antiviral activity against both HCMV and most animal cytomegaloviruses (9). Furthermore, the metabolism of DHPG and its activation and its mechanisms of inhibition of viral DNA replication appear to be similar (T. Matthews, personal communication, Syntex Research, Palo Alto, California). In contrast, acyclovir was found to have little activity against HCMV, a virus that lacks a viral-specified thymidine kinase (12), while it is very active in inhibiting murine CMV (MCMV), which also lacks thymidine kinase (12). The molecular aspects responsible for the activity of acyclovir against MCMV are not completely understood. It appears to be related to sensitivity of viral DNA polymerase to acyclovir, which has been activated by pathways other than thymidine kinase (13).

For an animal model to be useful in the in vivo evaluation of a drug, the pathogenesis of virus infection and disease induction should mimic those seen with HCMV. CMV infections in animals vary in degree to which they mimic the human virus. For example, guinea pig CMV (GPCMV) has been found to be an excellent animal model system for congenital CMV infection (14). Similarly, MCMV adrenalitis in the athymic nude mouse mimics the virus tissue interactions of HCMV in individuals with AIDS (15,16). While it is arguable that the CMV of animals are not perfect analogs for HCMV, significant insight into the pathogenesis of CMV infection has been gained using these systems. The role of antiviral therapy in the modification of infections and diseases due to CMV can be understood by studying these systems.

III. METHODS OF ANTIVIRAL TESTING IN ANIMALS

The activity of an antiviral agent, such as ganciclovir, against a nonhuman CMV may be assessed by a number of in vitro and in vivo methods (Table 1). In vitro, the ability of an agent to inhibit viral replication in cell culture can be measured by several means, including viral yield reduction or the reduction of virus infectivity. Viral yield reduction is assessed by the quantity or titer of virus produced in cell culture over time in the presence of varying concentrations of antiviral agents. Alternatively, antiviral activity can be measured by the reduction in the number of plaques formed or by the reduction in virus titer of a standard virus pool in the presence of graded doses of drug. Recently, the inhibition of viral DNA synthesis by drug, measured by DNA hybridization, has become a useful method for assessing antiviral compounds, especially for viral agents with slow replication cycles (17). The antiviral activity of an agent is generally reported as the μm or μg/ml concentration of drug that reduces viral yield or replication by 50%. Comparisons of the sensitivity of a given animal virus and HCMV to a given antiviral agent generally set the stage for further comparisons in vivo.

For in vivo testing of an antiviral agent, a number of endpoints for efficacy can be used (8). These include protection from lethal infection, suppression of virus replication in tissues, and the prevention of disease or tissue damage during viral infection. Protection from lethal infection most often

Table 1 Common Systems for the Assessment of Antiviral Activity of Agents Using Animal Cytomegaloviruses

In vitro
   Virus yield reduction
   Reduction of virus plaque formation
   Reduction of infectious dose$_{50}$
   Suppression of viral DNA synthesis

In vivo
   Reduction in mortality
   Reduction in virus replication
   Inhibition of disease production

involves administration of a lethal virus challenge. The survival of drug-treated animals is compared to that of placebo controls, and the efficacy is indicated by a reduction in mortality. This method indicates whether a drug will function against CMV in vivo. However, since HCMV rarely leads to overwhelming infection in the acute stage, lethality studies in animals do not have a clear correlate to human infection by HCMV.

The suppression of virus replication in a given tissue also indicates the ability of a drug to alter virus replication in vivo, and has clearer analogy to human infections by HCMV such as retinitis or adrenalitis. Drug efficacy is generally assessed by determining the virus content or titer in the tissues of infected animals at times after virus challenge. These values are then compared to those of placebo-treated controls. As with lethality studies, this method of drug assessment indicates whether an antiviral agent will function in vivo. Additionally, this method may also be used to determine if a drug or drug-delivery method has special tissue specificity.

Cytomegaloviruses are known to produce disease by both direct effects of virus on tissue and by immunopathological processes (18,19). Animal model systems of the latter situation often predict if antiviral therapy, which can inhibit virus replication, will concomitantly prevent tissue injury and disease. Examples of these situations will be discussed below.

IV. IN VITRO ASSESSMENT OF GANCICLOVIR

During development, ganciclovir was tested for its ability to inhibit in vitro replication of a number of animal cytomegaloviruses. Using a plaque reduction assay, we compared the activity of acyclovir and ganciclovir against the Smith strain of MCMV (20). Both acyclovir and ganciclovir were active against MCMV, producing 50% reduction of virus replication at 0.85 μm/ml (3.7 μM) and 3.8 μg/ml (14.0 μM), respectively. This level of activity of DPHG was comparable to the levels of activity reported for HCMV. The effective level of acyclovir required to inhibit MCMV is significantly lower than levels reported for HCMV.

Freitas et al. compared the activity of ganciclovir and acyclovir using two strains of HCMV, three monkey viruses, and two rodent viruses (Table 2) (21). In vitro, ganciclovir was active against all viruses at <15 μM, except GPCMV, which was inhibited at 70 μM. Ganciclovir was significantly more active than acyclovir against all viruses except MCMV. Both ganciclovir and acyclovir inhibited virus replication at drug concentrations well below the level that affected the cells' ability to proliferate (data not shown), yielding favorable therapeutic indices. In another report, Fong and co-workers also observed that GPCMV was somewhat resistant to ganciclovir in vitro (22). The 50% effective dose was 71 μM. Cumulatively, these data indicate

Table 2 Antiviral Activity of Ganciclovir (DHPG) and Acyclovir for Human, Simian, and Rodent Cytomegaloviruses Assayed by Viral Plaque Inhibition

CMV[a]	Plaque inhibition ED_{50} (μM)[b]		Cell type
	DHPG	Acyclovir	
Human (AD169)	7 ± 3	95 ± 10	MRC-5
	7 ± 2	55 ± 10	HET
Human (Davis)	7 ± 1	64 ± 4	MRC5
	5 ± 2	39 ± 10	HET
Vervet monkey (CSG)	13 ± 4	51 ± 1	MRC5
	9 ± 5	40 ± 22	HET
Rhesus monkey (68.1)	8 ± 2	39 ± 14	MRC5
	7 ± 2	40 ± 15	HET
Squirrel monkey	1.3 ± 1	28 ± 19	SML
GP CMV (22122)	70 ± 30	700 ± 230	GPE
MCMV (Smith)	11 ± 1	1 ± 0.8	SNC

[a]Strains in parentheses.
[b]The 50% effective dose (ED_{50}) ± SD was determined by three plaque assays for all virus except GPCMV. The endpoint for GPCMV was a 1 log reduction in virus yield.
Source: Data adapted from Ref. 21.

that most animal strains of CMV studied are comparable to HCMV in sensitivity to the antiviral effects of ganciclovir.

V. GANCICLOVIR AND LETHAL CMV INFECTION

The ability of ganciclovir to reduce mortality following lethal virus challenge has been reported by a number of laboratories using MCMV. MCMV will cause lethal infection when virus is inoculated either intraperitoneally (IP) or intravenously (IV) (23). These routes of infection favor virus replication in the spleen and liver, producing marked atrophy and necrosis of the spleen and a severe hepatitis (24). Tissue injury in this system seems to be the result of direct effects of virus infection rather than an immunopathological process. The mortality rate is influenced by virus dose, virus virulence, and the strain of mouse being employed (25-27).

Katzenstein et al. initially reported that mice treated with ganciclovir given subcutaneously (SC) has a lower mortality rate than placebo-treated controls following lethal virus challenge (28). The reductions in mortality were related to the dose of ganciclovir given. Antiviral treatment did not prevent the development of latent infection.

A more comprehensive analysis of the ability of ganciclovir and acyclovir to prevent virus-induced death was reported by Freitas et al. (Table 3) (21). Weanling mice were inoculated IP with MCMV in a dose that produced mortality in >90% of controls. Mice were treated with ganciclovir, 50 mg/kg per day given SC twice daily beginning 6, 24, 48, 72, or 96 hours after virus challenge. Antiviral treatment with both ganciclovir and acyclovir significantly reduced virus-induced death. Ganciclovir was more active at reducing mortality when treatment was initiated as late as 48 hours after virus challenge. The mean day to death was also increased in ganciclovir-treated mice, demonstrating a protective effect by drug treatment. Graded doses of ganciclovir and acyclovir were then studied. Ganciclovir improved survival in a dose-related fashion. Doses of ganciclovir as low as 10 mg/kg reduced mortality and prolonged survival if treatment was started within 24 hours of virus challenge. Acyclovir increased survival at higher doses, but a dose-related effect was not apparent. Virus content of organs was also reduced by treatment. Kern subsequently reported similar findings (8).

Ganciclovir was also found to prevent death in mice during immunosuppressive therapy (Table 4) (29). The protective effects of ganciclovir to lethal

Table 3 Effects of Ganciclovir (DHPG) and Acyclovir on Murine CMV-induced Mortality in Weanling BALB/c Mice

Drug (mg/kg)	Time (h) to first treatment[a]	No. of survivors/ total no. (% survival)	Mean survival time ± SD (days)[b]
Saline	6	2/19 (11)	5.2 ± 1.2
DHPG			
50	6	18/20 (90)[c]	6.5 ± 0.71
50	24	15/19 (79)[c]	10.7 ± 3.8[d]
50	48	9/19 (47)[c]	8.0 ± 2.5[d]
50	72	6/20 (30)	6.1 ± 1.6
50	96	1/20 (5)	4.8 ± 0.71
Acyclovir			
50	6	10/19 (53)[c]	7.0 ± 1.2[d]
50	24	12/20 (60)[c]	7.7 ± 1.9[d]
50	48	0/20 (0)	8.2 ± 2.2[d]
50	72	7/20 (35)	5.8 ± 2.9
50	96	4/19 (21)	4.3 ± 0.62

[a]Time of first treatment after virus inoculation.
[b]Mean survival time of the mice that died.
[c]Statistically significant ($p < 0.05$) by Mann-Whitney U-test.
[d]Statistically significant ($p < 0.05$) by Fisher exact test.
Source: Data adapted from Ref. 21.

Table 4 Effect of Ganciclovir (DHPG) on MCMV-Induced
Mortality in Normal and Immunosuppressed BALB/c Mice

Treatment group	Dose (U)	No. of survivors/total (%)
Normal mice		
DHPG (mg/kg/d)	20	13/13 (100)
	19.2	8/8 (100)
	12.8	8/8 (100)
	6.4	7/7 (100)
	5.0	6/7 (86)
	2.5	6/15 (40)
	1.25	2/8 (25)
	0.625	2/8 (25)
	0.3125	0/8 (0)
Saline	—	2/25 (8)
Immunosuppressed mice		
DHPG (mg/kg/d)	20	6/10 (60)
	15	4/5 (80)
	10	6/10 (60)
	7.5	1/10 1(10)
	5	0/9 (0)
Saline	—	1/10 (10)

Source: Data adapted from Ref. 29.

virus challenge in BALB/c mice was compared to those in mice receiving
cortisone acetate (125 mg/kg/day) and antithymocyte globulin (ATG) 0.2
ml twice weekly. Ganciclovir treatment reduced the mortality in both groups,
although a higher dose of drug was required to protect immunosuppressed
mice (3 mg/kg/day vs. 10 mg/kg/day to obtain 50% reduction in mortality).
Ganciclovir also reduced the virus content of the tissues but did not interfere
with the subsequent generation of an antibody response to MCMV.

Thus, these studies indicate that ganciclovir can modify acute lethal CMV
infection in animals and prevent the effects resulting from direct effects of
virus on host tissues.

VI. GANCICLOVIR AND VIRUS REPLICATION IN TISSUES

Another measure of antiviral activity is the degree of suppression of virus
replication in tissues. This is indicated by a decrease in virus titer in tissues
at times after infection. As in the lethality studies, a number of variables
must be considered to produce meaningful results. The replication of CMV
in tissues of most animal models is again influenced by the virus dose and

the route of administration. In mice, viral replication is also influenced by the strain of mouse being studied (30). For example, intranasal or intratracheal inoculation of virus favors replication of virus in the lungs while IP inoculation favors virus replication in the spleen and liver (23,25,31). Mice who possess the K phenotype of the major histocompatibility locus (e.g., C3H or CBA) are more resistant to virus replication than mice of the H2 B or D phenotype (e.g., C57Blk/10 or BALB/c AnN, respectively) (30). These variables can be manipulated to alter the tissue tropism of the virus for study purposes.

The ability of ganciclovir to suppress virus replication during acute infection has been reported by several laboratories. We initially demonstrated that ganciclovir can suppress MCMV replication in the lungs, salivary glands, and spleens of mice following intranasal inoculation (Table 5) (20). The drug

Table 5 Effect of oral and Parenteral Ganciclovir (DHPG) and Acyclovir (ACV) on MCMV Replication in Lungs and Salivary Glands of BALB/c Mice Following Intranasal Inoculation with MCMV

| | | MCMV titer ($\log_{10}$ PFU/ml) | | | |
| | | Salivary gland | | Lung | |
Drug	Dose	Titer	% Reduction	Titer	% Reduction
Oral administration					
None		6.23	—	4.64	—
ACV IG[a]	50	5.49	83	4.48	30
	500	4.20	99	3.28	97
ACV PO[b]	100	5.66	73	4.08	72
	300	4.84	96	3.64	90
DHPG PO	40	5.43	84	3.11	97
	100	4.72	97	3.00	98
	200	4.08	99	2.78	99
	300	3.23	99	2.36	99
Parenteral administration					
None		5.59	—	3.86	—
ACV SC[c]	5	5.65	0	4.26	0
	50	4.84	82	2.94	88
DHPG SC	5	4.11	97	3.00	86
	10	3.83	98	2.67	94
	50	1.83	99	2.48	96

[a]Gastric intubation.
[b]Given ad libitum in the drinking water.
[c]Given subcutaneously beginning 24 h after inoculation.
Source: Adapted from Ref. 20.

was effective when administered by the PO, SC, or intragastric routes. Suppression of virus replication in all tissues was related to the dose of drug administered. In subsequent studies from our laboratory, Debs et al. demonstrated that ganciclovir administered in a small-particle aerosol was effective in suppressing virus replication in the lungs of mice inoculated with MCMV intranasally (Table 6) (32). These studies also suggested that this route of administration was tissue-specific, since salivary gland titers were minimally altered.

Ganciclovir has also been shown to suppress GPCMV replication in vivo during acute infection (22), despite significant resistance of GPCMV to ganciclovir in vitro. Ganciclovir was administered SC at 50 mg/kg per day given in two doses. Ganciclovir significantly reduced the titer of GPCMV in the salivary gland, and there was a reduction in virus-induced lesions by histology. Interestingly, ganciclovir had no effect on GPCMV replication in spleen, lung, or blood, and there was no reduction in the histological lesions in these organs. Ganciclovir did not prevent antibody formation.

Ganciclovir was also shown to be effective in reducing MCMV replication in the presence of immunodeficiency, indicating that its effects are independent of host immunity (28). In BALB/c mice being treated with cortisone

Table 6 Effect of Ganciclovir (DHPG), Administered Either Orally or by Small Particle Aerosol, on MCMV Replication in the Lungs and Salivary Glands of BALB/c Mice Following Intranasal Inoculation with MCMV

Treatment	Dose (mg/kg/d)	Route	MCMV titer ($\log_{10}$ PFU/ml)	
			Salivary gland	Lung
Expt. 1				
None			5.2 ± 0.6	4.9 ± 0.4
DHPG	200	Oral[a]	2.5 ± 0.0 (>99)	1.9 ± 0.3 (>99)
DHPG	25	Aerosol[b]	5.3 ± 0.0 (0)	4.2 ± 0.0 (82)
Expt. 2				
Water			5.7 ± 0.4	3.9 ± 0.0
DHPG	200	Oral	4.4 ± 0.5 (95)	2.3 ± 0.5 (97)
DHPG	100	Aerosol	5.6 ± 0.9 (0)	2.7 ± 0.9 (93)
DHPG	200	Aerosol	5.4 ± 0.0 (42)	2.3 ± 0.3 (97)

[a]Ganciclovir (1.0 mg/ml) was provided in the drinking water ad libitum beginning 1 day after inoculation of virus.
[b]Ganciclovir was prepared at concentrations of 0.17, 0.68, or 1.36 mg/ml of water and was completely aerosolized over a 30-min period on 9 successive days, beginning 1 day after inoculation of virus.
Source: Data adapted from Ref. 32.

acetate (125 mg/kg/day) and antithymocyte globulin (ATG) 0.2 ml twice weekly, ganciclovir reduced the titers of MCMV in the hearts, livers, and salivary glands.

In unpublished data, we found that ganciclovir and acyclovir suppressed MCMV replication in athymic nude mice. Virus titers of the salivary gland and adrenal glands were reduced by ganciclovir given SC. These data indicate that ganciclovir is able to inhibit virus replication during acute infection in vivo, even in the presence of natural or iatrogenic immunosuppression. These data predicted the subsequent efficacy of ganciclovir in treating retinitis and GI infection in patients with AIDS (33).

VII. GANCICLOVIR AND LATENT CMV INFECTION

Following acute infection, both humans and animal viruses persist in the host indefinitely (34). Most often this is in a latent state, i.e., where replicating virus cannot be recovered. In some situations, chronic low-level replication occurs. Periodically, infection may return to an active state. Alterations of host immunity due to iatrogenic measures, such as immunosuppressive treatment, or diseases such as AIDS will induce latent virus to reactivate to a productive state, frequently with tissue injury. The effects of ganciclovir on viral latency have been reported. In a murine model, Katzenstein and colleagues demonstrated that ganciclovir treatment during acute infection, while reducing titers of virus below the level of detection, did not prevent the development of latent infection (28). Wilson et al. demonstrated that ganciclovir treatment during immunosuppression with cortisone acetate and ATG did not prevent reactivation of latent virus (29). Thus, ganciclovir, while altering acute virus replication, does not affect latency.

VIII. GANCICLOVIR AND DISEASES OF
ANIMAL CYTOMEGALOVIRUS

Animal models have proven valuable in our understanding of acute, chronic, and latent CMV infections and contributed to our concepts of the pathogenesis of CMV-induced diseases (10,11,34). CMV appears to induce disease by two mechanisms: direct effects of virus on host tissues and immunopathogenetic mechanisms (19,20). A number of animal models of tissue injury by direct viral effects have been developed. As mentioned, the lethal infection following IP infection is thought to be due to the direct consequences of viral injury, presumably damage to the liver. Similarly, MCMV-induced adrenalitis in athymic mice appears to be the consequence of direct viral effects on cells of the adrenal cortex and medulla (16,17). In both model systems, ganciclovir has been shown to be effective in treating CMV infections.

There is growing evidence from both human and animal studies that CMV is also able to produce disease by immunopathological mechanisms (18,19). Our laboratory has developed two models of MCMV-associated pneumonitis that appear to be mediated by immune-mediated injury. In initial studies, we observed that BALB/c mice inoculated intranasally with MCMV developed MCMV replication in lung tissue without evidence of pneumonitis (35). The addition of a single dose of cyclophosphamide, one day after virus challenge, induced diffuse interstitial pneumonitis not seen with MCMV or cyclophosphamide alone. Pneumonitis occurred in >90% of mice beginning 10 days after virus challenge and was characterized by an increase in the wet weight of the lung as well as histological evidence of both diffuse interstitial infiltration by lymphocytes and severe alveolitis. Analysis of the cells recovered by bronchoalveolar lavage demonstrated a marked influx of T lymphocytes (36). Virus content in the lungs of mice with pneumonitis was not significantly different from that in mice with MCMV infection alone. Using this model, we analyzed the effects of acyclovir and ganciclovir on the genesis of lung infection (Table 7) (20). Antiviral treatment suppressed virus replication in the salivary gland, lung, and spleens by >95%. Despite this reduction in virus content in the lungs, there was no decrease in the frequency of pneumonitis, suggesting that this process is not due to direct viral damage. However, continued immunosuppression with cortisone or cyclophosphamide or in vivo depletion of T lymphocytes with monoclonal antibody prevented

Table 7 Effects of Subcutaneous Acyclovir (ACV) or Ganciclovir (DHPG) on Occurrence and Severity of MCMV Interstitial Pneumonitis in BALB/c Mice 14 Days After Infection

| | | MCMV titer ($\log_{10}$ PFU/ml) | | | |
| | | Salivary | | | Interstitial |
Group[a]	Drug[b]	gland	Lung	Lung index[c]	pneumonitis[d]
Sham-CP	None			5.8 ± 0.6	2/9
Sham-CP	ACV			6.6 ± 0.7	—
Sham-CP	DHPG			5.8 ± 1.0	—
MCMV-CP	None	6.80	5.04	10.3 ± 0.2	8/9
MCMV-CP	ACV	5.52	4.08	7.6 ± 1.0	12/13
MCMV-CP	DHPG	2.52	2.48	7.8 ± 0.9	10/11

[a]Mice were given CP (200 mg/kg of body weight) 24 hours after either sham or virus inoculation.
[b]Antiviral drugs (50 mg/kg of body weight per day) were given SC in two doses beginning 1 day after virus or sham inoculation.
[c]Mean ± standard deviation of the wet weight of the right lung (mg) per body weight (g).
[d]Number of mice with histologic evidence of interstitial pneumonitis per total at risk.
Source: Adapted from Ref. 20.

pneumonitis. Thus, MCMV, in conjunction with cyclophosphamide, appears to trigger a process in the lungs that produces pneumonitis but does not require continued viral replication. The mechanism of injury is currently under investigation.

We also observed the genesis of pneumonitis in mice with acute MCMV infection and graft vs. host (GVH) reaction. These studies employed a murine model of interstitial pneumonitis seen with combined MCMV infection and GVH to the major histocompatibility (MHC) antigens (37). Unirradiated F1 (B10xB10.BR) mice develop GVH reaction to major MHC antigens when given spleen cells from the B10.BR parent (38). When MCMV infection is combined with the GVH challenge, there is a significant augmentation of the GVH reaction. In addition, mice with combined MCMV and GVH develop severe and diffuse pneumonitis, not seen with either MCMV or GVH alone. This process is similar in nature to that seen with HCMV and cyclophosphamide. It is characterized by increased lung weight and histological evidence of diffuse interstitial pneumonitis and alveolitis. As one index of immune processes in lung tissue, we characterized the types of host immune cells recoverable by bronchoalveolar lavage during pneumonitis (39). During MCMV/GVH pneumonitis, the total number of cells recovered by BAL significantly increased (8.8 $\pm$ 1.0 $\times$ 10^4 Sham/GVH vs. 58.2 $\pm$ 7.0 $\times$ 10^4 MCMV/GVH), due primarily to an influx of Thy 1.2 lymphocytes (4.3 $\times$ 10^4 Sham/GVH vs. 50.0 $\times$ 10^4 MCMV/GVH). Characterization of cells using multiparameter FACS analysis revealed that >80% of all BAL cells were Thy 1.2+ of donor origin. In addition, Thy 1.2 cells were of both L3T4+ (43%) and Lyt 2+ (38%) phenotype. Thus, MCMV/GVH pneumonitis is marked by an influx of donor T lymphocytes. Nonspecific immunosuppression with cyclophosphamide or cortisone or in vivo depletion of T lymphocytes prevented the pneumonitis.

In order to examine the contribution of virus replication in the development of tissue injury, we examined the effect of inhibitors of MCMV on the frequency and severity of pneumonitis (Table 8) (40). Prior studies have demonstrated that treatment with either acyclovir and ganciclovir inhibited MCMV replication in lung tissue during acute infection (20). Similarly, after virus and GVH challenge, ganciclovir reduced MCMV titers in lung tissue by >99%, although MCMV could be recovered by prolonged cocultivation of explants (40). Despite this fact, antiviral treatment did not alter the frequency and only moderately altered the severity of pneumonitis. These data indicate that MCMV is able to trigger pneumonitis, but factors other than direct damage by the virus to the lungs are responsible for pneumonitis. Ganciclovir successfully suppresses replication of virus, but does not affect the progression of disease. The data obtained from these two models correlate with the observations of ganciclovir treatment of pneumonitis in BMT patients.

Table 8 The Effect of Parenteral Ganciclovir (DHPG) on MCMV Replication and the Frequency of Pneumonitis in Mice 14 Days After MCMV or Sham Infection and GVH Challenge

| | | MCMV titer ($\log_{10}$PFU/ml) | | | |
| | | Salivary | | Lung | |
Group	Drug[a]	gland	Lung	index[b]	Pneumonitis[c]
Sham GVH	PBS	—	—	4.8 ± 0.5	1/10
Sham GVH	DHPG	—	—	4.8 ± 0.8	0/5
MCMV/GVH	PBS	5.7	2.2	6.1 ± 1.0	10/10
MCMV/GVH	DHPG	3.6	<0.5	6.1 ± 0.7	9/10

[a]Antiviral drugs (50 mg/kg of body weight per day) were given SC in two doses beginning 1 day after virus or sham inoculation.
[b]Mean ± standard deviation of the wet weight of the right lung (mg) per body weight (g).
[c]Number of mice with histologic evidence of interstitial pneumonitis per total at risk.
Source: Data adapted from Ref. 39.

Ganciclovir limited the replication of HCMV but could not prevent the progression of tissue damage culminating in pneumonitis and death (41). However, recent studies indicate that when ganciclovir is combined with intravenous gammaglobulin there is improved survival in bone marrow transplant recipients with CMV pneumonitis (see Chapter 11 for a complete discussion).

IX. CONCLUSIONS

Animal models are proving increasingly valuable in studies of the pathogenesis of viral infections and the preclinical evaluation of antiviral agents. If model systems are carefully selected, in vitro data and in vivo observations on both virus replication and disease production are important indicators of drug efficacy in humans. Animal models played a significant role in the development of ganciclovir. Many of the insights derived from animal systems regarding antiviral effects and the evolution of disease were substantiated in subsequent human studies. These systems should prove useful for the evaluation of agents in the future.

REFERENCES

1. Weller TH. The cytomegaloviruses: Ubiquitous agents with protean clinical manifestations. N Engl J Med 1971; 285:203-214, 267-274.
2. Zaia JA. Epidemiology and pathogenesis of cytomegalovirus disease. Sems Hematol 1990; 27(1S):5-10.
3. Stagno S, Pass RF, Alford CA. Perinatal infections and maldevelopment. Birth Defects 1981; 17:31-50.

4. Betts RF. Cytomegalovirus (CMV) in the compromised host(s). Ann Rev Med 1977; 28:103-110.

5. Zaia JA. The biology of human cytomegalovirus infection after bone marrow transplantation. Intern J Cell Cloning 1986; 4(S):135-154.

6. Pollard RB. Cytomegalovirus infections in renal, heart, heart-lung and liver transplantation. Ped Infect Dis J 1988; 7(S):97-102.

7. Jacobson MA, Mills J. Serious cytomegalovirus disease in the acquired immunodeficiency syndrome: Clinical findings, diagnosis, and treatment. Ann Intern Med 1988; 108:585-594.

8. Kern ER. Animal models as assay systems for the development of antivirals. In DeClercq E, Walker RT (Eds), Antiviral Drug Development. Plenum, New York, 1988, pp 149-172.

9. Matthews T, Boehme R. Antiviral activity and mechanism of action of ganciclovir. Rev Infect Dis 1988; 10(suppl 3):490-494.

10. Rapp F. The biology of cytomegaloviruses. In Roizman B (Ed), The Herpesviruses, Vol. 3. Plenum, New York, 1983, pp 1-66.

11. Plummer G. Cytomegalovirus of man and animals. Prog Med Virol 1973; 15:92-125.

12. Plotkin SA, Stan SE, Bryan CK. In vitro and in vivo responses of cytomegalovirus to acyclovir. Am J Med 1986; 73:257-261.

13. Burns WH, Wingard JR, Sandford GR, Bender WJ, Saral R. Acyclovir in mouse cytomegalovirus infection. Am J Med 1982; 73:118-124.

14. Bia FJ, Griffith BP, Fong KY, Hsuing GD. Cytomegalovirus infections in the guinea pig: Experimental models for human disease. Rev Infect Dis 1983; 5:177-195.

15. Shanley JD, Pesanti EL. Murine cytomegalovirus adrenalitis in athymic nude mice. Arch Virol 1986; 88:27-35.

16. Shanley JD. The modification of acute murine cytomegalovirus adrenal gland infection by adoptive spleen cell transfer. J Virol 1987; 61:23-28.

17. Stanberry L, Myers MG. Evaluation of varicella-zoster antiviral drugs by a nucleic acid hybridization assay. Antivir Res 1988; 9:367-377.

18. Grundy JE, Shanley JD, Griffiths P. Cytomegalovirus pneumonitis in transplant patients—A hypothesis. Lancet 1987; ii:996-999.

19. Zaia JA. Understanding human cytomegalovirus infection. In Gale RP, Champlin R (Eds), New Strategies in Bone Marrow Transplantation, UCLA Symposium on Molecular and Cellular Biology. Allan R Liss, New York, 1990, in press.

20. Shanley JD, Morningstar J, Jordan MC. Inhibition of murine cytomegalovirus lung infection and interstitial pneumonitis by acyclovir and 9-(1,3-dihydroxy-2-propoxymethyl)guanine. Antimicrob Agents Chemother 1985; 28:172-175.

21. Freitas VR, Smee DF, Chernow M, Boehme R, Matthews TR. Activity of 9-(1,3Dihydroxy-2-propoxymethyl)guanine compared with that of acyclovir against human, monkey, and rodent cytomegalovirus. Antimicob Agents Chemother 1985; 28:240-245.

22. Fong CKY, Cohen SD, McCormick S, Hsuing GD. Antiviral effect of 9-(1,3-Dihydroxy-2-propoxymethyl)guanine against cytomegalovirus infection in a guinea pig model. Antivir Research 1987; 7:11-23.

23. Selgrade MK, Collier AM, Saxton L, Daniels MJ, Graham JA. Comparison of the pathogenesis of murine cytomegalovirus in lung and liver following intra-peritoneal or intra tracheal infection. J Gen Virol 1984; 65:515-523.
24. Mannini A, Medearis DN. Mouse salivary gland virus infection. Am J Hyg 1961; 73:329-343.
25. Shanley JD, Pesanti EL. The relationship of virus replication and interstitial pneumonitis in murine cytomegalovirus lung infection. J Infect Dis 1985; 151: 454-458.
26. Henson D, Smith RD, Gehrke J. Nonfatal mouse cytomegalovirus hepatitis. Am J Pathol 1966; 49:871-887.
27. Grundy (Chalmer) JE, Mackenzie JS, Stanley NF. Influence of H-2 and Non-H-2 genes on resistance to murine cytomegalovirus infection. Infect Immunol 1981; 32:277-286.
28. Katzenstein DA, Crane RT, Jordan MC. Successful treatment of murine cytomegalovirus disease does not prevent latent virus infection. J Lab Clin Med 1986; 108:155-160.
29. Wilson EJ, Medearis DN, Hansen LA, Rubin RH. 9-(1,3Dihydroxy-2-propoxy-methyl)guanine prevents death but not immunity in murine cytomegalovirus infected normal and immunosuppressed BALB/c mice. Antimicrob Agents Chemother 1987; 31:1017-1020.
30. Shanley JD. Host genetic factors influence murine cytomegalovirus lung infection and interstitial pneumonitis. J Gen Virol 1985; 65:2121-2128.
31. Jordan MC. Interstitial pneumonia and subclinical infection after intranasal inoculation of murine cytomegalovirus. Infect Immunol 1978; 21:275-280.
32. Debs RJ, Montgomery AB, Brunnette EN, DeBruin M, Shanley JD. Aerosol administration of antiviral agents to treat lung infection due to murine cytomegalovirus. J Infect Dis 1988; 157:327-331.
33. Koretz H, et al. Treatment of serious cytomegalovirus infections with 9-(1,3-dihydroxy-2-propoxymethyl)guanine in patients with AIDS and other immuno-deficiencies. N Engl J Mcd 1986; 314:801-805.
34. Jordan MC. Latent infection and the elusive cytomegalovirus. Rev Infect Dis 1983; 5:205-215.
35. Shanley JD, Pesanti EL, Nugent K. Pathogenesis of pneumonitis due to murine cytomegalovirus. J Infect Dis 1982; 146:388-396.
36. Shanley JD, Ballas ZK. Alteration of bronchoalveolar cells during murine cytomegalovirus interstitial pneumonitis. Am Rev Resp Dis 1985; 132:77-81.
37. Grundy JE, Shanley JD, Shearer GM. Augmentation of GVH reaction by cytomegalovirus infection resulting in interstitial pneumonitis. Transplantation 1985; 39:548.
38. Shearer GM, Levy RB, Graft-vs-host associated immune suppression is activated by recognition of allogeneic murine I-A antigens. J Exp Med 1983; 157: 936-946.
39. Shanley JD, et al. Interstitial pneumonitis during murine cytomegalovirus infection and graft-vs-host reaction. characterization of bronchoalveolar lavage cells. Transplantation 1987; 44:658-662.

40. Shanley JD, Pomeroy C, Via CS, Shearer GM. Interstitial pneumonitis during murine cytomegalovirus infection and graft vs host reaction: effect of ganciclovir. J Infect Dis 1988; 158:1391-1394.

41. Shepp DH, Dandliker PS, deMiranda P, et al. Activity of 9-[2-hydroxy-1-(hydroxymethyl)ethoxymethyl]guanine in the treatment of cytomegalovirus pneumonia. Ann Intern Med 1985; 103:368-373.

3

Clinical Safety of
Intravenous Ganciclovir

William C. Buhles, Jr.
Syntex Research
Palo Alto, California

I. INTRODUCTION

Early in the 1980s chemists working independently at four laboratories synthesized a novel nucleoside analog of 2'deoxyguanosine. This compound, with the chemical name of 9-(1,3-dihydroxy-2-propoxymethyl)guanine, was found to have significantly greater antiviral potency in vitro against the human herpesvirus group than acyclovir, also a nucleoside analog (1,2). The compound came to be known as DHPG, and later as ganciclovir. In vitro and animal testing defined the antiviral activity, toxicity, and safety profile of ganciclovir (1-12), and in 1984 clinical use of ganciclovir for the treatment of serious cytomegalovirus (CMV) infections was initiated (13). This chapter will summarize both the preclinical and clinical information that is available regarding the safety of ganciclovir.

II. STUDIES AT THE CELLULAR LEVEL

A. Mechanism of Action

Ganciclovir is phosphorylated intracellularly to ganciclovir monophosphate (GCV-MP), and further phosphorylation occurs by cellular enxymes, leading

Table 1 In Vitro Inhibition of Human and Animal Cells by Ganciclovir

Cell type	ID_{50} of ganciclovir (μM)	Reference
Human cells		
Human foreskin fibroblast	40-280	3
Human fibroblast strain (WI-38)	>50	4
HeLa S3	125	14
Human embryonic lung	110	14
Human embryonic tonsil	250	15
Raji cells	200	16
Hematopoietic progenitor (CFU-GM)	2.7	16
Hematopoietic progenitor (BFU-E)	1.6	16
Animal cells		
Squirrel monkey lung	1500	14
Guinea pig embryo	2900	14
African green monkey kidney	135-850	2,3
Mouse embryo fibroblast	210	14

to the accumulation of GCV-triphosphate (GCV-TP). GCV-TP preferentially inhibits viral DNA polymerase and, to a lesser extent, cellular polymerases (1,4,9). The initial phosphorylation is accomplished by one or more cellular guanosine kinases, which in virus-infected cells are induced to higher levels than in noninfected cells. Even in the absence of virus infection, however, normal, uninduced levels of this enxyme system are sufficient to phosphorylate ganciclovir. Thus, ganciclovir has some toxicity for uninfected cells, and based on in vivo animal safety studies appears to primarily effect rapidly dividing cell populations.

B. Cytotoxicity for Uninfected Cells In Vitro

The in vitro cytotoxicity of GCV for a variety of uninfected human and animal cells, as measured by inhibition of replication, has been reported. There is considerable variation in sensitivity, with human bone marrow progenitor cells being the most sensitive (Table 1).

III. SAFETY STUDIES IN ANIMALS (17)

A. Single-Dose Toxicity Studies in Animals

At high doses, single intravenous (IV) boluses of ganciclovir caused mortality in mice and dogs. The median lethal dose was approximately 900 mg/kg in mice and between 150 and 500 mg/kg in dogs. In mice, the cause of death was related to pathological changes in the intestines, and in dogs death was related to suppression of hematopoietic and renal function along with pathological changes of the gastrointestinal tract.

B. Chronic (1- and 3-Month) Toxicity Studies in Animals

One-month toxicity studies with IV ganciclovir were carried out in mice and dogs. Mice were given once-daily bolus injections of ganciclovir of 15, 45, or 135 mg/kg per day for 1 month. Testicular atrophy was the principal finding at 15 mg/kg per day. At doses of 45 and 135 mg/kg per day, mice exhibited decreased numbers of erythrocytes, increased levels of blood urea nitrogen (BUN), glutamate-oxaloacetate transminase and glutamate-pyruvate transaminase (females only), thymic involution and atrophy, and atrophy of male and female reproductive organs.

Dogs received IV bolus injections of ganciclovir at 10, 30, or 90 mg/kg per day given in equal doses twice daily (i.e., 5, 15, and 45 mg/kg/dose) for 1 month. A dose of 10 mg/kg per day resulted in decreased leukocyte counts, decreased bone marrow cellularity, and atrophic sebaceous glands and testes. In addition to these changes, dogs receiving ganciclovir at 30 or 90 mg/kg per day exhibited decreased body weight, anorexia, hypothermia, decreased numbers of reticulocytes and platelets, decreased bone marrow cellularity, renal tubular dilatation (high-dose only), and atrophy of the testes, sebaceous glands, and hair follicles. The dose of 90 mg/kg per day was lethal to all the dogs tested.

A second study in dogs using lower ganciclovir doses of 0.4, 1.2, or 3.6 mg/kg per day in equal twice-daily doses revealed dose-related testicular atrophy with hypospermatogenesis at all dose levels. No other treatment-related changes were noted.

C. Reproductive Toxicity

Female mice given daily IV ganciclovir up to 20 mg/kg for 2 weeks prior to mating did not show impaired fertility. However, female mice dosed with 90 mg/kg per day for 2 weeks prior to mating exhibited decreased fertility, decreased mating behavior, and increased embryolethality. These effects were reversible after a recovery period. The month-old male offspring of the high-dose females had hypoplastic testes and seminal vesicles.

In male mice, fertility was reversibly decreased after IV ganciclovir at a dose of 2.0 mg/kg per day for 2 months. This effect was irreversible at a dose of 10 mg/kg per day for 2 months. Ganciclovir caused hypospermatogenesis in mice and dogs after single IV doses of >30 mg/kg per day, and in dogs after IV doses of >0.4 mg/kg per day for 1 month.

D. Teratogenicity

Ganciclovir has been shown to be teratogenic in rabbits and embryotoxic in mice when given in doses approximately equivalent to the human dose (calculated on the basis of the body surface area). It would therefore be expected that the drug may be teratogenic and/or embryotoxic at the dose levels recommended for human use.

In mice, ganciclovir at 36 mg/kg per day (154 mg/m^2) IV had no effect on the developing fetuses. However, 108 mg/kg per day (463 mg/m^2) caused maternal/fetal toxicity and embryolethality.

In rabbits, ganciclovir 6.0 mg/kg per day IV had no effect on the developing fetuses. However, 20 and 60 mg/kg per day (442 and 1326 mg/m^2) during gestation caused fetal growth retardation, embryolethality, and teratogenicity, particularly 60 mg/kg per day, which also caused maternal toxicity. Teratogenic changes seen include cleft palate, anophthalmia/microphthalmia, aplastic kidney, aplastic pancreas, hydrocephaly, and brachygnathia.

E. Mutagenicity and Carcinogenicity Studies

Mutagenicity

Ganciclovir did not cause point mutations when evaluated in bacterial and yeast indicator organisms. In cultured mammalian cells, ganciclovir elicited point mutations in L5178YTK $\pm$ mouse lymphoma cells and caused chromosomal damage in human lymphocytes, but did not cause morphological transformation of BALB/c $-$3T3 cells. Single doses of ganciclovir given IV to mice did not induce chromosomal damage at 50 mg/kg, but did cause chromosomal damage at doses of 150 and 500 mg/kg. When further evaluated in vivo in mice, ganciclovir did not cause dominant lethality in any of three studies (one IV, two oral) that evaluated male fertility.

Carcinogenicity

Mice were dosed with 1, 20, or 1000 mg/kg per day of ganciclovir by oral gavage for 18 months in a bioassay for carcinogenicity. Treatment-related tumors were observed in the animals dosed with 20 and 1000 mg/kg per day. These tumors included epithelial tumors of the preputial gland, forestomach, clitoral gland, pancreas, skin, vagina, and mammary gland; vascular tumors of the ovaries, uterus, lymph node, and liver; and histiocytic sarcoma of the liver. No increased incidence of tumors was present in mice dosed with 1 mg/kg per day. The 1000-mg/kg-per-day oral dose in mice results in plasma ganciclovir levels approximately equivalent to levels resulting from an intravenous dose of 10 mg/kg per day.

F. Local Tolerance

Injection of ganciclovir at a concentration of 46 mg/ml (pH 11.2 ± 0.2) into the marginal ear veins of rabbits did not cause vascular irritation.

G. Intravitreal Safety Studies in Animals

Several groups have reported on the safety of ganciclovir injected intravitreally. Pulido et al. (18) reported that single intravitreal doses of 10 to 400 μg of ganciclovir to rabbit eyes (at concentrations of 0.4 to 2.0 mg/ml) resulted in no retinal toxicity, no ophthalmoscopic changes, and no changes in electro-retinography. Likewise, Schulman et al. (19) reported no adverse effects of 50 to 450 μg of ganciclovir injected into the vitreous of rabbits.

Syntex (17) has evaluated the safety or intravitreal injections in rabbits. Eyes injected with doses of ganciclovir of 100 to 400 μg per injection one to three times per week for 4 weeks showed no drug-related microscopic or ophthalmoscopic changes.

H. Safety in a Canine Model of Autologous Bone Marrow Transplantation

Appelbaum et al. (20) studied the hematological toxicity of ganciclovir in dogs given total body irradiation of 9.2 Gy and infused with autologous marrow cells. Ganciclovir was given intravenously at 1.0, 3.0, or 5.0 mg/kg per day starting on the day of marrow infusion. Doses of 5.0, but not 1.0 or 3.0, mg/kg per day were associated with a delayed time to platelet recovery. No effect was seen on time to recovery to an absolute neutrophil count (ANC) of >500 cells per μl.

IV. CLINICAL SAFETY OF GANCICLOVIR IN PEOPLE WITH HIV INFECTION

Between 1984 and 1990, more than ten thousand people were treated with ganciclovir under various investigational protocols. The safety data from these clinical studies will be reviewed. Clinical safety data are presented based on underlying immunodeficiency rather than type of CMV infection, because the safety profile of ganciclovir has been found to vary more as a function of immunodeficiency.

A. Hematological Toxicity

The most common adverse effect related to ganciclovir administration in humans has been hematological toxicity (21). This effect was predicted from animal safety studies, and involves both the leukocyte and the platelet cell lines. It has been difficult to quantify with accuracy the extent to which cytopenias occurring during the administration of ganciclovir are attributable to ganciclovir treatment, since infection with the human immunodeficiency virus (HIV) can result in cytopenia. In addition, persons receiving ganciclovir are often receiving other potentially myelotoxic therapy, making it difficult to attribute cause to one or a combination of drugs. The data summarized below are divided arbitrarily into clinical information from uncontrolled, nonrandomized studies or case series, and separately from randomized, controlled studies.

Results from Nonrandomized Studies

Leukopenia/Neutropenia. Leukopenia and neutropenia are almost always seen simultaneously when they occur, and there is depression of all leukocyte types. Leukopenia and neutropenia will be considered synonomous in the following analysis.

Some of the most complete data with regard to hematological toxicity were gathered during detailed data collection on the first set of patients given open-label treatment under "compassionate use" release protocols in the United States between May of 1984 and January of 1987 (22). A total of 427 people with the diagnosis of AIDS had sufficient hematological data reported to allow characterization of the severity, duration, and frequency of neutropenia during treatment with ganciclovir. Most of these patients received doses of either 5 mg/kg BID or 2.5 mg/kg TID for 14 to 21 days, and more than 50% continued to receive maintenance ganciclovir treatment at doses between 25 and 35 mg/kg per week, given five or seven times per week. Severe neutropenia, defined as an ANC $<500/\mu l$, occurred in 16.2%. Most treating physicians chose to interrupt ganciclovir treatment temporarily at this threshold ANC value. Moderate neutropenia (ANC of 500 to $<1000/\mu l$) occurred in 24.3% of the patients with AIDS and less often resulted in interruption of treatment.

An analysis of a subset of these 427 people with AIDS, specifically the first 262 (23), revealed no association between the mean daily ganciclovir dose and the frequency of neutropenia across the dose range of 5 to 15 mg/kg per day. In this same group of patients, baseline ANC did not seem to be related to risk of neutropenia following an induction treatment course; patients with a starting ANC $<1000/\mu l$ did not have a higher frequency of neutropenia (defined here as an ANC $<1000/\mu l$ or a drop of ANC to $<50\%$ of baseline ANC) than patients with a baseline ANC of $>4000/\mu l$. Seventy-five percent of the patients who did eventually develop neutropenia (30% of all treated patients) did so by the time they had received a cumulative ganciclovir dose of about 140 mg/kg, during which time they were receiving induction doses (7.5 to 10.0 mg/kg/day) (21). The median time to first neutropenia was 12 days. A Kaplan-Meier-type survival analysis of the risk of developing neutropenia with continued ganciclovir treatment (induction followed by maintenance) indicated that up to 54% of patients who remain on therapy will eventually develop neutropenia at some time during their therapy. It is not known if this estimate is affected by concomitant medications, but it is not affected by zidovudine toxicity as these patients were evaluated before zidovudine became available. Thus, ~40% of AIDS patients treated with ganciclovir will develop some neutropenia (ANC <1000/μl) during or shortly following induction treatment, and an additional 15% will probably manifest neutropenia for the first time during maintenance treatment.

Not all neutropenic episodes lead to discontinuation of treatment. Data from the 427 AIDS patients detailed above (22) indicate that approximately 20% require one or more interruptions of therapy because of neutropenia. The neutropenia is reversible in most cases. Upon discontinuation of ganciclovir treatment at an ANC of ~500/μl, the ANC increases within 3 to 7 days. Some individuals with marginal myelopoietic reserve may require several weeks for the ANC to return to >1000/μl. It is these patients who may not be able to tolerate therapeutic maintenance doses of ganciclovir for long periods of time.

A second excellent data set for evaluating the incidence of neutropenia in AIDS patients treated with ganciclovir is from the Treatment IND protocol conducted by the AIDS Collaborative Treatment Group Office of the National Institutes of Health (NIH). This study enrolled only patients with AIDS and immediately sight-threatening CMV retinitis (24). Data from the first 200 enrolled patients (the most complete reporting) indicated a rate of neutropenia of 26%. Of the total of 1125 enrolled in this study, neutropenia/leukopenia was reported in 12.7%, with one individual reported to have neutropenia with sepsis. The disparity in numbers most likely reflects incomplete reporting in the people enrolled later, and the first estimate is probably the most accurate.

Of the entire data set—4430 AIDS patients who received ganciclovir treatment in the Syntex Research-sponsored open-label protocols between May 1984 and January 1989—17% were reported to have leukopenia/neutropenia (25). It should be noted that this frequency of neutropenia reported by investigator physicians as an adverse event is lower than when actual cell counts are the basis of defining neutropenia (40%). The frequency of reports of neutropenia from physicians (17%) is similar to the frequency of severe neutropenia (ANC <500/μl) detected when actual cells counts are evaluated (16.2%). This suggests that physicians are reporting neutropenia to study sponsors as an adverse event only when the ANC approaches or drops below the $500/\mu l$ threshold, when decisions regarding drug discontinuation must be made.

Multiple reports of the treatment of life- or sight-threatening CMV disease in case series of persons with AIDS have appeared in the literature. Details as to the frequency of neutropenia, as well as the definition of neutropenia/leukopenia, vary from series to series. Table 2 summarizes the reported frequency of neutropenia in these published case series.

A minority of those who require treatment with ganciclovir will experience repeated episodes of neutropenia to the extent that adequate doses cannot be given to control CMV disease. Studies conducted by the sponsor of the drug, Syntex Research, do not provide an accurate measure of the incidence of such intolerance, since the sponsor's data set is more likely to include only persons who can tolerate some drug and thus remain in the study. Several published papers give data on the proportion of persons who cannot tolerate ganciclovir due to repeated episodes of severe neutropenia. Jabs et al. (33) reported that five of 31 patients (16%) with CMV retinitis and AIDS were not able to tolerate full-dose maintenance ganciclovir treatment because of recurrent neutropenia. Orellana et al. (34) reported that in a series of 25 people with CMV retinitis and AIDS who received maintenance ganciclovir treatment, three (12%) developed "profound" leukopenia (WBC $< 800/\mu l$).

The incidence of bacterial or fungal sepsis secondary to neutropenia and related to ganciclovir treatment is difficult to estimate because most persons treated with ganciclovir have underlying immunodeficiency which may render them more susceptible to such infections. In a data set of 427 cases of AIDS treated with ganciclovir, all those who were deceased were evaluated for

Table 2 Frequency of Reported Neutropenia/Leukopenia in Persons with AIDS Treated with Ganciclovir: Literature Reports of Case Series

Reference	CMV disease	Number of persons treated	Number of persons with neutropenia (%)
Masur et al. (26)	Retinitis	8	3 (38)
Kotler et al. (27)	Retinitis/colitis	18	2 (11)
Henderly et al. (28)	Retinitis	23	3 (13)
Holland et al. (29)	Retinitis	40[a]	12 (30)
		26[b]	10 (38)
Chachoua et al. (30)	Gastrointestinal	41	6 (15)
Laskin et al. (31)	Multiple	97	53 (55)
Jacobson et al. (32)	Retinitis/colitis	44[a]	2 (5)
		32[b]	10 (31)
Jabs et al. (33)	Retinitis	31	9 (29)

[a]Induction treatment.
[b]Maintenance treatment.

cause of death; those with cause of death listed as sepsis or bacterial or fungal infection were evaluated further to determine the neutrophil count prior to death (35). Two were identified who died of sepsis or disseminated infection and who had an ANC $<500/\mu l$ prior to death. In these two cases, the neutropenia persisted even though ganciclovir treatment was discontinued. Based on these data, it is estimated that the frequency of fatal infections secondary to neutropenia in persons treated with ganciclovir is less than 1%.

Sepsis was reported as an adverse event in 46 of 4430 individuals (1%) receiving ganciclovir under open-label protocols in the United States. In the Treatment IND protocol treatment series, four of 1125 people (0.4%) with CMV retinitis and AIDS were reported to have sepsis.

Thrombocytopenia. The data set consisting of 427 AIDS patients from the U.S. open-label trials provides information on the frequency of thrombocytopenia. In this group, the frequency of severe thrombocytopenia (platelet count $<20,000/\mu l$) was 5.3%. The frequency of moderate thrombocytopenia (defined for the purposes of this analysis as a platelet count of 20,000 to $<50,000/\mu l$) was 8.7%. Overall, 14% of persons with AIDS treated with ganciclovir experienced one or more episodes of thrombocytopenia with a platelet nadir $<50,000/\mu l$. Eight-six percent of persons with AIDS treated with ganciclovir did not have a platelet count below $50,000/\mu l$. For the entire open-label data set of persons with AIDS, thrombocytopenia (not defined as threshold platelet count) was reported in 162 (3.7%). As with severe neutropenia, it is likely that physicians reported thrombocytopenia as an adverse event in this clinical trial only when platelets counts became very low, since the rate of 3.7% is close to the rate of thrombocytopenia observed using a threshold platelet count of $<20,000/\mu l$ (5.3%).

In the Treatment IND study sponsored by the NIH (24), of the first 200 persons with AIDS treated with ganciclovir, 101 completed 28 days or more of therapy with ganciclovir and had laboratory data available for analysis. Of these 101, two (2%) had a platelet count less $<50,000/\mu l$ on day 28, and one of these patients started treatment with a platelet count below $50,000/\mu l$. Of the total 1125 individuals enrolled, 21 (1.9%) had thrombocytopenia reported as an adverse event.

Case series reported in the literature indicate a low frequency of thrombocytopenia in persons with AIDS treated with ganciclovir. Masur et al. (26) reported none of eight, Kotler et al. (27) reported none of 18, Henderly et al. (28) reported none of 23, Holland et al. (29) none of 40, Chachoua et al. (30) reported none of 41, Laskin et al. (31) reported four of 97 (4%), Jabs et al. (33) none of 31, and Orellana et al. (34) none of 41. Jacobson et al. (32) evaluated mean platelet counts in their series of patients. During induction ganciclovir treatment in 40 patients, the mean platelet count decreased from $230,000$ to $200,000/\mu l$. During maintenance treatment in 32 persons, the mean platelet count decreased from 228,000 to 173,000/μl. Two (4.5%) developed thrombocytopenia requiring modification of ganciclovir dosing.

In the U.S. open-label ganciclovir trials, hemorrhage was rarely reported. Hemorrhage of any type was reported in 38 of 4430 patients (0.9%). Robinson et al. (36) reported an individual with CMV retinitis and AIDS who developed severe thrombocytopenia after initiation of ganciclovir induction treatment. He developed bilateral vitreous hemorrhage and intracranial hemorrhage with hemiparesis in spite of multiple platelet transfusions.

Anemia. In open-label trials in the United States, of the first 427 persons with AIDS who were treated with ganciclovir, 5% had anemia reported as an adverse event. In a similar trial in Europe, six persons among 99 treated had anemia (6.1%) (37). Of the 4430 persons with AIDS treated under the U.S. open-label protocols, 536 had adequate laboratory data reported to evaluate anemia based on hemoglobin levels (25). The majority of these 536 are included in the data set of the first 427 treated and referenced above (Ref. 22). Among the 536 people, minimum hemoglobin values during ganciclovir treatment were: >8.0 g/dl, 342 patients (63.8%); 6.5 to 7.9 g/dl, 154 patients (28.7%); and <6.5 g/dl, 40 patients (7.5%).

Data from the first 200 patients treated under the NIH Treatment IND protocol indicate a low frequency of anemia in persons treated with ganciclovir (24). Of the first 200 treated patients, hemoglobin values were available after 28 days of treatment for 105 patients. Of these 105, eight patients (7.6%) had hemoglobin values <8.0 g/dl. At baseline, 7.2% of the patients (all with CMV retinitis and AIDS) had hemoglobin <8.0 g/dl, indicating little change over the first 28 days of treatment. After 60 days of ganciclovir, 85 patients had hemoglobin values reported, of whom four (4.7%) had hemoglobin <8.0 g/dl.

Since anemia may occur frequently in persons with AIDS, it is difficult to attribute anemia to ganciclovir treatment. Complicating this is the fact that, because the lifespan of erythrocytes is considerably longer in the peripheral circulation than that of either neutrophils or platelets, it is more difficult to observe temporal association of anemia with ganciclovir treatment. Zidovudine treatment for HIV infection is also associated with anemia (37). However, most of the 536 persons above who had hemoglobin values reported were treated with ganciclovir before zidovudine became available. In a placebo-controlled study of zidovudine in persons with HIV infection, the frequency of anemia (hemoglobin <7.5 g/dl) was 6% in the individuals receiving placebo who had CD4 lymphocyte counts <200/μl (38). Nearly all persons with AIDS and CMV retinitis have CD4 counts less than 200/μl (39); thus, underlying HIV disease may account for some of the reported anemia.

In the group of 4430 individuals treated under open-label protocols, 133 (3%) had anemia reported by the investigator as an adverse event.

Jacobson et al. (32) evaluated hemoglobin in 44 patients during treatment with ganciclovir. Of the 44 who received induction treatment, the mean baseline was 10.2 g/dl and the mean nadir during induction was 9.3 g/dl. During maintenance treatment, the starting mean hemoglobin was 10.3 g/dl for 33 persons, and the mean nadir was 8.7 g/dl. None of these patients was reported to have received concomitant zidovudine treatment. Thirty percent required red blood cell transfusions at some time during their ganciclovir therapy. The authors state that there were numerous other possible causes of anemia and that there was no apparent association between anemia and dose of ganciclovir.

Results from Randomized, Controlled Studies

Safety results from randomized, controlled studies are important to the assessment of clinical safety not only because they provide a comparison group to clarify events that are truly drug-related, but because they often demand more complete monitoring and reporting of safety data by participating physicians. The results below summarize hematological safety data from controlled studies of intravenous ganciclovir.

Leukopenia/Neutropenia. A recently reported double-blind, placebo-controlled study of intravenous ganciclovir in persons with CMV colitis and AIDS yields very clear data on the incidence of neutropenia associated with ganciclovir (40). Sixty-two persons were randomized, 32 to ganciclovir induction treatment at 5 mg/kg BID and 30 to intravenous placebo on the same schedule, for 14 days. The results are shown in Table 3. Individuals in the ganciclovir treatment group had neutropenia (ANC $<1000/\mu l$) more frequently than the placebo group (26% in the ganciclovir vs. 10% in the placebo groups). Data from this placebo controlled study indicate that the in-

Table 3 Minimum Neutrophil Count During Induction Ganciclovir Treatment in a Placebo-Controlled Study in Persons with AIDS and CMV Colitis

Minimum absolute neutrophil count (Cells/μl)	No. of subjects (%)	
	Ganciclovir $(n = 31)^a$	Placebo $(n = 30)$
>2000	9 (29.0)	15 (50.0)
1000 to <2000	14 (45.2)	12 (40.0)
500 to <1000	5 (16.2)	2 (6.7)
<500	3 (9.7)	1 (3.3)

[a]One subject had no ANC measured.

cremental increase in the frequency of neutropenia that occurs during ganciclovir induction treatment is approximately 15 to 20%.

One other prospectively randomized, controlled trial of induction ganciclovir in persons with AIDS has been reported (41). In addition, three randomized, controlled studies of ganciclovir maintenance treatment of CMV retinitis in AIDS have been conducted, two comparing ganciclovir to observation only (42,43) and one comparing ganciclovir maintenance treatment to one-half-dose ganciclovir maintenance treatment plus recombinant beta-interferon (44). Table 4 summarizes the incidence of neutropenia reported in these four studies.

The frequency of neutropenia reported in three of these controlled trials is similar to that observed in the open-label trials summarized above ($\leq 40\%$). In the two randomized trials utilizing an observation-only (no-treatment) maintenance arm, the incidence of neutropenia in untreated persons could not be determined since individuals so assigned had early progression of retinitis and were retreated with ganciclovir induction treatment. In the study reported by Rozenbaum et al. in Paris (42), the frequency of neutropenia (ANC $< 500/\mu l$) was 60%, if all induction, maintenance, and reinduction courses of therapy were evaluated. This is a higher frequency than has been observed in any other study, controlled or uncontrolled, and might be attributed to the fact that 11 of the 16 persons with neutropenia were also receiving zidovudine treatment.

Thrombocytopenia.   Thrombocytopenia was uncommon in persons treated in controlled clinical studies. In the double-blind, placebo-controlled study

Table 4   Frequency of Neutropenia Reported in Controlled Clinical Trials (Persons with CMV Retinitis and AIDS)

Reference	Treatment[a]	Total no. patients	No. with ANC of:		
			< 500	500 to 1000	> 1000
Gaub et al. (41)	I (5 mg/kg BID)	8	1	2	3
	I (2.5 mg/kg BID)	5	1	1	1
Jacobson et al. (43)	I (2.5 mg/kg TID)	11	0	3	8
	M (5 mg/kg 5×/wk)	9	2	2	2
Rozenbaum et al. (42)	I (5 mg/kg BID)	22	4	6	12
	M (5 mg/kg 5×/wk)[b]	20	12	4	4
Syntex (44)	I,M (6 mg/kg 5×/wk)	20	2	5	5
	I,M (5 mg/kg 3×/wk + beta-IFN)	7	3	2	2

[a]I = induction ganciclovir treatment; M = maintenance ganciclovir treatment.
[b]Eleven of the 16 with neutropenia were also treated with zidovudine.

in patients with CMV colitis and AIDS, one ganciclovir-treated person (3.1%) and no placebo-treated person developed a platelet count of less than 25,000/μl. None of the other 61 in the study had a platelet count less than 50,000/μl during the 14-day treatment period or for 7 days afterward.

In the other four controlled trials detailed above, two of 94 (2.1%) had a platelet count less than 25,000/μl and one of 94 (1.1%) had a platelet nadir between 25,000 and 50,000 cells/μl.

Anemia. Data from the double-blind, placebo-controlled study of ganciclovir induction treatment in persons with CMV colitis and AIDS indicate little association of ganciclovir treatment with anemia (40). Table 5 summarizes the hemoglobin values in the two treatment groups. Note that this protocol excluded concomitant zidovudine therapy, and all persons treated in this study were hospitalized, reducing the likelihood of surreptitious zidovudine administration. As stated earlier, it is difficult to draw conclusions about the effects of ganciclovir on red blood cell production if counts are followed for only 21 days, as was the case in the above controlled study. Clearly, ganciclovir induction caused no acute reduction in hemoglobin.

Of the other controlled studies referenced above, only the randomized comparison of ganciclovir maintenance treatment to low-dose ganciclovir maintenance plus beta-interferon followed an adequate number of individuals for more than 30 days, at a time when anemia would become apparent secondary to decreased erythropoiesis. Of the 19 subjects available for hematologic analysis, the median time of follow-up was greater than 77 days for both groups (range of 25 to 139 days). During this period, which included induction treatment followed immediately by maintenance treatment at the assigned regimen, seven of 19 (36.8%) had a minimum hemoglobin <8.0 g/dl, and one of these (5.3%) had a hemoglobin <6.5 g/dl. There was no significant difference between the treatment groups at this interim analysis.

Table 5 Minimum Hemoglobin Values in Persons with AIDS Receiving a 14-Day Induction Treatment Course of Ganciclovir

Minimum hemoglobin (g/dl)	No. of persons (%)	
	Ganciclovir $n = 32$	Placebo $n = 30$
≥9.5	16 (50)	10 (33)
8.0 to <9.5	13 (41)	14 (47)
6.5 to <8.0	3 (9)	6 (20)
<6.5	0	0

B. Hematological Toxicity of Ganciclovir/Zidovudine Concomitant Therapy

A formal clinical evaluation of the tolerability of concomitant ganciclovir and zidovudine was undertaken by Hochster et al. (45). Forty-one persons with life- or sight-threatening CMV infections and AIDS were enrolled. Persons with prior full-dose zidovudine (1200 mg/day), reduced dose zidovudine (600 mg/day), prior ganciclovir treatment, or no prior therapy were enrolled. A baseline ANC of $\geq 1500/\mu l$ was required for entry. Zidovudine was dose-reduced for grade 3 hematological toxicity (ANC <7.9 g/dl) and both zidovudine and ganciclovir were discontinued for any grade 4 hematological toxicity (ANC $<500/\mu l$, Hgb <6.5 g/dl).

Pharmacokinetic studies showed no apparent pharmacokinetic interactions between the two drugs (46). Of 10 patients treated with 1200 mg/day zidovudine and ganciclovir maintenance treatment at 5 mg/kg, 5 days per week, nine (90%) required dose reduction because of hematological toxicity. The median ANC nadir was $828/\mu l$ (range 320-2250), and the median hemoglobin nadir was 8.0 g/dl (range 6.0-11.2), indicating that approximately three of the 10 (30%) had grade 4 neutropenia requiring discontinuation of ganciclovir. The remaining six requiring dose reductions had the dose of zidovudine reduced. An additional 11 patients, all of whom had been on ganciclovir maintenance therapy, were started on zidovudine treatment at 600 mg/day. Nine of the 11 (81%) required a dose reduction. Again, it can be estimated from the published data that three of the 11 had grade 4 neutropenia, and none had grade 4 anemia; thus, three of 11 (27%) would have required discontinuation of ganciclovir.

This frequency of severe and dose-limiting neutropenia (ANC $<500/\mu l$) is no different from that seen in the study of ganciclovir vs. ganciclovir plus beta-interferon discussed above (44) in which patients were not taking zidovudine. Since the ganciclovir plus zidovudine protocol called for dose modifications at grade 3 neutropenia or anemia (ANC $<750/\mu l$, Hgb <7.9 g/dl), it is not possible to determine if more people could have been maintained on maintenance ganciclovir treatment plus zidovudine at 600 mg/day if doses had been maintained until grade 4 toxicity occurred.

A study by Nussbaum et al. (47), which reported on 26 individuals treated with both ganciclovir and zidovudine, may address this issue. Ganciclovir was given at a dose of 5 mg/kg daily either 7 days per week (17 patients) or 5 days per week (nine patients). Zidovudine was initiated at 1200 mg/day. For grade 3 neutropenia, the zidovudine dose was reduced to 600 mg/day, and only for grade 4 neutropenia were drugs interrupted. Anemia was treated by transfusion and no dose modifications were made for anemia. Mean duration of follow-up was 12.1 weeks. Full doses were tolerated for 48% of the person-weeks, and ganciclovir plus 600 mg/day zidovudine was tolerated for an additional 26% of the person-weeks. The currently recommended dose of zidovudine (600 mg/day) plus maintenance ganciclovir was therefore tolerated for approximately 75% of the person-weeks evaluated. Everyone had at least one grade 3 neutropenia (ANC 750/μl) and there were 19 episodes of grade 4 neutropenia. One person developed bacteremia during a neutropenic episode. There was one episode of grade 4 thrombocytopenia ($<25,000/\mu$l). The authors stated that persons who require ganciclovir therapy should not be denied zidovudine treatment because the toxicity is tolerable.

C. Use of Granulocyte-Macrophage Colony Stimulating Factor with Ganciclovir

Because of the incidence of neutropenia observed in persons receiving ganciclovir or concomitant treatment with ganciclovir and zidovudine, in February 1988 a pilot evaluation of colony stimulating factor was initiated. Recombinant human granulocyte-macrophage colony stimulating factor (rhGM-CSF) was administered IV or subcutaneously to 32 persons who had AIDS and life- or sight-threatening CMV infections (48,49). All had experienced severe and dose-limiting neutropenia during previous treatment with ganciclovir. Twenty-eight of the 32 persons had an ANC $<$ 500 cells/μl at study entry, and all had an ANC less than 1000 cells/μl. After receiving daily administration of rhGM-CSF for as few as 5 days, all 32 had a dramatic and sustained increase in ANC to $>$1000 cells/μl concurrent with reinstitution of ganciclovir treatment. Twenty-six of the 32 (81.3%) had an increase in the ANC to $>$2000/μl. Ninety-two percent were able to tolerate full-dose ganciclovir maintenance treatment. Although the majority had some progression of retinitis secondary to interruptions in ganciclovir treatment prior to initiation of rhGM-CSF therapy, 30 of the 32 had stabilization or improvement of retinitis during combined treatment with rhGM-CSF and ganciclovir. Thirteen were able to tolerate combined ganciclovir and zidovudine while receiving rhGM-CSF.

The availability of the recombinant CSFs will clearly have a clinically significant impact on the myelotoxicity observed in persons receiving zidovudine or ganciclovir therapy, or combined treatment with these two drugs, since dose interruptions for neutropenia may become less frequent.

D. Changes in Clinical Chemistry Values

Renal Function

Changes in Serum Creatinine/BUN. Renal function as measured by serum creatinine was evaluated in a subset of 366 persons with AIDS who were enrolled under open-label protocols in the United States between 1984 and 1987 and had adequate lab data. Of the 366, 55 (15%) had an increase in serum creatinine to a level >1.5 g/dl at some time during ganciclovir treatment. In most cases this elevation was transient. Three (0.8%) were discontinued from ganciclovir due to decreased renal function. Using the database of all 4430 persons with AIDS who were treated under open-label protocol in the United States, decreased renal function was reported as an adverse event in 92 (2.1%).

The NIAID Treatment IND study also specifically tracked renal function. Among the first 200 entered (most complete reporting), 175 had creatinine values reported, and 12 of the 175 (6.9%) reported a serum creatinine >1.5 g/dl at some point in the study.

In the placebo-controlled study of induction ganciclovir treatment of persons with CMV colitis and AIDS, eight of 24 ganciclovir-treated individuals (25%) and six of 30 placebo-treated individuals (20%) had a maximum serum creatinine value >1.5 g/dl at any time during the study. This was not a statistically significant difference and indicates that both treated and untreated persons with AIDS may frequently have serum creatinine levels >1.5 g/dl.

Among the other controlled studies of ganciclovir treatment in persons with AIDS, neither Jacobson et al. (43) nor Gaub et al. (41) mention renal impairment or increases in serum creatinine. In the randomized study of ganciclovir vs. ganciclovir plus beta-interferon, four of 19 individuals (21%) had a maximum serum creatinine >1.5 g/dl at some time during the study.

Relationship of Renal Function to Neutropenia. Since up to 25% of AIDS patients may experience upward transient fluctuations of serum creatinine, and since ganciclovir is excreted unmetabolized by kidneys, the relationship between serum creatinine and incidence of neutropenia was studied. It is not known if there is a relationship between tissue levels or plasma levels of ganciclovir and myelotoxicity, but it could be hypothesized that such a direct relationship exists.

A total of 366 persons with AIDS who were treated with ganciclovir under open-label protocols and who had detailed laboratory data were evaluated. Participants had to have an ANC value and a concurrent serum creatinine measurement. Among those whose maximum serum creatinine was >1.5 g/dl, 18.1% had neutropenia (ANC <1000/μl) at the same time. Among those whose maximum serum creatinine was ⩽ 1.5 g/dl, 8.8% were neutropenic. This modest association between elevated serum creatinine and neutropenia does not prove a causal relationship, as these individuals may have been taking concomitant medications characterized as having both renal and marrow toxicity. The data do indicate that laboratory monitoring in persons treated with ganciclovir is essential to ensure safety and to dose appropriately.

Hepatic Function

Among 4430 persons with AIDS who were treated with intravenous ganciclovir under open-label protocols in the United States, 140 patients (3.2%) had liver dysfunction or elevated liver function tests reported as an adverse event. In an analysis of the first 427 treated between May 1984 and January 1987, nine (2.1%) had ganciclovir treatment discontinued due to liver dysfunction or rising liver function tests. Similar data collected from the Treatment IND study indicate that three of 200 persons (1.5%) had increased liver function test results. Deaths were reported for 64 of these 200 Treatment IND participants within the follow-up period of the study (17 months), and none of the 64 had liver failure or liver dysfunction listed as a cause of death.

Some data are also available from controlled trials of ganciclovir. Among the 22 persons with CMV retinitis randomized to maintenance or no-maintenance ganciclovir in Paris, one person (4.5%) had liver dysfunction listed as an adverse event with markedly elevated SGPT, SGOT, glutamyl transpeptidase (GGT), and alkaline phosphatase upon initiation of induction ganciclovir treatment (38).

Analysis of all liver function test values for the 62 persons with CMV colitis and AIDS who were randomized to ganciclovir induction treatment or placebo was undertaken. The results are shown in Table 6. There was no difference between treatment groups in the proportion of persons with an abnormal alkaline phosphatase, SGOT, SGPT, or total bilirubin value at any time during study drug administration. Clearly, these HIV-infected individuals frequently have elevated liver function test values, as nearly two-thirds of the placebo-treated individuals had abnormal values.

Shea et al. (50) reported a suspected case of ganciclovir-induced hepatotoxicity in a person with AIDS and CMV retinitis who was treated with intra-

Table 6 Frequency of Abnormal Liver Function Test Values in Placebo-Controlled Study of Induction Ganciclovir Treatment

Laboratory parameter	Number of persons with abnormal value during study drug administration (%)	
	Ganciclovir $n = 32$	Placebo $n = 30$
Alkaline phosphatase	20 (62.5)	20 (66.7)
SGOT	17 (53.1)	21 (70.0)
SGPT	15 (46.9)	18 (60.0)
Total bilirubin	0 (0.0)	2 (6.7)

Source: Ref. 40.

venous ganciclovir. This person had rises in SGOT, SGPT, GGT, and alkaline phosphatase upon institution of ganciclovir induction treatment. When the ganciclovir was discontinued, values for SGPT and SGOT decreased (although they remained abnormal), while GGT and alkaline phosphatase continued to rise. The person was being treated with sulfadoxine-pyrimethamine concomitant with the ganciclovir, and it also was discontinued. Upon rechallenge with ganciclovir and sulfadoxine-pyrimethamine, values for SGPT and SGOT again rose, and ganciclovir was again discontinued with a modest decrease in the SGOT and SGPT values. Biopsy of the liver showed acid-fast granulomas, no evidence of chronic hepatitis, and was culture-positive for *Mycobacterium avium intracellulare.*

E. Other Clinical Adverse Events in Persons with HIV Infection

During the clinical trials of intravenous ganciclovir, treatment was interrupted or discontinued due to adverse events in approximately 32% of persons at some point in the treatment course. In some instances, treatment was restarted and the adverse event reappeared. The majority of these discontinuations ($\sim 65\%$) were due to leukopenia/neutropenia.

Adverse events other than those discussed above (which are evaluable by reference to some quantifiable laboratory parameter) are more difficult to evaluate because the population involved is so very ill, with protean manifestations of underlying disease. Additionally, these persons were being treated with numerous concomitant medications, many with the potential for significant toxicity.

Other than the laboratory abnormalities noted above, two clinical adverse events have been reported to occur with a frequency greater than 2% in persons with AIDS: rash and fever (25). Fever is most likely a manifestation of underlying disease in these persons. Detailed measurement of temperature was undertaken in the double-blind, placebo-controlled study in persons with CMV colitis and AIDS (40). During induction ganciclovir treatment for 14 days, persons in the ganciclovir group had lower body temperatures than placebo-treated individuals. Although the difference was not statistically significant ($p = 0.11$), these data indicate that ganciclovir probably does not cause a drug-induced fever, at least in most persons, and may reduce fever in this group.

Rash was reported to occur in 2% of individuals treated with intravenous ganciclovir (25). In most cases, this was reported as a maculopapular rash of the trunk, arms, and or legs. It was pruritic and often disappeared upon withdrawal of ganciclovir. In several instances where persons were rechallenged with intravenous ganciclovir, the rash recurred.

Table 7 Listing of Clinical Adverse Events Thought to Be "Possibly" Related to Ganciclovir Treatment: Open-Label Studies (Adverse Events Reported in Less than 1% of Treated Persons)

Body as a whole	Chills, edema, infections, malaise
Cardiovascular system	Arrhythmia, hypertension, hypotension
Nervous system	Abnormal thoughts or dreams, ataxia, coma, confusion, dizziness, headache, nervousness, paresthesia, psychosis, somnolence, tremor
Digestive system	Nausea, vomiting, anorexia, diarrhea, hemorrhage, abdominal pain
Respiratory system	Dyspnea
Skin	Alopecia, pruritus, urticaria
Special senses	Retinal detachment
Urogenital system	Hematuria
Injection site	Inflammation, pain, phlebitis

Other adverse events that have been reported in patients treated with intravenous ganciclovir and were thought by the treating physician to be "possibly or probably related" to ganciclovir treatment are listed by body system in Table 7. In the placebo-controlled study of ganciclovir treatment of CMV colitis in persons with AIDS (40), no adverse event other than neutropenia occurred more frequently in the ganciclovir group than among placebo-treated individuals.

F. Retinal Detachment

Rhegmatogenous retinal detachments have been reported with varying frequency in persons with CMV retinitis and AIDS who were treated with ganciclovir. The following series include documentation of retinal detachments: Henderly et al. (28), five of 23 persons (21.7%); Orellana et al. (34), eight of 50 eyes (16%); Holland et al. (29), seven of 40 persons (17.5%); Jabs et al. (33), seven of 46 persons (15.2%); and Freeman et al. (51), five of 17 persons (29.4%). Detachments were attributed to breaks in areas of scarred and healed retinopathy.

Retinal detachment has not been reported in persons treated with ganciclovir who did not have CMV retinitis. It has not been reported in anyone with an immunodeficiency other than AIDS.

V. CLINICAL SAFETY OF INTRAVENOUS GANCICLOVIR IN TRANSPLANT PATIENTS

Clinical safety data from transplant patients treated with ganciclovir is presented separately from those for persons infected with HIV. Transplant patients clearly constitute a different population with regard to manifestations of toxicity to ganciclovir, underlying disease processes, immunosuppression, and concomitant medications. Hematological changes have been further divided into those occurring in bone marrow transplant patients and those in patients receiving solid-organ allografts.

A. Hematological Changes

Hematological Changes in Bone Marrow Transplant Patients

Considerable attention has been paid to the safety of intravenous ganciclovir in bone marrow transplant patients. Such patients are at considerable risk of developing CMV pneumonia or other life-threatening CMV infections, and thus are often treated with ganciclovir. However, the hematological toxicity of ganciclovir may be exacerbated in these patients with little or no marrow reserve.

The frequency of leukopenia and neutropenia observed in bone marrow transplant patients as reported in the literature is summarized in Table 8. Shepp et al. (52) noted that neutropenia occurred after more than 10 days of treatment with ganciclovir in all but one patient, and was reversible upon interruption of therapy. Neither Shepp et al. (52), Erice et al. (53), nor Reed et al. (54) noted a strong correlation between creatinine clearance or plasma levels of ganciclovir and occurrence of neutropenia. Reed et al. (54) reported that the nadir of the neutrophil count occurred a median of 4 days after ganciclovir was discontinued. Severe neutropenia (ANC $< 500/\mu$l) lasted for a median of 4 days in the seven patients who were severely neutropenic. Emanuel et al. (55) reported that the neutropenia (ANC $< 500/\mu$l) was observed after

Table 8 Leukopenia/Neutropenia Reported in Bone Marrow Transplant Patients Receiving Intravenous Ganciclovir

Reference	Dose of GCV	No. patients neutropenic/treated (%)
Shepp et al. (52)	5 mg/kg TID	2/5 (40%)
	2.5 mg/kg TID	2/5 (40%)
Erice et al. (53)	1.25-5 mg/kg TID	9/15 (60%)
Reed et al. (54)	1-2.5 g/kg TID	7/15 (46%)
Emanuel et al. (55)	2.5 mg/kg TID, then 5 g/kg QD	8/10 (80%)
Reed et al. (56)	2.5 mg/kg TID	12/18 (67%)
Verdonck et al. (57)	2.5 mg/kg TID	0/6
Schmidt et al. (58)	5 mg/kg BID ×21 d, then 5 mg/kg QD	3/13 (23%)

a median of 12 days (range of 7 to 20 days), and that counts recovered after 7 to 10 days. Seven of the eight patients reported by Emanuel et al. to have had neutropenia could resume ganciclovir treatment after recovery of the ANC. Reed et al. (56) also reported that neutropenia did not appear until day 14 of induction ganciclovir treatment in the eight patients who developed low counts. Only three of these patients discontinued ganciclovir due to an ANC $< 500/\mu l$ during induction treatment, but six of eight patients receiving maintenance treatment were neutropenic.

Table 9 shows interim results from an ongoing double-blind, placebo-controlled trial of prophylactic ganciclovir treatment for the prevention of CMV disease in bone marrow transplant patients (59). Patients in this study must be seropositive for CMV pretransplant. They are randomized to receive either intravenous ganciclovir or placebo for 7 days, at 5 mg/kg BID from day -7 to the day before transplant, then after engraftment (WBC $>1000/\mu l$) continue treatment with the originally assigned study drug at 6 mg/kg QD 5 days per week. Patients are treated until day 120 following transplant. Based on the results from this interim analysis, more ganciclovir-treated patients than placebo-treated patients had an ANC $<1000/\mu l$ on day 56, but not at 14 or 28 days of therapy.

In their double-blind, placebo-controlled study of the efficacy of ganciclovir in treating bone marrow transplant recipients with CMV gastrointestinal disease, Reed et al. (60) reported no apparent effect of ganciclovir on neu-

Table 9 Minimum Absolute Neutrophil Counts in Bone Marrow Transplant Patients Treated with Ganciclovir or Placebo

Treatment (minimum ANC, cells/μl)	Time after ganciclovir started (postengraftment) No. of persons (%)		
	Day 14	Day 28	Day 56
Ganciclovir			
$\geqslant 3000$	12 (41)	8 (31)	3 (14)
1000 to 2999	15 (51)	13 (50)	9 (43)
599 to 999	1 (4)	1 (4)	4 (19)
< 500	1 (4)	4 (15)	5 (24)
Placebo			
$\geqslant 3000$	7 (29)	9 (39)	5 (33)
1000 to 2999	15 (63)	11 (48)	9 (50)
599 to 999	0	0	1 (7)
< 500	2 (8)	3 (13)	0

Source: Ref. 59.

trophil counts compared to placebo. In total, they treated 18 patients with ganciclovir (2.5 mg/kg TID for 14 days) and 19 with placebo on the same schedule. Treatment was discontinued in one ganciclovir patient and in four placebo patients because of a >50% decrease in ANC. The mean ANC for the placebo group showed a greater decrease than the mean ANC of the ganciclovir group, although this difference was not statistically significant. These results, along with those from the prophylactic study (Table 9), suggest that a 14- to 28-day course of ganciclovir is less likely to result in neutropenia than treatment for a longer period in bone marrow transplant patients.

Changes in platelet counts and red blood cell indices are difficult to interpret and ascribe to a single drug treatment. Engraftment following bone marrow transplantation occurs first with the leukocytes and later for the platelet and erythroid series, which usually recover or engraft around the time that patients are most likely to be receiving ganciclovir treatment. Thus, low counts may be due to therapy or merely to variances in rate of engraftment. In addition, these patients frequently receive platelet and erythrocyte transfusions during this posttransplant period, further confounding evaluation of drug effects. The interim data from the placebo-controlled prophylactic study in bone marrow transplant patients indicate an increase in the frequency of thrombocytopenia in patients treated with ganciclovir vs. placebo (Table 10).

Emanuel et al. (55) reported that one patient developed pure red cell aplasia after receiving ganciclovir plus intravenous immunoglobulin treatment for CMV pneumonia. After 9 days of therapy, the patient developed erythroid

Table 10 Minimum Platelet Counts in Bone Marrow Transplant Patients Treated with Ganciclovir or Placebo

Treatment (minimum) platelet count (cells/μl)	Time after ganciclovir started No. of persons (%)		
	Day 14	Day 28	Day 56
Ganciclovir			
≥100,000	9 (31)	9 (35)	8 (38)
25,000 to 99,999	10 (34)	11 (42)	6 (29)
<25,000	10 (35)	6 (23)	7 (33)
Placebo			
≥100,000	11 (42)	12 (50)	8 (53)
25,000 to 99,999	11 (42)	8 (33)	6 (40)
<25,000	4 (16)	4 (17	1 (7)

Source: Ref. 59.

aplasia with a duration of 4 weeks. Ganciclovir was not restarted in this patient, who eventually recovered normal erythropoietic function.

Use of GM-CSF with Ganciclovir in Bone Marrow Transplant Patients

Fouillard et al. (61) reported on the use of GM-CSF in 14 patients after autologous marrow transplantation, six of whom required treatment with ganciclovir for CMV infection. In three patients, the GM-CSF and ganciclovir were given together and no neutropenia was observed. In the other three (nonrandomized) patients, ganciclovir was given alone, and severe neutropenia (ANC $< 500/\mu l$) occurred in all three. When one of these patients was subsequently given GM-CSF, the ANC increased to $> 500/\mu l$ within 3 days.

Hematological Changes in Patients with Solid-Organ Allografts

Among 101 patients receiving solid-organ allographs (liver, kidney, heart, heart-lung) who were treated open-label with ganciclovir and reported in the literature, 11 (11%) were reported to have leukopenia/neutropenia (62-66). The largest single-center series of cases was by Stratta et al. (66), who reported leukopenia or thrombocytopenia in five of 69 (7%) liver allograft patients.

The best data available concerning the hematological effects of ganciclovir on peripheral cell counts in this patient population are from a double-blind, placebo-controlled study of ganciclovir prophylaxis in heart transplant patients (67). This study enrolled patients who were CMV-seropositive pretransplant or received an organ from a CMV-seropositive donor, or both. Patients were randomized to start treatment on the day after transplant, and received ganciclovir or placebo, 5 mg/kg BID for 14 days, then 5 mg/kg per day for 14 additional days. Total treatment duration was 28 days. Doses of ganciclovir were adjusted for renal impairment. Interim hematological data are available for comparison of 50 ganciclovir-treated and 46 placebo-treated patients. The results are shown in Table 11. In this patient population, unlike persons with AIDS, no hematological effects were observed after 4 weeks of treatment with ganciclovir. There was no statistically significant difference with regard to ANC between the ganciclovir and the placebo groups, and more placebo patients than ganciclovir patients had an ANC in the 1000-1999/μl range. This could be related to the possible efficacy of ganciclovir in preventing CMV syndrome, one manifestation of which is neutropenia. There were several more ganciclovir-treated patients who had thrombocytopenia than placebo patients, but this difference was not statistically significant and may have been an incidental finding. Values for minimum hemoglobin were also analyzed and did not show a difference between the treatment groups.

Table 11 Effects of a 28-Day Course of Intravenous Ganciclovir or Placebo on Hematological Indices in Heart Allograft Recipients

	Number of patients (%)	
Hematological index	Ganciclovir $n = 50$	Placebo $n = 46$
Minimum ANC (cells/μl)		
>3000	35 (70)	22 (49)
2000-2999	8 (16)	9 (20)
1000-1999	3 (6)	11 (24)
500-999	1 (2)	1 (2)
<500	3 (6)	2 (4)
Minimum platelets (cells/μl)		
>100,000	29 (58)	26 (57)
50,000-100,000	17 (34)	19 (41)
25,000-49,999	2 (4)	1 (2)
<25,000	2 (4)	0

Source: Ref. 67.

As has been observed in nonrandomized trials and patient series involving intravenous ganciclovir, the hematological toxicity of ganciclovir depends on the bone marrow reserve and hematopoietic status of the patient. In individuals with AIDS or those who have received a marrow graft, bone marrow function is abnormal and hematological toxicity is more common than in patients (such as solid-organ allograft recipients) in whom the marrow is quite normal. This same sensitivity of the marrow to potentially myelotoxic drugs is seen with zidovudine, where the rate of neutropenia (ANC <750) was 47% in persons with advanced AIDS but only 6 to 10% in persons with early HIV infection and more normal marrow (68,69).

B. Changes in Clinical Chemistry Values, Transplant Patients

Renal Function

Shepp et al. (52) reported that four of 10 patients had worsening of renal function while receiving ganciclovir for treatment of CMV pneumonia. In all cases there were other possible causes of the renal dysfunction. There is no mention in six other published reports (53-58) of renal toxicity, whether or not attributed to ganciclovir treatment.

In the interim analysis of safety results from the double-blind, placebo-controlled prophylaxis study in bone marrow transplant patients (59), fewer ganciclovir-treated patients than placebo-treated patients had an elevated serum creatinine (≥ 1.5 mg/dl), indicating no renal toxicity of ganciclovir in this patient population.

In solid-organ allograft recipients, Keay et al. (63) reported that two heart transplant patients developed significant decreases in creatinine clearance during treatment with ganciclovir. No other report in the literature documents occurrences of renal dysfunction (62,64-66).

Renal function was also evaluated in the placebo-controlled study of prophylactic ganciclovir in heart allograft recipients. There was a statistically significant increase in the frequency of patients with a serum creatinine greater than 2.5 mg/dl in the ganciclovir-treated group (22%) vs. the placebo group (4%). In the ganciclovir-treated group, five of 50 patients had creatinine >2.5 mg/dl during the first week of therapy, and six patients had this elevation during week 3 or 4 of the 28-day treatment period. However, the median time to elevated serum creatinine (≥ 1.5 mg/dl) was identical for the ganciclovir- and the placebo-treated groups, and the total proportion of patients with an elevated creatinine was not different between groups. All patients were receiving cyclosporine to prevent allograft rejection, and it is not known if the increased incidence of serum creatinine over 2.5 mg/dl in the ganciclovir-treated group of patients might be the result of the combined effects of these two drugs.

In dogs dosed intravenously with 90 mg/kg per day for 30 days, ganciclovir caused renal tubular dilatation with deposition of insoluble cast material in excretory tubules, and increased serum creatinine and BUN. This toxicity was not seen in any other animal safety study at lower doses.

Recommendations for Dosing in Renal Impairment (see Section VI.A)

C. Other Clinical Adverse Events in Transplant Patients

Evaluation of adverse events in the patient who has received a bone marrow transplant or solid-organ allograft is quite difficult, for reasons outlined earlier. Attribution of drug relatedness of such events is best made by comparing the frequency of a particular event in placebo-controlled situations. Fortunately, two placebo-controlled studies—one in bone marrow (allograft) recipients and one in heart allograft recipients, each involving about 100 patients total—have undergone interim analysis. The analysis and comparison of adverse events in these two studies are summarized in Table 12. Bone marrow transplant recipients who were treated with ganciclovir or placebo received a dose of 6 mg/kg per day, 5 days per week from engraftment (WBC $>1000/\mu l$) until day 120 posttransplant. Heart recipients received 5 mg/kg BID from the day after transplant until day 14, then 5 mg/kg once daily through day 28 after transplant.

Table 12 Frequency of Adverse Events Reports in Placebo-Controlled Prophylactic Studies of Ganciclovir

| | Number of patients reporting event (%) | | | |
| | Bone marrow transplant | | Heart transplant | |
Adverse event	Ganciclovir	Placebo	Ganciclovir	Placebo
Total patients	44	40	50	47
Digestive system				
GI pain	12 (27)	12 (30)	2 (4)	5 (11)
Diarrhea	19 (43)	17 (43)	3 (6)	4 (9)
Gastritis	0	0	2 (4)	4 (9)
Sore mouth	16 (36)	16 (40)	0	1 (2)
Nausea	19 (43)	18 (45)	2 (4)	3 (6)
Abnormal LFTs	12 (27)	10 (25)	0	1 (2)
Body as a whole				
Fever	18 (41)	17 (43)	5 (10)	8 (17)
Chills	7 (16)	5 (13)	0	0
Myalgia	5 (11)	2 (5)	0	4 (9)
Edema	14 (32)	16 (40)	0	3 (6)
Skin and appendages				
Injection site reaction	2 (5)	5 (13)	0	0
Rash	17 (39)	17 (43)	2 (4)	1 (2)
Nervous system				
Headache	12 (27)	13 (33)	9 (18)	5 (11)
Convulsion/seizure	1 (2)	3 (8)	3 (6)	4 (9)
Cardiovascular system				
Hypertension	15 (34)	16 (40)	7 (14)	2 (4)
Hypotension	11 (25)	8 (20)	2 (4)	5 (11)
Tachycardia	17 (39)	17 (43)	0	2 (4)

As noted, when elevated serum creatinine was used as a measure of renal dysfunction, ganciclovir-treated heart transplant patients more commonly had renal abnormalities reported, perhaps due to concomitant dosing with cyclosporine. Four ganciclovir-treated patients had sepsis, compared with none of the placebo controls, but none of these septic episodes was associated with neutropenia. Placebo-treated heart transplant recipients tended to have increased herpesvirus infections of the skin.

VI. OTHER CLINICAL SAFETY DATA

A. Safety of Long-Term Dosing

Since many patients remain on ganciclovir treatment for prolonged periods of time (months), the long-term safety of intravenous ganciclovir is important.

The best long-term safety information is an analysis done in 1988 of data collected during the open-label protocol of ganciclovir in the United States (70). A total of 522 patients were considered, and only patients who received 120 days or more of ganciclovir dosing were included in the analysis. The time of first onset of any adverse event was tabulated, as was the Kaplan-Meier estimate of the median time to event onset and the proportion of events occurring within any given time after dosing was initiated. The majority of these persons had a diagnosis of AIDS.

A total of 60 patients were treated for 120 or more days. Fifty-one of the 60 reported one or more adverse events, and there were a total of 142 events reported. The results are summarized in Table 13. Events were more likely to be reported during the first 30 days of dosing in these patients. However, the data clearly indicate that the first occurrence of many adverse events, most notably leukopenia and thrombocytopenia, can occur after 60 or more days of dosing. For this reason, frequent laboratory and clinical monitoring of patients being dosed long-term with intravenous ganciclovir is imperative.

B. Safety in Pediatric and Geriatric Patients

Since ganciclovir causes cancer in animals and is mutagenic in in vitro tests, it may be a carcinogen in humans. Careful consideration must be given to the benefit to risk assessment in pediatric patients before initiating treatment with ganciclovir in this population.

From data collected during open-label studies in the United States between 1984 and 1988, an analysis of adverse events reported for pediatric patients was undertaken (68). During this 4-year period, 120 pediatric patients (age less than 13 years) were treated with intravenous ganciclovir. Ninety-eight

Table 13 Long-Term Safety of Intravenous Ganciclovir: Data from 60 Patients Treated for 120 Days or More

Adverse event	Cumulative probability (percent of patients) of first occurrence of event by				Median days to first event
	30 Days	60 Days	90 Days	120 Days	
Leukopenia	33	43	49	55	12
Thrombocytopenia	6	8	10	15	12
Anemia	3	6	6	7	30
Nausea	5	5	6	8	5
Emesis	2	3	7	9	49
Fever	5	7	8	11	13
Rash	4	5	7	7	9

Table summarizes events occurring at a cumulative frequency of 5% or more.

of the 120 patients (82%) were less than 6 years old, and 36 of the 120 (30%) were less than 1 year old. Of the 120 patients, 26 (22%) had AIDS and 94 had immunodeficiencies other than AIDS.

Overall, fewer adverse events were reported in the pediatric patients than in adult patients, and adverse events were less often reported as "probably related" to ganciclovir treatment. The prevalence of a few adverse events was higher (twofold or more increased frequency) in pediatric patients than in adult patients treated: abnormalities of renal function (6%), thrombocytopenia in pediatric persons with AIDS (12%), rash in pediatric persons with AIDS (12%), urticaria (8%), and abnormal dreams (2%). These comparisons were analyzed by comparing pediatric to adult patients in the same immunodeficiency category.

No specific studies of the safety and efficacy of intravenous ganciclovir in geriatric patients have been reported. Since elderly individuals may have reduced creatinine clearance, careful attention should be paid to assessing renal function and making appropriate dose adjustments in these patients (see Section VII.A).

C. Drug Interactions and Concomitant Medications

Concomitant administration of ganciclovir and zidovudine, and of ganciclovir and GM-CSF, has been discussed in Sections III.B and III.C (see also Chapter 13).

Hartman et al. (72) reported on the concomitant administration of 2',3'-dideoxyinosine (ddI) and intravenous ganciclovir. Ganciclovir administration resulted in no apparent change in the pharmacokinetics of ddI. In vitro studies by the same authors revealed that preincubation of cells with ganciclovir did not alter the intracellular phosphorylation of ddI. Liebman et al. (73) reported on five patients who were receiving intravenous ganciclovir maintenance treatment (6 mg/kg, 5 days per week) and were then started on treatment with ddI orally at 375 mg BID. Over a mean follow-up period of 5 weeks, no intolerance to either drug and no neutropenia were observed.

Concomitant administration of pentamidine, amphotericin, trimethoprimesulfamethoxizole, or acyclovir with intravenous ganciclovir was analyzed in 262 people with AIDS who were treated under open-label protocols between 1984 and 1987 (25). Use of any of these four medications was associated with a frequency of leukopenia 38 to 65% higher than in persons not taking such medications. Similarly, persons taking any one of these medications had a one- to fourfold higher reported frequency of thrombocytopenia. This observed association does not prove a causal relationship between concomitant medication and cytopenia, since severity of underlying illness or other factors may be causally related to both the cytopenia and the need for one of these medications. However, these data suggest that persons receiving intravenous ganciclovir with one or more of these medications should be monitored closely for toxicity.

Generalized seizures were observed in six persons who were receiving both intravenous ganciclovir and imipenem-cilastatin. Imipenem-cilastatin has been associated with seizures, and it is not known if ganciclovir potentiated this effect or not. These drugs should not be used together unless the potential benefit outweighs the risk.

Theoretically, drug interactions that involve inhibition or potentiation of metabolism are not likely with ganciclovir since, metabolically, ganciclovir is relatively inert. However, it is possible that intracellular interactions involving phosphorylation of nucleosides could occur between ganciclovir and other nucleoside analogs. Drugs that inhibit glomerular filtration would be expected to slow the excretion of ganciclovir and result in higher plasma and tissue levels. Drugs that have cytotoxic or cytostatic effects on rapidly dividing cell populations (alkylating agents, antimetabolites, other nucleoside analogs, folate inhibitors, or vinca alkyloids, for example) may theoretically have additive toxicity when administered concomitantly with ganciclovir.

D. Gonadal Function

In preclinical animal safety studies, ganciclovir was found to be a potent inhibitor of spermatogenesis (see Section III.C). Gonadal toxicity has been evaluated in humans in several clinical studies. Assessment of this data is confounded by the fact that the patients most likely to be receiving intravenous ganciclovir are people with HIV infection or transplant recipients. Males with advanced AIDS have testicular hypoplasia and hypo- or aspermatogenesis at autopsy (74,75), and transplant patients, particularly bone marrow transplant patients, are presumed to sustain irreversible toxicity to the spermatogonium. Any gonadal toxicity of ganciclovir would likely be difficult to detect when overlaid on this preexisting gonadal dysfunction.

In an evaluation of reproductive hormones in men with AIDS who received intravenous ganciclovir treatment during the first 2 years of the open-label studies, more than twice as many men had increases in testosterone, FSH, and LH than had decreases. Although these results could be secondary to inhibition of spermatogenesis (which results in an increase in FSH and LH), they could be secondary to other processes, including an improvement in pituitary and interstitial cell secretory function. In the placebo-controlled study of a 14-day course of induction ganciclovir treatment in people with CMV colitis and AIDS, interim results showed no effect of ganciclovir on testosterone, LH, FSH, or testicular volume over a 28-day period.

In an open-label study of ganciclovir treatment of CMV infection in renal transplant patients carried out in Europe (76), 10 men had sperm counts performed between 1 and 6 months after completing a 14-day course of induction ganciclovir treatment. Five of the 10 men had decreased sperm counts, but the other five had counts considered in the normal range. These data indicate that, at least in some individuals, treatment with ganciclovir does not result in irreversible aspermatogenesis.

Although it is likely that ganciclovir results in decreased spermatogenesis, assessment of interstitial cell histology in the testes of animals and observations of normal mating behavior in male and female rats dosed with ganciclovir (Section III.C) indicate no inhibition of potency or libido. Among 4430 people with AIDS who received ganciclovir under one or more open-label protocols between 1984 and 1989, impotence was reported in one individual.

E. Safety of Intravitreal Ganciclovir

The use of ganciclovir by intravitreal injection has been reported by several authors for the treatment of CMV retinitis. Table 14 summarizes the adverse events that have occurred in these cases. The adverse events reported by Cantrill et al. (77) occurred for the most part after a mean of 17 injections per eye over a 4-month period (see Chapter 7).

F. Immunosuppressive Effects

Bowden et al. (81) reported on the effects of ganciclovir on in vitro lymphocyte proliferative responses to antigen or mitogen. Peripheral blood lymphocytes from healthy adults were incubated in graded concentrations of ganciclovir in tissue culture media of 1.0 to 100 μg/ml. At concentrations of 5.0 μg/ml or more, ganciclovir inhibited lymphocyte proliferative responses to CMV antigen or PHA mitogen. However, ganciclovir did not

Table 14 Summary of Adverse Events Occurring in Persons Receiving Intravitreal Ganciclovir Injections

Reference	Number of eyes treated	Frequency of adverse event
Ussery et al. (78)	14	Retinal detachment (1)
Henry et al. (79)	1	None
Cantrill et al. (77)	15	Small conjunctival hemorrhage (''some'')
		Mild conjunctival scars (''some'')
		Scleral induration (''some'')
		Staphylococcic endophthalmitis (1)
Daikos et al. (80)	4	None

inhibit lymphocyte production of interleukin-2 or interferon gamma, nor did ganciclovir affect cytotoxicity. The data indicate that ganciclovir inhibits only those functions of lymphocytes requiring DNA synthesis and cellular proliferation.

VII. DOSING ADJUSTMENTS

A. Dose Adjustment for Renal Impairment

Ganciclovir is excreted essentially unmetabolized by the kidneys. The total clearance of ganciclovir is proportional to creatinine clearance, and thus dose modifications must be made in patients in whom creatinine clearance is significantly reduced. Table 15 gives the recommended dose reductions. Dose adjustments for maintenance treatment with intravenous ganciclovir have not been determined. Physicians may elect to reduce the dose for maintenance treatment to 50% of the induction dose given above and monitor carefully for efficacy and toxicity.

Creatinine clearance should be either measured or calculated based on serum creatinine, body weight, age, and sex using standard methods for estimating creatinine clearance. This is particularly important in persons who may have wasting or body weight markedly below the ideal. In people with AIDS whose body weight may be 20% or more below ideal, evaluating renal function by assessment of serum creatinine alone may overestimate both creatinine and ganciclovir clearance.

B. Overdosage

Overdosage with ganciclovir has been reported in five patients. In three patients who received seven doses of 22 mg/kg over a 3-day period, 9 mg/kg BID for 3 days, or two doses of 500 mg given to a 21-month-old child, no adverse events were observed after the dosing. One patient received ganciclovir at 5 mg/kg BID for 14 days, followed by treatment with 8 mg/kg once

Table 15 Recommended Doses of Intravenous Ganciclovir Induction Treatment in Renal Impairment

Creatinine clearance (ml/1.73 m²/min)	Ganciclovir dose (mg/kg)	Dosing interval (hours)
≥80	5.0	12
50-79	2.5	12
25-49	2.5	24
<25	1.25	24

daily for 4 days, and developed neutropenia of 17 days' duration. Another patient received a single dose of approximately 24 mg/kg (1675 mg) and developed neutropenia of 1 day's duration.

In open-label protocols, 25 persons received induction ganciclovir doses of 5 mg/kg TID or 15 mg/kg per day for 10 to 21 days. The frequency of neutropenia (defined as an ANC $<1000/\mu$l or a $>50\%$ decrease from baseline ANC) was six of 25 (24%), a figure no higher than that observed for the dose of 10 mg/kg per day.

VIII. SUMMARY

Ganciclovir (DHPG) is a nucleoside analog that is phosphorylated intracellularly even by uninfected mammalian cells and can inhibit cellular replication in more rapidly multiplying cell populations. In vitro testing reveals that the bone marrow progenitor cells are the most sensitive to the cytostatic effects of ganciclovir.

Preclinical animal studies conducted with ganciclovir indicate that ganciclovir toxicity is somewhat radiomimetic, affecting primarily the bone marrow, skin, and gastrointestinal mucosa as well as the reproductive tract. Ganciclovir causes hypospermatogenesis or aspermatogenesis in dogs at doses as low as 0.4 mg/kg per day and caused sterility in rodents. Ganciclovir resulted in teratogenicity in rabbits. Ganciclovir was found to be mutagenic in some in vitro/ex vivo assays and, in an 18-month lifetime bioassay for carcinogenicity, was found to be carcinogenic in mice. Because of its safety profile, ganciclovir should be limited to use for the treatment of life- or sight-threatening CMV infections where the expected benefits outweigh the risks.

The clinical safety of ganciclovir in persons with HIV infections has been studied. The most common toxicity seen is neutropenia that is dose-limiting (ANC $<500/\mu$l) in approximately 20% of treated patients. Neutropenia is usually reversible, although rare cases of irreversible neutropenia have been reported. Thrombocytopenia ($< 50,000/\mu$l) is less common in persons with HIV infection, approximately 15%. Hematological toxicity of ganciclovir may be enhanced when patients are concomitantly treated with zidovudine. However, as many as 75% of patients may tolerate ganciclovir for maintenance treatment with zidovudine at a dose of 500 to 600 mg/day. Granulocyte-macrophage colony stimulating factor has been shown to increase neutrophil counts in patients who are neutropenic secondary to ganciclovir therapy.

In persons with AIDS treated with ganciclovir, 2 to 7% of patients may have increases in serum creatinine to >1.5 g/dl sometime during treatment. Other adverse events that may be related to ganciclovir treatment in 2% of patients or less include hepatic dysfunction, rash, and fever.

Retinal detachment occurs at a frequency of between 15 and 30% of patients with CMV retinitis who are treated with intravenous ganciclovir. Detachment is believed to be secondary to healing and scarring of the retina following resolution of retinopathy after ganciclovir treatment. Retinal detachment has not been reported in patients treated with ganciclovir who do not have CMV retinitis.

The clinical safety of ganciclovir has also been studied in transplant patients. Neutropenia is frequently observed in bone marrow transplant patients treated with ganciclovir. Results from a double-blind, placebo-controlled trial indicate that severe neutropenia may occur in approximately 25% of patients after bone marrow transplantation as compared to placebo, but that this neutropenia is not seen until after 28 days of continuous ganciclovir treatment. Ganciclovir treatment may also delay time between engraftment of platelets in bone marrow transplant recipients. In patients receiving solid-organ allografts who have more bone marrow reserve, neutropenia is uncommon. Increases in serum creatinine and transient decreased renal function may occur in patients treated with ganciclovir more often than in patients treated with placebo following a solid-organ allograft. It is possible that this is the result of concomitant administration of both cyclosporine and intravenous ganciclovir. When clinical symptoms were compared between ganciclovir and placebo-treated bone marrow or heart transplant patients, only an increase in serum creatinine occurred more commonly in the ganciclovir group than the placebo group.

Ganciclovir appears to be safe when administered for 120 days or more; however, the probability of occurrence of hematological toxicity and other adverse events increases with time. It is estimated that up to 54% of persons with AIDS treated with ganciclovir may eventually develop neutropenia. In a study of the safety of ganciclovir in pediatric patients, no major differences between pediatric adverse events and those reported in adult patients were observed.

Care must be taken with the concomitant administration of ganciclovir with cytotoxic drugs or those that affect renal function. Since intravenous ganciclovir is excreted essentially unmetabolized by the kidneys, ganciclovir clearance is proportional to creatinine clearance, and dose modifications must be made in patients in whom creatinine clearance is reduced.

Ganciclovir is an effective and potent nucleoside antiviral. It has been shown to be effective in the treatment of CMV retinitis in immunocompromised persons and when given concomitantly with intravenous immunoglobulin in the treatment of CMV pneumonia in bone marrow transplant recipients. It has recently been shown that intravenous ganciclovir is effective for the prevention of CMV pneumonia and CMV disease in both bone marrow transplant and heart allograft recipients. In every instance in which ganciclovir is considered for use, the potential benefits must be weighed against the possible risks of administration.

ACKNOWLEDGMENTS

The author wishes to thank Ms. Regina Lino for invaluable assistance with the preparation of the manuscript, and Dr. Charles Du Mond for statistical analysis. A special thanks to Ms. Barbara Mastre, Ms. Patricia Cheney, and Dr. Bernadette DeArmond for assistance with monitoring and evaluation of clinical data.

REFERENCES

1. Field AK, Davies ME, DeWitt C, Perry C, Liou R, Germershausen J, Tolman RL. 9-{[2-Hydroxy-1-(hydroxymethyl)ethoxy]methyl}guanine: A selective inhibitor of herpes group virus replication. Proc Natl Acad Sci USA 1983; 50: 4139-4143.
2. Smee DF, Martin JC, Verheyden JPH, Matthews TR. Anti-herpesvirus activity of the acyclic nucleoside 9-(1,3-dihydroxy-2-propoxymethyl)guanine. Antimicrob Agents Chemother 1983; 23:676-682.
3. Smith KO, Galloway KS, Kennell WL, Ogilvie KK. A new nucleoside analog, 9-{2-hydroxy-1-(hydroxymethyl)ethoxy}guanine, highly active in vitro against herpes simplex virus types 1 and 2. Antimicrob Agents Chemother 1982; 22:55-61.
4. Cheng Y, Huang E, Lin J, Mar E, Pagano JS, Dutschman GE, Grill SP. Unique spectrum of activity of 9-[1-3-dihydroxy-2-propoxy)methyl-guanine against herpesviruses in vitro and its mode of action against herpes simplex virus type 1. Proc Natl Acad Sci USA 1983; 50:2767-2770.
5. Fraser-Smith EB, Smee DF, Matthews TR. Efficacy of the acyclic nucleoside 9-(1,3-dihydroxy-2-propoxymethyl)guanine against primary and recrudescent genital herpes simplex virus type 2 infections in guinea pigs. Antimicrob Agents Chemother 1983; 883-887.
6. Tocci MJ, Livelli TJ, Perry HC, Crumpacker CS, Field AK. Effects of the nucleoside analog 2'-nor-2'-deoxyguanosine on human cytomegalovirus replication. Antimicrob Agents Chemother 1984; 25:247-252.
7. Davies MM, Bondi JV, Field K. Efficacy of 2'-nor-2'-deoxyguanosine treatment for orofacial herpes simplex virus type 1 skin infections in mice. Antimicrob Agents Chemother 1984; 25:238-241.
8. Collins P, Oliver NM. Comparison of the in vitro and in vivo antiherpes virus activities of the acyclic nucleosides, acyclovir (Zovirax) and 9-[(2-hydroxy-1-hydroxymethyl-ethyoxy)methyl]guanine (BWB759U). Antiviral Res 1985; 5:145-156.
9. Biron KK, Stanat SC, Sorrell JB, Fyfe JA, Keller PM, Lambe CU, Nelson DJ. Metabolic activation of the nucleoside analog 9-{[2-hydroxy-1-(hydroxymethyl)-

ethoxy]methyl}guanine in human diploid fibroblasts infected with human cyto-megalovirus. Proc Natl Acad Sci USA 1985; 82:2473-2477.

10. Shanley JD, Morningstar J, Jordan MC. Inhibition of pneumonitis by acyclovir and 9-(1,3-dihydroxy-2-propoxymethyl)guanine. Antimicrob Agents Chemother 1985; 28:172-175.

11. Plotkin SA, Drew WL, Felsenstein D, Hirsch MS. Sensitivity of clinical isolates of human cytomegalovirus to 9-(1,3-dihydroxy-2-propoxymethyl)guanine. J Infec Dis 1985; 152:833-834.

12. Wilson EJ, Medearis Jr DN, Hansen LA, Rubin AH. 9-(1,3-Dihydroxy-2-prop-oxymethyl)guanine prevents death but not immunity in murine cytomegalovirus-infected normal and immunosuppressed BALB/c mice. Antimicrob Agents Chemother 1987; 31:1017-1020.

13. Koretz SH, Buhles WC, Roe RL, Brewin A, Merigan T, Eisenberg MP, Masur H, Bissett L, Lane HC, Fauci AS. Treatment of serious cytomegalovirus infections with AIDS and other immunodeficiencies. N Engl J Med 1986; 314:801-905.

14. Freitas VR, Smee DF, Chernow M, Boehme R, Matthews TR. Activity of 9-(1,3-dihydroxy-2-propoxymethyl)guanine compared with that of acyclovir against human, monkey and rodent cytomegalovirus. Antimicrob Agents Chemother 1985; 28:240-245.

15. Lin JC, Smith MC, Pagano JS. Prolonged inhibitory effect of 9-(1,3-dihydroxy-2-propoxymethyl)guanine against replication of Epstein-Barr virus. J Virol 1984; 50:50-58.

16. Sommadossi J, Carlisle R. Toxicity of 3'-azido-3'-deoxythymidine and 9-(1,3-dihydroxy-2-propoxymethyl)guanine for normal human hematopoietic progenitor cells in vitro. Antimicrob Agents Chemother 1987; 31:452-454.

17. Cytovene® (ganciclovir sodium) Product Monograph. Syntex Laboratories, Palo Alto, CA, 1989.

18. Pulido J, Peyman GA, Lesar T, Vernot J. Intravitreal toxicity of hydroxyacy-clovir (BW-B759U), a new antiviral agent. Arch Ophthalmol 1985; 103:840-841.

19. Schulman J, Peyman GA, Horton MB, Liu J, Barber JC, Fiscella R, de Miranda P. Intraocular penetration of new antiviral agent, hydroxyacyclovir (BW-B759U). Jpn J Ophthalmol 1986; 30:116-124.

20. Appelbaum F, Meyers J, Deeg H, Graham T, Schuening F, Storb R. Toxicity trial of prophylactic 9-[2-hydroxy-1-(hydroxymethyl)ethoxymethyl]guanine (ganciclovir) after marrow transplantation in dogs. Antimicrob Agents Chemother 1988; 32:271-273.

21. Buhles WC, Mastre BJ, Tinker AJ, Strand V, Koretz SH, Syntex Collaborative Treatment Study Group. Ganciclovir treatment of life- or sight-threatening cytomegalovirus infection: experience in 314 immunocompromised patients. Rev Infec Dis 1988; 10:S495-S504.

22. Syntex, unpublished data, CL 4737.

23. Syntex, unpublished data, CL 2793.

24. Katz D, Mastre B, De Armond B. Ganciclovir (GCV) in AIDS patients with immediately sight-threatening CMV retinitis (ISTCR): initial summary of "Treatment IND" data. VI International Conference on AIDS, San Francisco, June 1990, abstract B.432.

25. Unpublished data, Syntex Research Study no. 1257, 1990.
26. Masur H, Lane HC, Palestine A, Smith PD, Manischewitz J, Sevens G, Fujikawa L, Macher AM, Nussenblatt R, Baird B, Megill M, Wittek A, Quinnan V, Parrilo JE, Rook AH, Eron LJ, Poretz DM, Goldenberg RI, Fauci AS, Gelmann EP. Effect of 9-(1,3-dihydroxy-2-propoxymethyl)guanine on serius cytomegalovirus disease in eight immunocompromised homosexual men. Ann Intern Med 1986; 104:41-44.
27. Kotler DP, Culpepper-Morgan JA, Tierney AR, Klein EB. Treatment of disseminated cytomegalovirus infection with 9-(1,3-dihydroxy-2-propoxymethyl)guanine: evidence of prolonged survival in patients with the acquired immunodeficiency syndrome. AIDS Res 1986; 299-308.
28. Henderly DE, Freeman WR, Causey DM, Rao NA. Cytomegalovirus retinitis and response to therapy with ganciclovir. Ophthalmology 1987; 94:425-434.
29. Holland GN, Sidikaro Y, Krieger AE, Hardy D, Sakamoto J, Frenkel LM, Winston DJ, Gottleib S, Bryson YJ, Champlin RE, Ho WG, Winters RE, Wolfe PR, Cherry JD. Retinopathy with ganciclovir. Ophthalmology 1987; 94:815-823.
30. Chachoua A, Dieterich D, Krasinski K, Greene J, Laubenstein L, Wernz J, Buhles W, Koretz S. 9-(1,3-Dihydroxy-2-propoxymethyl)guanine (ganciclovir) in the treatment of cytomegalovirus gastrointestinal disease with the acquired immunodeficiency syndrome. Ann Intern Med 1987; 107:133-137.
31. Laskin OL, Cederberg DM, Mills J, Eron LJ, Mildvan D, Spector SA. Ganciclovir for the treatment and suppression of serious infections caused by cytomegalovirus. Am J Med 1987; 83:201-207.
32. Jacobson MA, O'Donnell JJ, Porteous D, Brodie HR, Fiegal D, Mills J. Retinal and gastrointestinal disease due to cytomegalovirus in patients with the acquired immune deficiency syndrome: prevalence, natural history, and response to ganciclovir therapy. Qtly J Med 1988; 67:473-486.
33. Jabs DA, Enger C, Bartlett JG. Cytomegalovirus retinitis and acquired immunodeficiency syndrome. Arch Ophthalmol 1989; 107:75-80.
34. Orellana J, Teich SA, Friedman AH, Lerebours F, Winterkorn J, Mildvan D. Combined short- and long-term therapy for the treatment of cytomegalovirus retinitis using ganciclovir (BW B759U). Ophthalmology 1987; 94:831-838.
35. Syntex Research, unpublished data, CL 4194.
36. Robinson MR, Teitelbaum C, Taylor-Findlay C. Thrombocytopenia and vitreous hemorrhage complicating ganciclovir treatment. Am J Ophthalmol 1989; 560-561.
37. Walker RE, Parker RI, Kovacs JA, Masur H, Lane HC, Carleton S, Kirk LE, Gralnick HR, Fauci S. Anemia and erythropoiesis in patients with the acquired immunodeficiency syndrome (AIDS) and Kaposi sarcoma treated with zidovudine. Ann Intern Med 1988; 108:372-376.
38. Richman DD, Fischl MA, Grieco MH, Gottlieb MS, Volberding PA, Laskin OL, Leedom JM, Groopman JE, Mildvan D, Hirsch MS, Jackson GG, Durack DT, Nusinoff-Lerhman S, AZT Collaborative Working Group. The toxicity of azidothymidine (AZT) in the treatment of patients with AIDS and AIDS-related complex. N Engl J Med 1987; 317:192-197.
39. Unpublished data, Syntex Research studies no. 1697, 1692 (study chairs: DeArmond B, Spector S).

40. Dieterich D, Kotler D, Busch D, Crumpacker C, Mastre B, Du Mond C, DeArmond B, Buhles W. Randomized, placebo-controlled study of ganciclovir treatment of cytomegalovirus (CMV) colitis in AIDS patients (PTS). VI International Conference on AIDS, San Francisco, June 1990.

41. Gaub J, Poulson A, Pedersen C, Tinning S, Hojgaard K, Thomson MH, Faber V, Nielsen JO. Efficacy and safety of two different dose levels of ganciclovir for the treatment of cytomegalovirus chorioretinitis in AIDS patients. Scand J Infec Dis 1988; 20:479-482.

42. Rozenbaum W, Gherakhanian S, Zazoun L, Veseghi M, De Sahb R, Thomson M. Efficacy and toxicity of ganciclovir treatment in AIDS-related CMV retinitis. V International Conference on AIDS, Montreal, June 1989, MBP.132.

43. Jacobson MA, O'Donnell JJ, Brodie HR, Wofsy C, Mills J. Randomized prospective trial of ganciclovir maintenance therapy for cytomegalovirus retinitis. J Med Virol 1988; 25:339-349.

44. Unpublished data, Syntex Research study no. 1285 (study chairs: Merigan TC, Wolitz R, DeArmond B, Buhles W).

45. Hochster H, Dieterich D, Bozzete D, Reichman RC, Connor JD, Liebes L, Sonke RL, Spector SA, Valentine F, Pettinelli C, Richman D. Toxicity of combined ganciclovir and zidovudine for cytomegalovirus disease associated with AIDS. Ann Intern Med 1990; 113:111-117.

46. Hochster H, Liebes L, Connor J, Reichman D, Richman D. Pharmacokinetics of combined AZT and DHPG (ganciclovir): results of a multicenter Phase I study (ACTG 004).

47. Nussbaum J, Antoniskis D, Causey D, Leedom JM. Toxicity of combined AZT ganciclovir (DHPG) therapy in AIDS patients. V International Conference on AIDS, Montreal, June 1989, p 195.

48. Grossberg H. Schering Plough Research, unpublished data (study no. E87-004).

49. Grossberg H, Bonnem E, Buhles W (letter). N Engl J Med 1989; 320:1560.

50. Shea BF, Hoffman S, Sesin GP, Hammer SM. Ganciclovir hepatotoxicity. Pharmacotherapy 1987; 7(6):223-226.

51. Freeman WR, Henderly DE, Wan WL, Causey D, Trousdale M, Green RL, Rao NA. Prevalence, pathophysiology, and treatment of rhegmatogenous retinal detachment in treated cytomegalovirus retinitis. Am J Ophthalmol 1987; 103: 527-536.

52. Shepp DH, Dandliker PS, Miranda P, Burnette TC, Cederberg DM, Kirk LE, Meyers JD. Activity of 9-[2-hydroxy-1-(hydroxymethyl)ethoxymethyl]guanine in the treatment of cytomegalovirus pneumonia. Ann Intern Med 1985; 103: 368-373.

53. Erice A, Jordan C, Chace BA, Fletcher C, Chinnock B, Balfour HH Jr. Ganciclovir treatment of cytomegalovirus disease in transplant recipients and other immunocompromised hosts. JAMA 1987; 257:3082-3087.

54. Reed EC, Shepp DH, Dandliker PS, Meyers JD. Ganciclovir treatment of cytomegalovirus infection of the gastrointestinal tract after marrow transplantation. Bone Marrow Transpl 1988; 3:169.

55. Emanuel D, Cunningham I, Julyes-Elysee K, Brochstein JA, Kerman NA, Laver J, Stover D, White DA, Fels A, Polsky B, Castro Malaspina H, Peppard JR, Bartus P, Hammerling U, O'Reilly RJ. Ann Intern Med 1988; 109:777-782.

56. Reed E, Bowden RA, Dandiliker PS, Lilleby KE, Meyers JD. Treatment of cytomegalovirus pneumonia with ganciclovir and intravenous cytomegalovirus immunoglobulin in patients with bone marrow transplants. Ann Intern Med 1988; 109:783-788.
57. Verdonck LF, de Gast GC, Dekker AW, de Weger, Schuurman, Rozenberg-Arska M. Treatment of cytomegalovirus pneumonia after bone marrow transplantation with cytomegalovirus immunoglobulin combined with ganciclovir. Bone Marrow Transpl 1989; 4:187-189.
58. Schmidt GM, Kovacs A, Zaia JA, Horak DA, Blume KG, Nademanee AP, O'Donnell MR, Snyder DS, Forman SJ. Ganciclovir/immunoglobulin combination therapy for the treatment of human cytomegalovirus-associated interstitial pneumonia in bone marrow allograft recipients. Transplantation 1988; 46:905-907.
59. Unpublished data, Syntex Research. Interim results 1308, April 1989 (study chairs: Champlin R, Winston D, DeArmond B).
60. Reed EC, Wolford JL, Kopecky KJ, Lilleby KE, Dandliker PS, Todaro JL, McDonald GB, Meyers JD. Ganciclovir for the treatment of cytomegalovirus enteritis in bone marrow transplant patients. Ann Intern Med 1990; 112:505-510.
61. Fouillard L, Gorin NC, Laporte JPh, Eugene-Jolchine I, Isnard F, Najman A. GM-CSF and ganciclovir for cytomegalovirus infection after autologous bone-marrow transplantation. Lancet 1989; 2:1273.
62. Icenogle TB, Peterson E, Ray G, Minnich L, Copeland JG. DHPG effectively treats CMV infection in heart and heart-lung transplant patients: a preliminary report. J Heart Transpl 1987; 6:199-203.
63. Keay S, Bissett J, Merigan TC. Ganciclovir treatment of cytomegalovirus infections in iatrogenically immunocompromised patients. J Infec Dis 1987; 156:1016-1021.
64. Hecht DW, Snydman DR, Crumpacker CS, Werner BG, Heinze-Lacey B, Boston Renal Transplant CMV Study Group. J Infec Dis 1988; 157:187-190.
65. Mai M, Nery J, Sutker W, Husberg B, Klintmalm G, Gonwa T. DHPG (gancyclovir) improves survival in CMV pneumonia. Transpl Proc 1989; 21:2263-2265.
66. Stratta RJ, Shaefer MS, Markin RS, Wood PR, Kennedy EM, Langnas AN, Reed EC, Woods GL, Donovan JP, Pillen TJ, Duckworth RM, Shaw B. Clinical patterns of cytomegalovirus disease after liver transplantation. Arch Surg 1989; 124:1443-1449.
67. Unpublished data, Syntex Research ICM study no. 1496, interim report, June 1990 (study chairs: Merigan TC, Keay S, DeArmond B, Bristow M).
68. Burroughs Wellcome Co. Retrovir™ package insert, March 1987.
69. Volberding PA, Lagakos SW, Koch MA, Pettinelli C, Myers MW, Booth DK, Balfour HH, Reichman RC, Bartlett JA, Hirsch MS, Murphy RL, Hardy WD, Soeiro R, Fischl MA, Bartlett JG, Merigan TC, Hyslop NE, Richman DD, Valentine FT, Corey L. AIDS Clinical Trials Group of the NIAID. Zidovudine in asymptomatic human immunodeficiency virus infection. N Engl J Med 1990; 322:941-949.
70. Unpublished data, Syntex Research. Long-term safety analysis, October 1988.
71. Unpublished data, Syntex Research. Interim safety report: tolerance of pediatric patients to intravenous ganciclovir, CL 4373.

72. Hartman NR, Yarchoan R, Thomas RV, Pluda JM, Marczyk KS, Broder S, Johns DG, NCI. Effect of different oral preparations and presence of other medications on the pharmacokinetics of 2′,3′-dideoxyinosine. VI International Conference on AIDS, San Francisco, June 1990, S.B.470.

73. Liebman HA, Kunches LM, Saunders CA, Kelley SL, McCaffrey RP, Cooley TP. Treatment with 2′,3′-dideoxyinosine (ddI) given twice daily to patients with cytomegalovirus (CMV) retinitis receiving maintenance DHPG (ganciclovir). VI International Conference on AIDS, San Francisco, June 1990, S.B.474.

74. Reichert CM, O'Leary TJ, Levens DL, Simrell CR, Maecher AM. Autopsy pathology in the acquired immune deficiency syndrome. Am J Pathol 1983; 112:357-382.

75. Welch K, Finkbeiner W, Alpers CE, Blumenfeld W, Davis RL, Smuckler EA, Beckstead JH. Autopsy findings in the acquired immune deficiency syndrome. JAMA 1984; 252:1152-1159.

76. Unpublished data, Syntex Research. Interim results of AV002 (study chair: Thomson M).

77. Cantrill HL, Henry K, Melroe H, Knobloch WH, Ramsay RC, Balfour HH. Treatment of cytomegalovirus retinitis with intravitreal ganciclovir. Ophthalmology 1989; 96:367-374.

78. Ussery FM. Personal communication, Oct. 23, 1987.

79. Henry K, Cantrill H, Fletcher C, Chinnock BJ, Balfour HH. Use of intravitreal ganciclovir (dihydroxy propoxymethyl guanine) for cytomegalovirus retinitis in a patient with AIDS. Am J Ophthalmol 1987; 103:17-23.

80. Daikos GL, Pulido J, Kathpalia SB, Jackson GG. Intravenous and intraocular ganciclovir for CMV retinitis in patients with AIDS or chemotherapeutic immunosuppression. Br J Ophthalmol 1988; 72:521-524.

81. Bowden RA, Digel J, Reed EC, Meyers JD. Immunosuppressive effects of ganciclovir in in vitro lymphocyte responses. J Infec Dis 1987; 156:899-903.

82. Unpublished data, Syntex Research AV003 final report, CL4204 (study chair: Thomson M).

4

Ganciclovir Pharmacokinetics

**Edmund V. Capparelli, James R. Lane, Robert L. Sonke,
and James D. Connor**
*University of California, San Diego
San Diego, California*

I. INTRODUCTION

Ganciclovir [9-(1,3-dihydroxy-2-propoxymethyl)guanine] (DHPG) is a synthetic acyclic nucleoside of guanine. Ganciclovir has antiviral activity against all members of the human herpesvirus family, but has more toxicity than acyclovir, of which it is a congener. Fortunately, ganciclovir has 8-20-fold higher antiviral activity against human cytomegaloviruses (HCMV) in vitro than does acyclovir, which is generally ineffective against diseases caused by human CMV. For these reasons, ganciclovir is currently the preferred choice among newer antivirals in treating CMV retinitis, pneumonitis, and gastroenteritis in immunocompromised adults and children, including those with acquired immunodeficiency syndrome (AIDS).

A. Physical and Chemical Characteristics

Ganciclovir is a crystalline white to off-white solid that melts and decomposes at 243°C and has a MW of 255. The compound has a solubility of 3 mg/ml in 0.04 M acetate buffer, pH 4.7, and 0.2 M ionic strength. The solubility is constant between pH 3.5 and 8.5; the solubility increases markedly in strongly acidic and basic solutions. Formulated for clinical use, ganciclovir is concentrated in solution that is chemically stable for 6 months in glass ampules (50 mg/ml). It is also stable for 24 months at room temperature in a lyophilized formulation. Following dilution in saline (or other diluents for intravenous use), it is stable at room temperature for at least 5 days. Because of the low solubility of ganciclovir at more neutral pH, concentrated solutions (greater than 10 mg/ml) must be maintained at high pH or crystallization may occur.

B. Activation of Ganciclovir

Ganciclovir is thought to be activated to its antiviral form, ganciclovir triphosphate, through action of viral and host-specific enzymes. It is monophosphorylated by both HSV-1 and HSV-2 viral thymidine kinase (TK). However, CMV does not specify a viral TK, but it probably does induce an enzyme (a cellular deoxyguanosine kinase) for which ganciclovir is a substrate. Ganciclovir di- and triphosphorylated forms are the result of action by cellular kinases (1).

C. Mechanism of Action

The antiviral activity of ganciclovir triphosphate occurs as a result of inhibition of viral DNA synthesis in infected cells. DNA synthesis is interrupted through two mechanisms: 1) competitive inhibition of dGTP incorporation into new DNA and 2) incorporation of ganciclovir-TP into new viral DNA, causing subsequent termination of viral DNA elongation due to defectiveness.

D. In Vitro Pharmacodynamics

There is an approximately 10-fold increase in intracellular ganciclovir-TP concentration in CMV-infected cells compared to uninfected cells, so there is a preferential gradient for antiviral activity at the site of viral infection. Likewise, there is less toxicity to uninfected cell populations (compared to infected cells) due to decreased intracellular pools of ganciclovir-TP. Also relative to acyclovir, there is slower catabolism and excretion of ganciclovir from CMV-infected cells. These factors may influence the potency of ganciclovir in treating HCMV-caused diseases.

II. GANCICLOVIR ASSAYS

A. HPLC

High-performance liquid chromatography (HPLC) has been used extensively to measure ganciclovir in serum, plasma, cerebrospinal fluid (CSF), and urine of patients receiving ganciclovir in phase I, II, and III trials. HPLC methods are similar, varying in column selection and extraction-preparation of the biological samples to be assayed (2-5). Sensitivity of the HPLC methods are generally reported to be equal to or greater than 0.1 μg/ml; however, our most recent procedural adaptations allow quantitation at 0.02-0.05 μg/ml, starting with 400 μl of biological sample. We have found that approximately 95% of human serum/plasma specimens are free of interfering compounds, and that the occasional serum/plasma specimens that present with a "ganciclovir ghost" can be cleaned up and run successfully with adjustments in the mobile phase of the HPLC procedure.

B. RIA

Radioimmunoassay (RIA) quantitation of ganciclovir has the inherent problem of cross-reacting with acyclovir, of which it is a congener (6). RIA analysis can be utilized in studies in which patients are known to be free of acyclovir.

C. ELISA

An enzyme-linked immunosorbent assay (ELISA) has been used for quantitation of the antiherpes compound acyclovir. This assay also cross-reacts with ganciclovir and for that reason has also been used to measure ganciclovir in animals and humans free of acyclovir (7).

III. ABSORPTION

The oral absorption of ganciclovir is incomplete (this is based on a low bioavailability following oral doses and the assumption that ganciclovir is not metabolized in humans). A single-dose comparison of intravenous (200 mg) and oral (1000 mg) ganciclovir in eight patients with CMV retinitis and AIDS resulted in a bioavailability (F) of 6% (8). The peak concentration (C_{max}) was 0.6 μg/ml, and the time to peak concentration (T_{max}) was 2.5 hours after the 1000-mg dose. Following 14 days of oral therapy with 1000 mg every 8 hours, the C_{max}, T_{max}, and F were 1.2 μg/ml, 1.5 hours, and 9%, respectively (8). The mean trough concentration was 0.67 μg/ml. Other single-dose studies (9,10) reported similar results: F 5.6-13.4%, and T_{max} 1-5 hours.

Following 10 mg/kg and 20 mg/kg orally every 6 hours in four patients with CMV retinitis and AIDS, T_{max} was ~1-2 hours for both regimens (based on visual inspections of the graphs), and C_{max} were ~2 and 3 μg/ml, for the 10-mg/kg and 20-mg/kg doses, respectively (9). The F values were determined from 6-hour urinary recovery of unchanged ganciclovir following the last dose of each regimen. The authors assumed steady-state and 100% urinary excretion of unchanged drug. Bioavailability decreased from 4.6% (3.5% when AUC_{PO} is compared to AUC_{IV} from previous studies) to 3.0% (2.5%

when AUC_{PO} is compared to AUC_{IV} from previous studies) when the patients were increased from 10 mg/kg to 20 mg/kg. This suggests a limited absorptive capacity in the gastrointestinal tract.

There are currently no reports on the effects of food or drugs on the rate and extent of ganciclovir absorption.

Systemic absorption of ganciclovir following intravitreal administration of 200 μg (five doses over 15 days) appears to be insignificant (11). Ganciclovir serum concentrations were below the lower limit of the assay (0.1 μg/ml) at all time points. Intravitreal concentrations were 1.17 μg/ml at 51.4 hours following dose administration. The authors predicted that the intravitreal concentration should remain above the typical ID_{50} for CMV for 62 hours following a single 200-μg dose.

In CMV patients with normal renal function, mean peak and trough ganciclovir concentrations increased in proportion to dose. Following 1-2.5 mg/kg intravenous every 8 hours, peak concentrations were 1.75-4.75 and trough concentrations were 0.15-0.48 μg/ml (12). Mean steady-state serum ganciclovir peak and trough concentrations have averaged 11.5 (range 4.8-24.1) and 1.36 (range 0.11-3.50) μg/ml, respectively, following 5 mg/kg intravenous every 12 hours (13). More frequent administration, 5 mg/kg intravenous every 8 hours, resulted in peak and trough concentrations of 12.1 (range 6.2-19.2) and 2.8 (range <0.2 and 5.5) μg/ml, respectively.

IV. DISTRIBUTION

Following intravenous administration, ganciclovir exhibits biexponential decay from the systemic circulation (3,12,14,15). Autopsy findings in six bone marrow transplant (BMT) patients revealed the following tissue to blood ratios: kidney, 2.9-6.7; brain, 0.34-0.44; lungs, liver, and testes, ~ 0.09-1.0 (16).

Other reports confirm ganciclovir's capacity to cross the blood-brain barrier. The CSF to plasma ratios were 0.41 (1 hour after a 1-mg/kg intravenous dose), 0.24 (0.25 hours into the infusion, CSF/model-predicted plasma), 0.67 (5.6 hours postinfusion, CSF/model-predicted plasma), and 0.70 (5.5 hours postinfusion, 2.5 mg/kg) (3,12). The CSF/plasma ratio increased with time during the dosing interval, suggesting a slower rate of loss from the CSF than from the systemic circulation.

Subretinal fluid concentrations following a 5-mg/kg intravenous dose of ganciclovir in a 13-year-old BMT patient resulted in subretinal/plasma ratios of 0.88 and 2.03 at 5.5 and 8 hours postdose, respectively (17). In another patient, aqueous humor and subretinal to plasma ratios 2.5 hours following a 6-mg/kg 1-hour infusion of ganciclovir were 0.4 and 0.6, respectively. The vitreous humor concentration in this patient 21 hours after the 6-mg/kg dose was 0.2 μg/ml, while the plasma concentration was undetectable (18). These data suggest that the rate of loss from the eye, as from the CSF, is slower than the loss from the plasma. Intravitreal distribution kinetics support this observation (11).

Animal studies suggest that ganciclovir distributes into breast milk and crosses the placenta (19).

The plasma protein binding of ganciclovir is 1-2% (19). This is expected, as its congener, acyclovir, is only 15% bound to plasma proteins and ganciclovir is more hydrophilic than acyclovir.

The volume of distribution at steady-state (Vd_{SS}) via model-independent and model-dependent analysis varied in adults between 32.8 and 44.8 L/1.73 m² (3,15). The average V_{SS} in three neonates was 25 L/1.73 m² (J. Lane, unpublished data). The mean apparent volume of distribution (two-compartment, V_{beta}) was 1.17 L/kg in 12 patients with normal renal function and 1.04 L/kg in 7 patients with renal dysfunction (14). Newborns, and perhaps patients with renal dysfunction, may demonstrate decreased distribution volumes of ganciclovir when compared to other patients with CMV. The intravitreal V_{beta} (one-compartment) in a 29-year-old AIDS patient with CMV retinitis was 11.7 ml (11). The authors suggest that this volume, being larger than the volume of human vitreous humor, may represent distribution into the retina.

V. ELIMINATION

A. Metabolism

A minor metabolite of ganciclovir, 8-hydroxy-ganciclovir, has been identified in monkeys (M. Chaplin, Syntex Research, data on file). No metabolites of ganciclovir have been identified in man.

B. Excretion

The primary route of ganciclovir elimination is renal excretion. In two studies during steady-state dosing, recovery of unchanged drug in the urine averaged over 91% (range 86-102%) and 93.9 ± 12.6% of the drug administered during that 24-hour period (16,20). Similar results were obtained in another study (14), in which urine excretion accounted for 73.2 ± 31% of administered ganciclovir over a 72-hour period.

C. Clearance

Several reports have estimated clearance during ganciclovir administration in patients. In the largest published study to date (15), the total ganciclovir clearance was 203 ± 77 ml/min/1.73 m^2 in 51 patients following first dose and steady-state administration. The elimination half-life was found to be 3.5 ± 1.6 hours. In a smaller study by Fletcher et al. (3), six patients receiving chronic ganciclovir had a ganciclovir clearance of 208 ± 105 ml/min/ 1.73 m^2. A strong correlation was found between creatinine clearance and ganciclovir clearance using orthogonal regression analysis; the total ganciclovir clearance was equal to 2.4 × creatinine clearance (Cl_{Cr}) ($r = 0.96$) in patients with a range of creatinine clearance from 60 to 146 ml/min/1.73 m^2 (3) estimated by the method of Cockcroft and Gault (21).

In a report by Sommadossi et al. (14), ganciclovir clearance averaged 4.20 ± 2.13 ml/min/kg and half-life averaged 3.6 ± 1.4 hours in 12 patients with normal renal function. The relationship between renal function and ganciclovir clearance in a subgroup of patients was also examined. In a subgroup of seven patients with varying degrees of renal function (creatinine clearance ranging from ~15 to 180 ml/min), linear regression analysis showed that the relationship between ganciclovir clearance and creatinine clearance was 1.25 × Cl_{Cr} + 8.57 ml/min/1.8 m^2 ($r = 0.923$). Due to the nature of this patient population, there were a number of AIDS patients with depressed creatinine concentrations (≤0.5 mg/dl). This was probably due to reduced muscle mass (i.e., creatinine production), and in these patients renal function may have been overpredicted using this method. Laskin et al. (20) also estimated a similar relationship between renal function and ganciclovir clearance and found them related by the following equation: Ganciclovir clearance = 1.8 × Cl_{Cr} ($r = 0.88$). No study has determined renal clearance from urinary data or calculated nonrenal clearance due to the large proportion of unchanged ganciclovir collected in the urine.

VI. RENAL DYSFUNCTION

Seven patients with elevated serum creatinine (≥1.4 mg/dl, mean 3.4 mg/ dl) had reduced ganciclovir clearance of 1.20 ± 87 ml/min/kg and prolonged elimination half-life of 11.5 ± 3.9 hours (14). Two other patients with moderate renal dysfunction (estimated creatinine clearance 22 and 46 ml/min/1.73 m^2) were shown to have prolonged elimination half-lives of 9.5 and 29 hours. Lake et al. (22) reported ganciclovir clearance to be 10 ml/min/1.73 m^2 in a patient with an artificial heart requiring hemodialysis. This patient's elimination half-life was reported to be 28.3 hours. In patients with renal dysfunction, several of the elimination half-life determinations have been subject to low precision due to the relatively short sample-collection interval (12 hours) utilized in some of the studies. This may account for discrepancies observed among these patients with regard to elimination half-life.

Ganciclovir appears to be well cleared by hemodialysis and to a lesser extent by continuous arteriovenous hemodialysis (CAVHD). In one report, hemodialysis was required in two patients receiving ganciclovir. Four-hour hemodialysis sessions (average blood flow ~300 ml/min) resulted in 53 ± 11% reduction in total body amount of ganciclovir (14). While samples were not obtained a few hours postdialysis to ensure that no rebound phenomena postdialysis occurred, patients were given approximately 60% of the loading dose and achieved similar peak plasma concentrations. An extensive evaluation was performed by Lake et al. (22) in a patient with a Jarvis 7-70 artificial heart and end-stage renal failure who received ganciclovir for 6 weeks. They demonstrated clearance by the dialyzer of 68 ml/min/1.73 m² (with an average blood fow of 250 ml/min). The arteriovenous extraction coefficient (AV/A) was calculated to be 0.29 and the half-life during dialysis was approximately 4 hours. Ganciclovir clearance has been determined in one patient on CAVHD. This patient's half-life was 24 hours and sieve coefficient (ultrafiltrate/arterial drug concentration) for ganciclovir was 0.69 (23).

VII. OTHER PATIENT POPULATIONS

Currently there is no information regarding ganciclovir clearance in hepatic dysfunction. However, hepatic dysfunction is expected to have minimal effect on ganciclovir clearance due to the primary renal elimination. Thus far no significant difference in ganciclovir pharmacokinetics has been observed between transplant and AIDS patients. Our limited experience with neonates demonstrate an average clearance of 120 ml/min/1.73 m² in full-term infants (greater than 3500 g).

VIII. SINGLE-DOSE VS. CHRONIC ADMINISTRATION

No obvious diffcrences between acute and chronic dosing have been ob served in ganciclovir pharmacokinetics. Little difference was noticed between day-1 and day-14 plasma concentrations (peak, 5.7 ± 1.6 and 5.3 ± 2.8 μg/ml; trough, 0.7 ± 0.5 and 1.1 ± 0.4 μg/ml, respectively) (3,14). Fletcher et al. (3) used pharmacokinetic parameters following the first dose to predict the subsequent peak (0.25 hour postdose) and trough concentrations at steady state. The individual root mean squared error was 0.84 μg/ml (95% confidence limit 0.73 to 0.93 μg/ml) and there was slight bias to overpredict subsequent concentrations (mean error, −0.37 μg/ml; 95% confidence limit, −0.73 to −0.24) (3). Our own experience with seven patients who had pharmacokinetic analysis determined after single-dose and steady-state therapy demonstrated no change in clearance (246 ± 71 vs. 237 ± 56 ml/min/1.73 m²) or Vd_{SS} (44.8 ± 14.9 vs. 43.8 ± 6.2 L/1.73 m²). However, the elimination half-life appeared to be significantly increased from 2.7 ± 0.5 to 3.5 ± 0.4 hours during chronic therapy ($p < 0.01$). This may be related to changes in the proportionality between plasma and tissuc when calculating elimination half-life using compartmental (single-dose) vs. non-compartmental (steady-state) methods.

IX. DOSE/RESPONSE

A. Efficacy

There is scant information regarding the dose or plasma concentration associated with beneficial outcome as no definitive dose ranging studies have been performed. Additionally, little can be drawn from the clinical studies available due in part to the small number of patients involved in the published studies and the high overall response rates for most infections (13,24). Even in pulmonary infections where ganciclovir appears to be less effective (13), there is no information to suggest that one dosing regimen is superior to another.

In vitro studies have shown that the concentration of ganciclovir required to reduce plaque formation in most human strains of CMV by 50% (ID_{50}) ranges from <0.25 to 2.75 μg/ml (25-27). Furthermore, the ID_{90}s for many isolates (mean 2.0, range 0.15 to 4 μg/ml) are also exceeded by the peaks produced by conventional ganciclovir dosing.

B. Toxicity

The primary toxicity of ganciclovir is bone marrow suppression. This is a direct extension of its antiviral properties, and one might expect a useful correlation between drug concentrations and toxicity. There appears to be an enhancement of toxicity from ganciclovir in infected cells. Uninfected cells show 5-15 times less sensitivity to ganciclovir and have shown no inhibition at concentrations up to 25 μg/ml (25). Cytotoxic effects occur at higher concentrations (25-75 μg/ml) in uninfected cells where protein synthesis is reduced by 50% (12,25).

Clinical toxicity, specifically neutropenia defined as ANC <1000 or 50% decrease from baseline, occurs more frequently in AIDS patients than in transplant recipients. In one report using doses of 5 mg/kg every 12 hours, more than half of all AIDS patients developed neutropenia while only 20% of transplant patients incurred toxicity (13). This may result from the additive effects of other myelosuppressive therapies that AIDS patients often receive and makes causal assessment of blood dyscrasias from ganciclovir difficult in these patients. In a relatively small study with bone marrow transplant patients, all three patients who developed neutropenia had peak and trough ganciclovir concentrations of greater than 12.5 μg/ml and 2.5 μg/ml, respectively. Patients who did not develop neutropenia had peak and trough ganciclovir concentrations less than 8.25 μg/ml and 1.25 μg/ml, respectively (18). However, neutropenia has been reported in transplant recipients who had extrapolated peak and trough ganciclovir concentrations less than 5 μg/ml and 0.25 μg/ml, respectively.

X. DRUG INTERACTIONS

At present, no pharmacokinetic drug interactions have been reported with ganciclovir. However, since renal clearance exceeds glomerulofiltration and elimination probably involves some tubular secretion, agents that compete with or block secretion of bases, such as probenecid, may impede ganciclovir clearance as it does with acyclovir (28). Studies investigating combined therapy with zidovudine suggest no significant pharmacokinetic interactions between the two agents (29).

REFERENCES

1. Biron KK, Stanat SC, Sorrel JB, Fyfe JA, Keller PM, Lambe CU. Metabolic activation of the nucleoside analog 9-[(2-hydroxy-1-(hydroxymethyl)ethoxy)-methyl]guanine in human diploid fibroblasts infected with human cytomegalovirus. Proc Natl Acad Sci USA 1985; 82:2473-2477.
2. Woolf NK, Ochi JW, Silva EJ, Sharp PA, Harris JP, Richman DD. Ganciclovir prophylaxis for cochlear pathophysiologic during experimental guinea pig cytomegalovirus labyrinthitis. Antimicrob Agents Chemother 1988; 32:865-872.
3. Fletcher C, Sawchuk R, Chinnock B, De Miranda P, Balfour HH. Human pharmacokinetics of the antiviral drug DHPG. Clin Pharmacol Ther 1986; 40:281-286.
4. Sommadossi JP, Bevan R. High performance liquid chromatographic method for the determination of 9-(1,3-dihydroxy-2-propoxymethyl)guanine in human plasma. J Chromatogr 1987; 414:429-433.
5. Wiltink EHH, Stekkinger P, Brakenhoff JAC, Danner SA. Determination of 9-(1,3-dihydroxy-2-propoxymethyl)guanine (DHPG) in biological fluids by reversed phase high performance liquid chromatography. Pharmaceutisch Weekblad Scientific Edition 1987; 9:261-264.
6. Nerenberg C, McClung S, Martin J, Fass M, LaFargue J, Kushinsky S. A radioimmunoassay procedure for the determination of the antiviral nucleoside DHPG 9-[(1,3-dihydroxy-2-propoxy)methyl]guanine in plasma or serum. Pharm Res 1986; 3:112-115.
7. Tadepalli SM, Quinn RP, Averett. A competitive enzyme-linked immunosorbent assay to quantitate acyclovir and BW B759U in human plasma and urine. Antimicrob Agents Chemother 1986; 29:93-98.
8. Follansbee S, Busch D, Connor J, Jung D, Mastre B, Buhles W. Phase I study of the safety and pharmacokinetics of oral ganciclovir. International AIDS Conference IV, San Francisco, 1990.
9. Jacobson MA, De Miranda P, Cederberg DM, Burnette T, Cobb E, Brodie HR, Mills J. Human pharmacokinetics and tolerance of oral ganciclovir. Antimicrob Agents Chemother 1987; 31:1251-1254.

10. De Miranda P, Burnette T, Cederberg D, Blum MR, Brodie HR, Mills J. Absorption and pharmacokinetics of the antiviral 9-[{2-Hydroxy-1-(hydroxymethyl)-ethoxy}methyl]-guanine (BW 759U) in humans. In Twenty-Sixth Interscience Conference on Antimicrobial Agents and Chemotherapy, Washington D.C., 1986, p 300.

11. Henry K, Cantrill H, Fletcher C, et al. Use of intravitreal ganciclovir (dihydroxy propoxymethyl guanine) for cytomegalovirus retinitis in a patient with AIDS. Am J Ophthalmol 1987; 103:17-23.

12. Laskin OL, Stahl-Bayliss CM, Kalman CM, Rosecan LR. Use of ganciclovir to treat serious cytomegalovirus infection in patients with AIDS. J Infect Dis 1987; 155:323-327.

13. Winston DJ, Ho WG, Bartoni K, Holland GN, Mitsuyasu RT, Gale RP, Busuttil RW, Champlin RE. Ganciclovir therapy for cytomegalovirus infections in recipients of bone marrow transplants and other immunosuppressed patients. Rev Infect Dis 1988; 10(suppl 3):S547-553.

14. Sommadossi JP, Bevan R, Ling T, Lee F, Mastre B, Chaplin MD, Nerenberg C, Koretz S, Buhles WC. Clinical pharmacokinetics of ganciclovir in patients with normal and impaired renal function. Rev Infect Dis 1988; 10(suppl 3):S507-513.

15. Weller S, Liao SHT, Cederberg DM, de Miranda P, Blum MR. The pharmacokinetics of ganciclovir in patients with cytomegalovirus (CMV) infections. J Pharm Sci 1987; 75:S120.

16. Shepp DH, Dandliker PS, De Miranda P, Burnette TC, Cederberg DM, Kirk LE, Meyers JD. Activity of 9-[2-hydroxy-1-(hydroxymethyl)ethoxymethyl]-guanine in the treatment of cytomegalovirus pneumonia. Ann Intern Med 1985; 103:368-372.

17. Jabs DA, Wingard JR, De Bustros S, De Miranda P, Saral R, Santos GW. BW B759U for cytomegalovirus retinitis: intraocular drug penetration. Arch Ophthalmol 1986; 104:1436-1437.

18. Jabs DA, Newman C, de Bustros S, Polk BF. Treatment of cytomegalovirus retinitis with ganciclovir. Ophthalmol 1987; 94:824-830.

19. Faulds D, Heel RC. Ganciclovir: a review of its antiviral activity, pharmacokinetic properties and therapeutic efficacy in cytomegalovirus infections. Drugs 1990; 39:597-638.

20. Laskin OL, Cederberg DM, Mills J, Eron LJ, Mildvan D, Spector SA. Ganciclovir for the treatment and suppression of serious infections caused by cytomegalovirus. Am J Med 1987; 83:201-207.

21. Cockcroft DW, Gault MH. Prediction of creatinine clearance from serum creatinine. Nephron 1976; 16:31-41.

22. Lake KD, Fletcher CV, Love KR, Brown DC, Joyce LD, Pritzker MR. Ganciclovir pharmacokinetics during renal impairment. Antimicrob Agents Chemother 1988; 32:1899-1900.

23. Rello, Roglan A, Garcia-Cases C, Jane F, Net A. Effect of continuous arteriovenous hemodialysis on ganciclovir pharmacokinetics. DICP, Ann of Pharmacother 1990; 24:544-545.

24. Shanley JD, Morningstar J, Jordan MC. Inhibition of murine cytomegalovirus lung infection and interstitial pneumonitis by acyclovir and 9-(1,3-dihydroxy-2-propoxymethyl)guanine. Antimicrob Agents Chemother 1985; 28:172-175.

25. Mar EC, Cheng YC, Huang ES. Effects of 9-[(1,3-dihydroxy-2-propoxy)methyl]-guanine on human cytomegalovirus replication in vitro. Antimicrob Agents Chemother 1983; 24:518-521.
26. Smee DF, Martin JC, Verheyden JPH, Mathews TR. Anti-herpes virus activity of acyclic nucleoside 9-(1,3-dihydroxy-2-propoxymethyl)guanine. Antimicrob Agents Chemother 1983; 23:676-682.
27. Plotkin SA, Drew WL, Felsenstein D, Hirsch MS. Sensitivity of clinical isolates of human cytomegalovirus to 9-(1,3-dihydroxy-2-propoxymethyl)guanine. J Infect Dis 1985; 152:833-834.
28. Laskin OL, de Miranda P, King DH, Page DA, Longstreth JA, Rocco L, Lietman PS. Effects of probenecid on the pharmacokinetics and elimination of acyclovir in humans. Antimicrob Agents Chemother 1982; 21:804-805.
29. Hochster H, Dierich D, Bozzette S, Reichman RC, Connor JD, Liebes L, Sonke RL, Spector SA, Valentine F, Pettinelli C, Richman DD. Toxicity of combined ganciclovir and zidovudine for cytomegalovirus disease associated with AIDS. Ann Intern Med 1990; 113:111-117.

5

Ganciclovir Treatment of Cytomegalovirus Retinitis in Patients with AIDS: Infectious Disease Perspective

Mark A. Jacobson
*San Francisco General Hospital
and University of California, San Francisco
San Francisco, California*

I. INTRODUCTION

Ganciclovir (DHPG; 9-[(1,3-dihydroxy-2-propoxy)methyl]guanine; Cytovene), a nucleoside analog closely related in structure to acyclovir, is the first antiviral drug to be licensed in the United States for the treatment of disease caused by cytomegalovirus (CMV) infection. The only indication for which ganciclovir therapy has been approved by the FDA to date is the treatment of CMV retinitis. Although this drug is clearly beneficial in preventing retinal necrosis and loss of vision, ganciclovir therapy is a double-edged sword. The drug as currently approved can be administered only by the intravenous route, and retinitis relapse occurs within a short time after therapy has been discontinued. Hence, a permanent indwelling central venous catheter is required for daily home intravenous administration. In addition, ganciclovir is myelosuppressive, which makes coadministration of other myelotoxic therapy, such as zidovudine or vinblastine, problematic. Nevertheless, as the first antiviral drug to demonstrate clinical efficacy in CMV

Parts of this chapter were originally published in Volberding PA, Jacobson MA (Eds), *AIDS Clinical Review 1990*, Marcel Dekker, New York, 1990.

retinitis, ganciclovir represents a major advance in the therapy of AIDS-related opportunistic infections.

II. IN VIVO ANTIVIRAL EFFECT

The activity of ganciclovir in in vitro and animal models of CMV infection is described in Chapters 1 and 2. In prospective clinical trials, intravenous ganciclovir has been associated with a dramatic decrease in recovery of CMV from blood, urine, and saliva. At least 80% of consecutive CMV retinitis patients treated with a single 2-3-week course of induction ganciclovir therapy have stopped shedding CMV (1,2). However, CMV could be isolated from most of these individuals soon after ganciclovir was discontinued. Prolonged maintenance ganciclovir therapy has also been associated with a persistent in vivo antiviral effect. For example, in a small, randomized, prospective study, CMV was isolated from only 9% of blood and urine cultures obtained from retinitis patients during chronic daily ganciclovir maintenance therapy, compared with 40% of cultures obtained from retinitis patients who had therapy stopped after an initial induction ganciclovir course ($p <$ 0.001) (3).

Generally, the susceptibilities of CMV strains isolated before and after ganciclovir therapy in prospective studies remained unchanged (4,5), suggesting that emergence of CMV resistance to ganciclovir would not become a serious clinical problem. However, CMV strains resistant to ganciclovir were recovered from the blood of three patients with CMV disease refractory to ganciclovir therapy (6). The mechanism of ganciclovir resistance in these cases appeared to be due to a failure of cells infected with the resistant CMV strains to phosphorylate ganciclovir (7). This phenomenon is discussed in more detail in Chapter 11. The emergence of ganciclovir-resistant CMV may be particularly relevant to retinitis patients receiving long-term maintenance ganciclovir therapy. Of 13 patients who had ganciclovir susceptibility compared in paired isolates obtained before and 1-15 months after initiating chronic ganciclovir therapy, 38% developed in vitro evidence of ganciclovir resistance (8).

III. EFFICACY OF GANCICLOVIR IN CMV RETINITIS

Prior to the introduction of ganciclovir therapy, the natural history of untreated AIDS-associated CMV retinitis was gradual, progressive retinal destruction by outward expansion of retinal inflammation into previously uninvolved retina as well as by simultaneous development of new lesions in other parts of the retina (9). Spontaneous remission was extremely rare.

In 1986 and early 1987, five phase 1 studies of intravenous ganciclovir therapy for AIDS-related CMV retinitis were published. A total of 86 patients were observed in these combined trials, and 74 (86%) patients had retinitis stabilize or improve during a 10-20-day course of ganciclovir (2,10-13). In nearly all these patients, clinical responses were associated with decreased isolation of CMV from blood and urine. However, most patients examined serially after therapy was discontinued had progression of retinal inflammation, often accompanied by increased recovery of CMV from body fluids.

Because of this clear pattern of clinical failure when ganciclovir therapy was discontinued, investigators began initiating a suppressive or maintenance treatment regimen (usually a single infusion of ganciclovir 5-6 mg/kg given 5-7 days per week) as soon as the initial or induction 10-21-day course (ganciclovir 2.5 mg/kg q 8 hr or 5 mg/kg q 12 hr) was completed.

Subsequently, two small, randomized, prospective phase 2 studies have evaluated the efficacy of chronic ganciclovir maintenance therapy. In these two studies, a total of 25 evaluable patients were given a 2-3-week course of ganciclovir induction therapy, after which patients were randomized to receive immediate daily maintenance therapy or to have maintenance therapy deferred until there was evidence of retinitis progression (3,14). Retinitis progression was defined by a set of objective ophthalmological criteria (e.g., increased size of lesions, new lesions, or involvement of an increased area of the retina). In both studies, time to retinitis progression was longer in the group that began daily maintenance ganciclovir therapy immediately after completing a course of induction therapy. No life-threatening adverse effects occurred in either of these small studies.

Although it has been clearly demonstrated that chronic maintenance ganciclovir therapy delays retinal destruction in patients with sight-threatening CMV retinitis, the optimal dose for chronic maintenance ganciclovir therapy is not well established. An early, nonrandomized trial of chronic maintenance ganciclovir demonstrated a trend toward improved efficacy with higher cumulative weekly doses (5). The median time to retinitis progression was 27 days in four individuals who received 10-15 mg/kg per week compared to 105 days in 10 individuals treated with 30 mg/kg per week (5). In another study, a group of 14 CMV retinitis patients received chronic maintenance ganciclovir therapy at a dose of 25 mg/kg per week, with a median time to retinitis progression of 53 days (15). For seven of these patients, hematological assessment permitted dose increase to 37.5 mg/kg per week after progression occurred. On this higher maintenance dose, retinitis remained stable for a median additional 28 days.

Deciding whether and when to initiate ganciclovir therapy entails knowledge of the anatomical location of retinitis; the patient's baseline absolute neutrophil count and marrow reserve; the necessity for therapy with other potentially myelosuppressive drugs such as zidovudine, antineoplastic chemotherapy, and sulfa congeners; and the feasibility and desirability of placing and caring for a chronic indwelling venous catheter.

Whether or not retinitis progression translates into functional visual loss depends on the anatomical location of any new retinal inflammation. If retinitis progresses into the posterior retina where central vision occurs or into the optic disc where the optic nerve enters the retina, then a symptomatic scotoma or even blindness may result. However, if progression occurs in the anterior retina, there may be no new subjective visual symptoms unless vitreous floaters or a retinal detachment complicates the peripheral retinal inflammation. Hence, blindness can result from a small increase in size of a macular CMV lesion. On the other hand, vision may remain 20/20 at the same time that massive anterior extension of retinitis occurs. Thus, the success with which ganciclovir prolongs time to retinitis (an anatomical measurement) progression does not always correlate with functional vision.

Thus, before initiating ganciclovir treatment for CMV retinitis, the clinician must consider the precise anatomical location of retinal CMV lesions. An active inflammatory CMV lesion adjacent to the macula in an eye with 20/100 or better corrected vision is a medical emergency. Barring any contraindications (e.g., absolute granulocytopenia), ganciclovir therapy should be initiated immediately in such a situation. If one eye is irreversibly blind due to macular or optic nerve head destruction and the other eye is uninvolved, the only reason to initiate ganciclovir therapy would be to prevent dissemination to the contralateral eye. Since the risk of spread to the other eye is significant (at least 50%), elective initiation of ganciclovir is reasonable. On the other hand, it might make just as much sense to follow the patient closely, deferring treatment with ganciclovir as well as placement of a permanent indwelling venous catheter until the contralateral eye is involved. If a patient has a single anterior retinal lesion, either immediate or deferred treatment could be appropriate. A multicenter randomized study is now under way to determine the optimal management in this latter situation. Patients with anterior retinal lesions that are not immediately sight-threatening are being randomized either to initiate ganciclovir therapy immediately or to defer treatment and be examined by an ophthalmologist at biweekly intervals, beginning treatment once retinitis progression occurs.

An important complication of CMV retinitis is retinal detachment. However, it is not known whether ganciclovir therapy increases or decreases the risk of retinal detachment in CMV retinitis. Detachments are often associated with anterior retinitis (the neural retina is bound down anteriorly to underlying structures). Anecdotally, detachments have occurred frequently in patients whose retinal inflammation has resolved with ganciclovir therapy (16). However, since most patients with CMV retinitis are treated, it cannot be concluded that retinal detachment is a complication of ganciclovir therapy.

IV. ADVERSE EFFECTS OF GANCICLOVIR

The most important adverse effect of ganciclovir is myelosuppression, which can result in neutropenia or, more rarely, thrombocytopenia. We observed absolute neutrophil counts <800 cells/μl in 10 of 32 (31%) patients receiving chronic daily maintenance ganciclovir therapy (15). However, truly dose-limiting neutropenia is probably less frequent. Retrospective studies have indicated that risk of bacterial infection does not increase in HIV-infected patients when absolute neutrophil counts are 500-1000 cells/μl compared with >1000 cells/μl (17). In a detailed analysis of 438 AIDS patients treated with ganciclovir, only 16% had a nadir absolute neutrophil count <500 cells/μl and 5% had a nadir platelet count $<20,000$ cells/μl (18). There is one case report of irreversible neutropenia and subsequent death due to pseudomonal bacteremia following induction ganciclovir therapy (1). (See Chapter 3 for an extensive review of ganciclovir-associated adverse effects.)

Ganciclovir has been reported to cause azoospermia in animal studies and probably decreases spermatogenesis, perhaps irreversibly, in humans. However, no apparent effect on gonadal function has been observed in humans (19). Anemia occurs frequently in ganciclovir-treated patients, but a clear relationship between dose and effect has not been demonstrated. Rarely, rash, nausea, and central nervous system adverse events have been associated with ganciclovir therapy.

Since chronic ganciclovir administration generally requires placement of a permanent indwelling central venous catheter, catheter-associated infections are a potential secondary adverse effect of ganciclovir therapy. Infection rates of 0.29-0.47 infections per 100 central venous catheter days have been reported in AIDS patients who have had central venous catheters placed for a variety of reasons, including ganciclovir therapy (20,21).

Both ganciclovir and zidovudine (AZT, Retrovir) are myelosuppressive, and the risk of severe neutropenia increases if the two drugs are coadministered. Cases of prolonged pancytopenia due to combined ganciclovir and zidovudine therapy have been reported (22). This phenomenon appears to be due to synergistic bone marrow toxicity since no pharmacokinetic interaction between the two drugs has been observed. Nevertheless, some patients are able to tolerate combined therapy when usual maintenance doses of ganciclovir are combined with reduced doses of zidovudine (300-600 mg/day) (23). If such combined therapy is to be attempted, careful patient monitoring with frequent blood counts is mandatory. Patients should have a stable absolute neutrophil count ≥ 1000 cells/μl after at least 2 weeks of ganciclovir therapy before zidovudine is initiated at a dose of 300 mg/day or less.

V. NEW STRATEGIES FOR GANCICLOVIR THERAPY

New strategies for improving ganciclovir therapy for CMV retinitis focus on either using different routes of administration or combining ganciclovir with other agents to improve efficacy and/or reduce toxicity. Intravitreal ganciclovir treatment is discussed in Chapter 13. In addition, the possibility of ganciclovir administration by the oral route is of particular interest since the comorbidity of intravenous or intravitreal administration could be avoided. There have been two studies of ganciclovir oral administration in humans. Oral bioavailability ranged from 3 to 16%, and peak plasma concentrations were 3-12 μM (24,25). Because the drug was administered for less than 1 week in both studies, long-term tolerance of oral ganciclovir is unknown. If oral ganciclovir is well tolerated and suppressive levels of drug can be achieved in plasma in subsequent longer phase 1 studies that are now in progress, then the oral route of administration might be a reasonable alternative maintenance regimen for quiescent CMV retinitis.

The strategy of combining ganciclovir with granulocyte-macrophage colony stimulating factor (GM-CSF) to reduce neutropenic toxicity and permit higher weekly maintenance ganciclovir doses is discussed in Chapter 12. Finally, combining ganciclovir with other new antiviral drugs with activity against CMV, such as foscarnet, is another promising strategy.

It may be possible to combine low doses of ganciclovir on a daily basis with low doses of foscarnet or to administer high doses of each drug on alternate days or weeks to improve efficacy and reduce toxicity. The basis for this hypothesis is recent in vitro evidence of an additive or synergistic antiviral effect when ganciclovir and foscarnet are combined (26,27). Studies in two independent laboratories have confirmed that a combination of ganciclovir and foscarnet can increase in vitro efficacy against human strains of CMV (26,27). The interaction between these two antiviral drugs, when used simultaneously, has been evaluated by the fractional inhibitory concentration (FIC) method in which the FIC for each combination of two specific drug concentrations is calculated by the formula FIC = (IC of drug X in combination/IC of drug X alone) + (IC of drug Y in combination/IC of drug Y alone) (26). Using this method, Manischewitz et al. reported a mean FIC of 0.72 (26), and Freitas et al. reported a mean FIC of 0.64 (27) when ganciclovir and foscarnet were combined to inhibit CMV replication in cell culture. These in vitro results are consistent with an additive or synergistic inhibition of CMV replication.

Since the major reported adverse effects of ganciclovir and foscarnet are mutually exclusive (i.e., myelosuppression for ganciclovir vs. nephrotoxicity and hypocalcemia for foscarnet), reduced-dose combination therapy or alternating high-dose therapy might provide a means to treat CMV retinitis patients with as much or more efficacy while reducing drug toxicity. Clinical trials of such a combined regimen are currently being planned.

In conclusion, the availability of intravenous ganciclovir therapy has already significantly improved quality of life for AIDS patients with CMV retinitis. Continued clinical research will likely improve the efficacy and tolerance of this drug in CMV retinitis and define the value of ganciclovir therapy for other CMV diseases as well.

REFERENCES

1. Buhles WC Jr, Mastre BJ, Tinker AJ, Strand V, Koretz SH. Ganciclovir treatment of life- or sight-threatening cytomegalovirus infection: experience in 314 immunocompromised patients. Rev Infect Dis 1988; 10S:495-504.
2. Masur H, Lane HC, Palestine A, Smith PD, et al. Effect of 9-(1,3-dihydroxy-2-propoxymethyl)guanine on serious cytomegalovirus disease in eight immunosuppressed homosexual men. Ann Intern Med 1986; 104:41-44.
3. Jacobson MA, O'Donnell JJ, Brodie HR, Wofsy CB, Mills J. Randomized prospective trial of ganciclovir maintenance therapy for cytomegalovirus retinitis. J Med Virol 1988; 25:339-349.
4. Cole NL, Balfour HH Jr. Does cytomegalovirus (CMV) become more resistant during antiviral therapy? 25th Interscience Conference on Antimicrobial Agents and Chemotherapy, Minneopolis, MN, 1985, abstract 128.
5. Drew WL, Buhles WC, Busch D, Mills J, Follansbee S, Merigan TC. Maintenance treatment of CMV retinitis using 9-(1,3-dihydroxy-2-propoxymethyl)guanine (DHPH). 26th Interscience Conference on Antimicrobial Agents and Chemotherapy, New Orleans, LA, 1986, abstract 569.
6. Erice A, Chou S, Biron KK, Stanat SC, Balfour HH Jr, Jordan MC. Progressive disease due to ganciclovir-resistant cytomegalovirus in immunocompromised patients. N Engl J Med 1989; 320:289-293.
7. Biron KK, Stanat SC, Reardon J, Erice A, Balfour HH Jr, Jordan MC. Ganciclovir-resistant isolates of CMV: antiviral susceptibility profiles and mode of resistance studies. Second International Cytomegalovirus Workshop, San Diego, CA, 1989, abstract 65.
8. Drew WL, Miner RC, Mehalko S, Gullett J. CMV resistance in patients receiving ganciclovir. 29th Interscience Conference on Antimicrobial Agents and Chemotherapy, Los Angeles, CA, 1989, abstract 61.
9. Bloom JN, Palestine AG. The diagnosis of cytomegalovirus retinitis. Ann Intern Med 1988; 109:963-969.
10. Collaborative DHPG Study Group. Treatment of serious cytomegalovirus infections with 9-(1,3-dihydroxy-2-propoxymethyl)guanine in patients with AIDS and other immunodeficiencies. N Engl J Med 1986; 314:801-805.
11. Holland GN, Sakamoto MJ, Hardy D, Sidikaro Y, Kreiger AE, Frenkel LM, and the UCLA CMV Retinopathy Study Group. Treatment of cytomegalovirus retinopathy in patients with acquired immunodeficiency syndrome: use of the experimental drug 9-[2-hydroxy-1-(hydroxymethyl)ethoxymethyl]guanine. Arch Opthalmol 1986; 104:1794-1800.

12. Laskin OL, Stahl-Bayliss CM, Kalman CM, Rosecan LR. Use of ganciclovir to treat serious cytomegalovirus infections in patients with AIDS. J Infect Dis 1987; 155:323-327.

13. Cederberg DM, Laskin OL, Mills J, Creagh-Kirk T. Efficacy and safety of 9-[2-hydroxy-1-(hydroxymethyl)ethoxymethyl]guanine (BW B759U) in AIDS patients with *Cytomegalovirus* retinitis. 26th Interscience Conference on Antimicrobial Agents and Chemotherapy, New Orleans, LA, 1986, abstract 565.

14. Rozenbaum W, Gharakhanian S, Zazoun L, et al. Efficacy and toxicity of ganciclovir maintenance treatment in AIDS-related CMV retinitis. V International Conference on AIDS, Montreal, Canada, 1989, abstract M.B.P.132.

15. Jacobson MA, O'Donnell JJ, Porteous D, Brodie HR, Feigal D, Mills J. Retinal and gastrointestinal disease due to cytomegalovirus in patients with the acquired immune deficiency syndrome: prevalence, natural history, and response to ganciclovir therapy. Quart J Med 1988; 254:473-486.

16. Causey DM, Freeman WR, Henderly DE, Wan WL, Rao NA, Leedom JM, et al. Retinal detachment in treated cytomegalovirus retinitis. III International Conference on AIDS, Washington, DC, 1987, abstract TP.160.

17. Farber BF, Woltmann J, Lesser M, Kaplan MH, Napolitano B. Clinical significance of neutropenia in patients with HIV disease. 28th Interscience Conference on Antimicrobial Agents and Chemotherapy, Los Angeles, CA, 1988, abstract 1248.

18. DeArmond B. Syntex Research, unpublished data.

19. Chachoua A, Dieterich D, Krasinski K, Greene J, Laubenstein L, Wernz J, Buhles W, Koretz S. 9-(1,3-Dihydroxy-2-propoxymethyl)guanine (ganciclovir) in the treatment of cytomegalovirus gastrointestinal disease with the acquired immunodeficiency syndrome. Ann Intern Med 1987; 107:133-137.

20. Thurn JR, Miller C, Johnson S, et al. Experience with central venous catheters (CVCs) in patients with AIDS. V International Conference on AIDS, Montreal, Canada, 1989, abstract M.B.P.85.

21. Raviglione MC, Battan R, Pablos-Mendez A, et al. Hickman catheter infections in AIDS. V International Conference on AIDS, Montreal, Canada, 1989, abstract M.B.P.89.

22. Jacobson MA, de Miranda P, Gordon SM, Blum MR, Volberding P, Mills J. Prolonged pancytopenia due to combined ganciclovir and zidovudine therapy. J Infect Dis 1988; 158:489-490.

23. Nussbaum J, Antoniskis D, Causey D, Leedom JM. Toxicity of combined AZT/ganciclovir (DHPG) therapy in AIDS patients. V International Conference on AIDS, Montreal, Canada, 1989, abstract M.B.O.49.

24. Jacobson MA, de Miranda P, Cederberg DM, Burnette T, Cobb E, Brodie HR, Mills J. Human pharmacokinetics and tolerance of oral ganciclovir. Antimicrob Agents Chemother 1987; 31:1251-1254.

25. Buhles WC. Unpublished data.

26. Manischewitz JF, Quinnan GV, Lane HC, Wittek AE. Synergistic effect of ganciclovir and foscarnet on cytomegalovirus replication in vitro. Antimicrob Agents Chemother 1990; 34:373-375.

27. Freitas VR, Fraser-Smith EB, Matthews TR. Increased efficacy of ganciclovir in combination with foscarnet against cytomegalovirus and herpes simplex virus type 2 in vitro and in vivo. Antivir Res 1989; 12:205-212.

6

Ganciclovir Treatment of Cytomegalovirus Retinitis in Patients with AIDS

Douglas A. Jabs
The Johns Hopkins University School of Medicine
Baltimore, Maryland

I. INTRODUCTION

Cytomegalovirus (CMV) retinitis is the most common intraocular infection in patients with the acquired immunodeficiency syndrome (AIDS) (1). Prior to the AIDS epidemic, CMV retinitis was a rare disease seen primarily in transplant patients, who were immunosuppressed (2-5). However, with the advent of the AIDS epidemic, CMV retinitis has become a common disease and now represents the most common intraocular infection seen at major urban hospitals. Ganciclovir, previously known as 9-(1,3-dihydroxy-2-prop-oxymethyl)guanine, was approved by the Food and Drug Administration for the treatment of CMV retinitis in immunocompromised patients in June 1989, and is the first drug available for the treatment of CMV retinitis.

II. CMV RETINITIS AND AIDS: EPIDEMIOLOGY

CMV retinitis is by far the most common intraocular infection in patients with AIDS (1). Estimates of the frequency of CMV retinitis in patients with AIDS have varied from 6 to 38% (1,6-13). Series surveying ambulatory out-patients (6) have tended to give lower estimates, while autopsy series (11) have shown higher figures. The variability in these estimates is multifactoral, including underdetection in nonophthalmological series, referral bias in ophthalmological series, variability in patient populations, and the limitations of retrospective data analysis. However, one series (13), recognizing the potential for bias of ascertainment in its reported frequency of 29%, estimated a minimum frequency of 11% among all AIDS patients seen at its institution, and it surmised that the true frequency was somewhere between 11 and 29%. All the above data suggest that approximately 20-25% of patients with AIDS will ultimately develop CMV retinitis at some time during the course of their disease.

While it was initially suggested that CMV retinitis was a preterminal event (6), it subsequently became evident that CMV retinitis may occur at any time during the course of AIDS (13-15). Holland et al. (15) reported a median interval of 9 months from the diagnosis of AIDS to the diagnosis of CMV retinitis, but the range was wide, from 0 to 45 months. Furthermore, CMV retinitis has been reported as the initial AIDS-defining opportunistic infection (14) or as occurring at the same time as the initial AIDS-defining opportunistic infection (13-15). Of patients with CMV retinitis and AIDS, 11 to 15% (13,15) will have CMV retinitis either as their AIDS-defining opportunistic infection or present at the initial time of AIDS diagnosis. In one series (13), 3% of patients with AIDS had CMV retinitis as their initial AIDS-defining opportunistic infection.

In contrast to the broad interval between AIDS diagnosis and diagnosis of CMV retinitis, the relationship of CMV retinitis and the level of immunodeficiency seems more precisely defined in that CMV retinitis is associated with a profound immunodeficiency (8,16). The absolute number of CD4+ T helper cells is substantially lower among patients with CMV retinitis and AIDS than among AIDS patients without CMV retinitis (8). Palestine et al. (8) reported that patients with CMV retinitis had an average CD4+ cell count of 20 cells/μl, and Hoechst et al. (16) reported the median CD4+ cell count in patients with AIDS and CMV retinitis as 37 cells/μl, with 94% of patients having a CD4+ cell count less than 20 cells/μl.

Although it was initially suggested (8) that CMV retinitis was a preterminal event with survival generally limited to 6 weeks, subsequent series have demonstrated that the median survival among patients with AIDS is substantially longer. Four separate series (13,15,17,18) from different cities reported a median survival of 5 to 6 months after the diagnosis of CMV retinitis, and recently Gross et al. (19) reported a median survival of 8 months. Furthermore, Holland et al. (15) reported that the median survival has been increasing over time, and the range of survival after the diagnosis of CMV retinitis is wide, with some patients surviving up to 2 years (13,15).

III. CMV RETINITIS: DIAGNOSIS AND NATURAL HISTORY

The diagnosis of CMV retinitis can generally be made reliably on ophthalmoscopy. CMV retinitis may be asymptomatic, especially if the lesion is small and anterior. However, patients often complain of floaters or a vague sense of blurred vision. With posterior lesions, the patient is often aware of a scotoma or loss of vision. Ophthalmoscopically, CMV retinitis presents as a necrotic retinitis, sometimes admixed with hemorrhage (Figure 1). The characteristic feature of CMV retinitis is a yellowish-white area of retinal necrosis with a granular border extending into the surrounding retina. While CMV retinitis was classically described as hemorrhagic, in patients with AIDS hemorrhages are often not present. It is unknown why some lesions appear fulminant and hemorrhagic and others granular. We have seen the nonhemorrhagic or granular form of CMV retinitis evolve into a fulminant and hemorrhagic retinitis. Occasionally, a very small CMV retinitis lesion may be

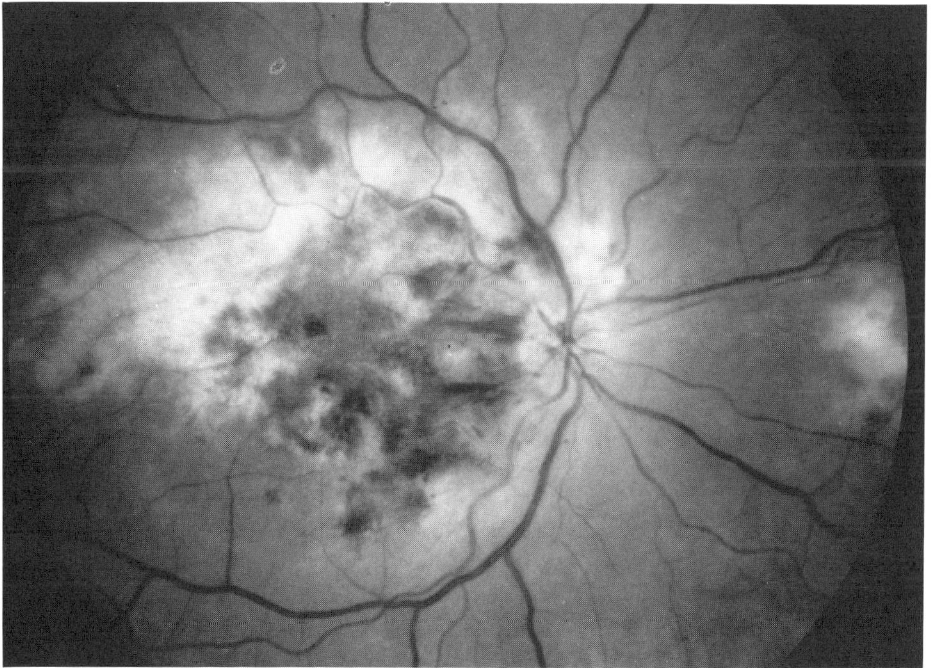

Figure 1 CMV retinitis in patients with AIDS. (From Ref. 1. Published courtesy of *Ophthalmology*.)

mistaken for a "cotton-wool" spot, the change seen in background AIDS retinopathy (1,10). However, follow-up examination generally reveals the diagnosis, since CMV retinitis will progress and enlarge over time. Other diseases that may occasionally look like CMV retinitis are fulminant toxoplasma retinitis and either herpes simplex retinitis or varicella zoster retinitis. All three of these infections are substantially less common than CMV retinitis in patients with AIDS.

Untreated CMV retinitis is a progressive disease (13). Cytomegalovirus is thought to be hematologically disseminated to the retina, where it invades the retinal cells and establishes a productive infection. Over 90% of patients with AIDS and CMV retinitis will have positive cultures for CMV from a nonocular source, primarily the blood or urine (13). The retinitis characteristically spreads outward from the periphery of the lesion. Areas previously infected with CMV show total destruction of the retinal architecture and replacement by a thin gliotic scar (11). There is often hyperpigmentation of the scarred lesion. Active CMV can be found at the border of the lesion. Occasionally a new focus of retinitis will be found as well. Untreated, the majority of patients will ultimately develop bilateral disease. Approximately one-third of patients will present with bilateral ocular involvement (13), and of those who present with unilateral disease, 60% will ultimately develop bilateral disease unless treated. The end stage of this process in the involved eye is a totally destroyed, often detached, retina and the loss of all vision.

A variety of criteria have been used to assess progression among patients who have CMV retinitis. The criterion most often in use currently is the time for the border of the retinitis to progress a specific distance (20). In the study reported by Holland et al. (20), 94% of untreated patients had a progression of their retinitis 500 μm or greater during a median follow-up period of 25 days. Given enough time, essentially all patients will suffer progression of their retinitis unless treated. Two case reports (21,22) of the resolution of CMV retinitis after the initiation of zidovudine (also known as azidothymidine) therapy have been reported. They are both noteworthy in that they are the rare exceptions (13). In both cases, zidovudine was instituted after the diagnosis of CMV retinitis, and a subsequent temporary arrest of the progression of the disease was achieved. In the case report by Guyer et al. (22) with follow-up until the patient's death, ultimate relapse of the retinitis occurred. Estimates of the median time to progression among untreated patients are generally on the order of 3 weeks.

IV. GANCICLOVIR THERAPY OF CMV RETINITIS: USE AND EFFICACY

Ganciclovir is a nucleoside analog that inhibits CMV by inhibiting DNA replication. Ganciclovir is triphosphorylated in the infected cell, and the triphosphorylated ganciclovir then inhibits DNA replication and the CMV infection. Autopsy studies of patients treated with ganciclovir (23) have demonstrated the presence of viral DNA at the border of the lesion but the absence of a productive infection.

Treatment of CMV retinitis is generally performed in a two-step fashion. Initially, a high dose of drug is given to control the infection (induction therapy) followed by long-term therapy to prevent relapse (maintenance). The phenomenon of relapse when an antibiotic is discontinued is characteristic of patients with AIDS and occurs with other infections as well (e.g., *Pneumocystis carinii* pneumonia, cryptococcal meningitis, and infections with *Toxoplasma gondii*). Initially, two different dosing schema were used for induction therapy, either 2.5 mg/kg every 8 hours intravenously (7.5 mg/kg per day) or 5 mg/kg intravenously every 12 hours (10 mg/kg per day). Subsequently, the 5 mg/kg every 12 hours has become the standard dose for induction therapy. Similarly, early studies used various durations of induction therapy for initial treatment. The most often used courses were 10, 14, and 21 days. Most investigators now use a 14-day induction course, and there have been no reported differences in efficacy between shorter and longer induction courses. Because relapse was easily detected when induction therapy was discontinued, maintenance ganciclovir became used early in the AIDS epidemic. The current dose of maintenance ganciclovir is generally 5 mg/kg per day intravenously once daily (35 mg/kg/week), although 6 mg/kg per day on 5 of 7 days is also used (30 mg/kg/week). Lower doses and every-other-day dosing schedules have been associated with unacceptably high rates of early relapse. Maintenance therapy is continued indefinitely and requires the placement of a permanent indwelling central venous catheter. Because ganciclovir is excreted in the urine, the dose must be adjusted for renal function according to the guidelines outlined in Table 1.

Table 1 Dose Adjustment of Ganciclovir for Renal Function

Creatinine clearance (ml/1.73 m²/min)[a]	Ganciclovir dose (mg/kg)	Dosing interval (hours)
≥80	5.0	12
50-79	2.5	12
25-49	2.5	24
<25	1.25	24

[a]Creatinine clearance can be related to serum creatine by the following formulas for men:

$$\frac{(140 - \text{age [yr]}) (\text{body wt [kg]})}{(72) (\text{serum creatinine [mg/dl]})} \times 1.73/\text{surface area (m}^2)$$

Creatinine clearance for women = 0.85 × the value for men.

Multiple series (Table 2) have reported the efficacy of ganciclovir for the treatment of CMV retinitis. Response rates have generally ranged from 80 to 100%, with 60 to 80% of patients achieving a remission (12,13,17,18, 24-29). These studies have all been retrospective and have not used identical standardized criteria for the analysis of the data. However, despite these limitations, these studies have derived similar definitions of response and complete response (remission) and reported similar response rates. Indeed, given the lack of preexisting standardized criteria, the agreement among various investigators is remarkably good.

In patients who are treated for CMV retinitis, the goal of treatment is the arrest of the progression of the disease to prevent further spread of the infection and maximize visual function. Retina previously infected by CMV is destroyed and will not recover function, and anti-CMV therapy will not halt the destruction of already infected retina. Therefore, immediately after anti-CMV therapy has been instituted, the borders of the lesion may be observed to progress slightly over the initial few days. This phenomenon represents the natural evolution of areas already infected by CMV rather than a failure of therapy. In patients successfully treated with ganciclovir, there is a subsequent arrest of the progression of the disease. Ultimately, the areas of necrotic retinitis will convert to a atrophic and gliotic scar, and the patient will be left with a nonprogressive atrophic lesion (Figure 2). We now use *remission* to describe the state of treated CMV infection at which only an atrophic and gliotic scar can be detected and there is no evidence of active necrotic retinitis. (Previously, many authors used the term *complete response* to refer to this state, and this term is synonymous with remission.) In patients treated with ganciclovir, the median time to remission has been reported as 21 to 31 days (13,18). Indeed, prior to the use of maintenance therapy, patients given only induction ganciclovir often achieved a remission

Table 2 Reported Response Rates of CMV Retinitis to Ganciclovir Therapy

Authors (ref.)	Response rate (remission) (%)
Palestine et al., 1986 (24)	88 (62)
DHPG Study Group, 1986 (25)	85
Henderly et al., 1987 (14)	100
Holland et al., 1987 (26)	97 (88)
Orellana et al., 1987 (18)	88
Laskin et al., 1987 (28)	91
Jacobson et al., 1988 (12)	81
Jabs et al., 1989 (13)	81 (61)

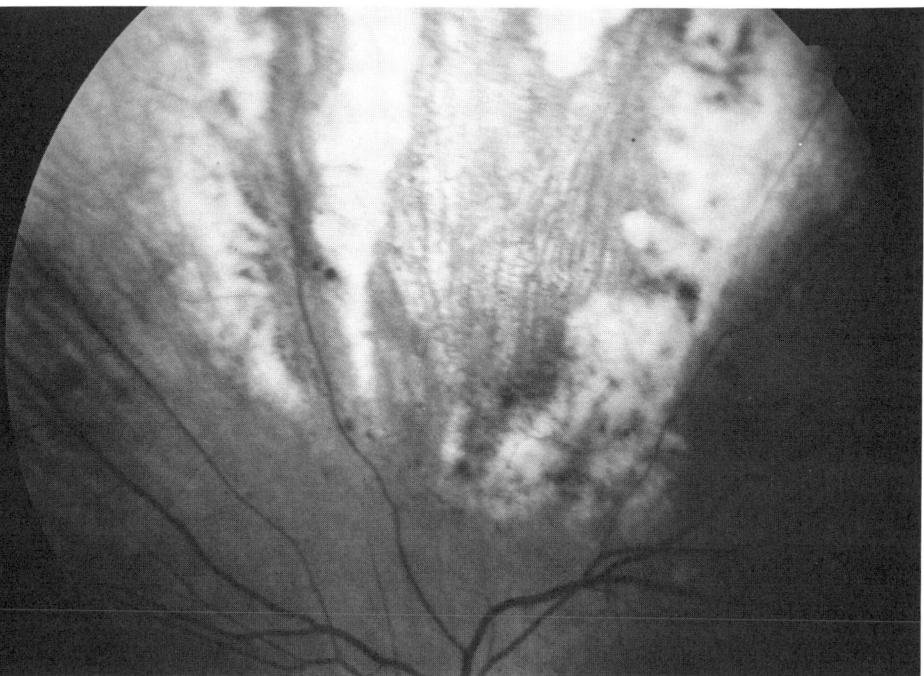

(a)

Figure 2   Response of CMV retinitis to ganciclovir therapy in a patient with AIDS. (a) CMV retinitis prior to the initiation of ganciclovir. (b) CMV retinitis 1 month after the initiation of ganciclovir therapy, demonstrating a good response to treatment. (c) Six months after the initiation of ganciclovir therapy, demonstrating no significant progression of the disease. [(a) and (b) from Ref. 27. Published courtesy of *Ophthalmology*.]

1 month after starting therapy only to subsequently suffer a relapse of active retinitis (24). The time lag between the institution of CMV therapy, the clearing of blood and/or urine cultures (which generally occurs by the seventh day of treatment), and the resolution of ophthalmoscopic evidence of active disease represents the time required for the areas of necrotic retinitis to resolve and leave a scar, and reflects the time to observe the clearing of necrotic material in the eye rather than a delay in the antiviral effect of ganciclovir on the CMV infection in the eye.

A conservative analysis of the results of ganciclovir therapy uses an "intent to treat" analysis in which all patients are included regardless of whether

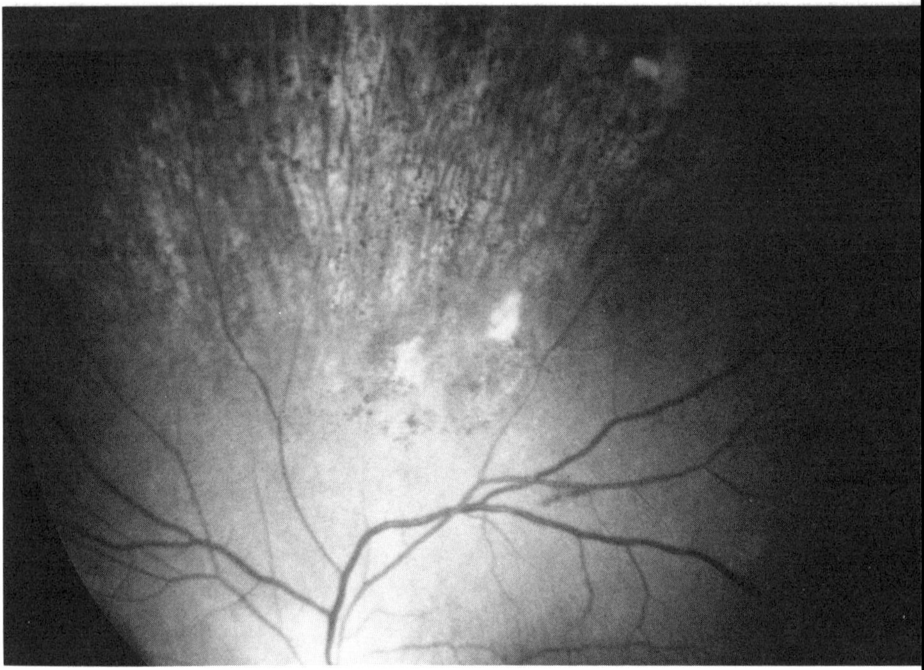

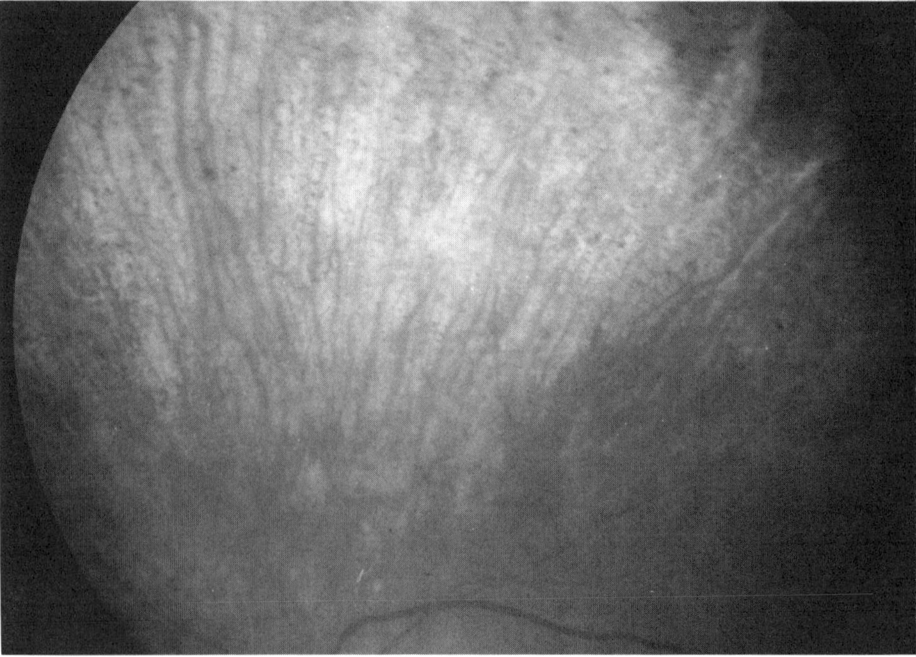

(b)

(c)   **Figure 2** *continued*

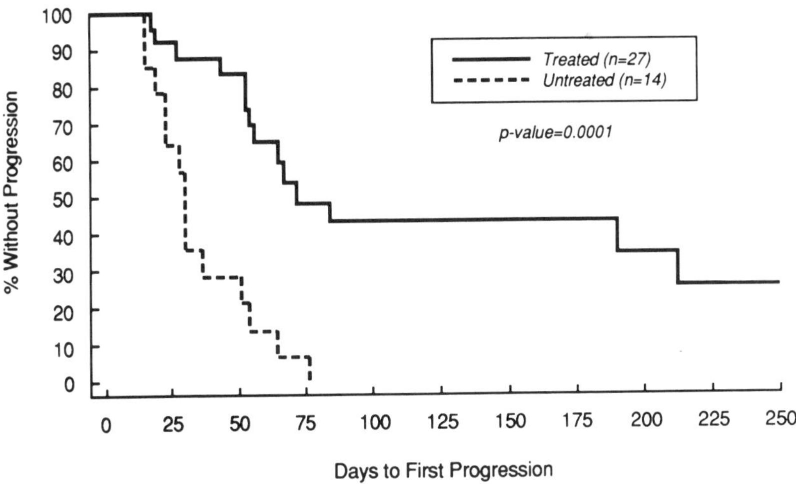

Figure 3   Kaplan-Meier analysis of the time to progression of CMV retinitis in patients with AIDS. Patients with treated CMV retinitis had a significantly longer time to progression than untreated patients.

the CMV relapses because of ganciclovir interolance or "breakthrough" while receiving maintenance ganciclovir. One such analysis revealed a median time to progression of 71 days in patients treated with ganciclovir compared to 29 days in those not treated (30) ($p < 0.0001$) (Figure 3). Similar results have been obtained in other series (12).

V. GANCICLOVIR THERAPY OF CMV RETINITIS: SIDE EFFECTS AND TOXICITY

A variety of side effects have been reported for ganciclovir, including granulocytopenia, thrombocytopenia, poorly characterized neurological side effects, and abnormal results of liver function tests. The most serious and frequent of these is granulocytopenia, which is often the dose-limiting side effect. Rates of granulocytopenia have varied from study to study, depending on the definition used. When granulocytopenia is defined as a 50% decrease in the granulocyte count, the reported rate of toxicity has been higher than in those studies in which granulocytopenia is defined as an absolute neutrophil count (ANC) of less than 500 cells/μl. When granulocytopenia is defined as an ANC of less than 500/μl, approximately one-third of patients (13) receiving ganciclovir will experience granulocytopenia sometime during the course of their disease. This granulocytopenia is almost always reversible, and the ANC recovers over several days. Often this fall in the

ANC occurs near or just after the completion of induction therapy; the ANC will rapidly recover with temporary interruption of therapy, and maintenance therapy may be started soon thereafter. Of patients who are treated with ganciclovir, 16% (13) are unable to tolerate the drug because of recurrent granulocytopenia whenever they are on treatment. Thrombocytopenia may occasionally limit the dose tolerated, but other side effects rarely lead to discontinuation of therapy. Because of the similar hematological toxicities, patients on ganciclovir do not tolerate concurrent zidovudine at the current standard doses (500 to 600 mg/day) (16). Investigators are now trying the concurrent use of zidovudine at a reduced dose (300 mg/day), but the long-term results are unknown at this time. Additionally, the use of GM-CSF in combination with zidovudine and ganciclovir maintenance appears promising (see Chapter 13).

VI. GANCICLOVIR THERAPY OF CMV RETINITIS: LONG-TERM OUTCOME

A. Relapse

When ganciclovir therapy is interrupted for a sufficiently prolonged period of time, relapse is essentially universal. The median time to relapse among patients who have had ganciclovir discontinued is approximately 3 to 4 weeks (13,29). Therefore, patients with AIDS treated for CMV retinitis are placed on lifetime maintenance therapy. CMV will often relapse while on maintenance—the phenomenon of breakthrough retinitis. Estimates of the relapse rate in patients receiving maintenance therapy vary from 18 to 50% (13,17, 18,26-29). Life table analysis shows an increasing cumulative rate of relapse over time among patients receiving continuous maintenance therapy, with approximately 35% of patients relapsing by 1 year of treatment (18). While relapse of retinitis on maintenance ganciclovir may be fulminant, it often appears as a slow, "smoldering," intermittent movement of the border (19), suggesting a partial effect of the maintenance dose.

Breakthrough of the retinitis appears to most often represent failure of the patient's immune system as the primary cause. One study demonstrated that patients who initially failed to respond to ganciclovir had a significantly shorter survival than patients who achieved a remission on ganciclovir (2.3 vs. 10 months; $p = 0.06$) (13). The authors interpreted this result as suggesting that patients with poorer immune systems, as evidenced by the shortened survival, were unlikely to respond to the drug, and patients with a better immune status, as evidenced by the longer survival, were able to respond to treatment and achieve a remission. Similarly, breakthrough of the retinitis has been associated with the lower lymphocyte count (19). While ganciclovir resistance has been described (31; Chapter 12), this situation currently appears to be an infrequent cause of relapse, and patients with relapse of the retinitis while on maintenance therapy will most often respond to a second course of induction therapy. The role of ganciclovir resistance in the future remains to be determined.

B. Visual Outcome

The visual outcome of patients with CMV retinitis is dependent on the location of the initial lesion. Involvement of vital ocular structures, such as the fovea or optic nerve, may result in permanent blindness despite a good response to treatment. Furthermore, patients with posterior, more immediately vision-threatening lesions are more apt to be treated than those with peripheral, less immediately vision-threatening lesions. Therefore, in retrospective series, there is a bias toward a better visual outcome in untreated patients, because of the initial location of their lesions. Despite these limitations on the interpretation of visual results, published series treating patients with ganciclovir suggest that the drug is able to preserve vision. Gross et al. (19) recently reported that 73% of eyes will maintain a visual acuity of 20/40 or better when treated with ganciclovir. Only 18% of eyes had a final visual acuity of 20/200 or worse. An earlier series (13) showed similar results with 55% of treated eyes attaining a final visual acuity of 20/40 or better and 34% of treated eyes a final acuity of 20/200. In this latter series, only 35% of untreated patients achieved a visual acuity of 20/40 or better, while 47% of patients ended up with a visual acuity of 20/200 or worse. Furthermore, in a small number of eyes in which visual acuity was grouped according to a classification of good (20/40 or better), impaired (20/50 to 20/100), or blind (20/200 or worse), the median time to decline of one level in the visual acuity was greater in patients who were treated with ganciclovir (173 days) than in those who were untreated (56 days) (Jabs DA, unpublished observations). Because of the limitations of retrospective data, these analyses must be interpreted with caution; however, collectively they suggest that ganciclovir is effective in preserving visual acuity.

Retinal detachment may complicate the course of CMV retinitis and alter the long-term visual outcome. Detachments occur as a consequence of the retinitis (13) due to the damage to the retina. The detachment rate among patients with CMV retinitis has been reported as 15 to 19% (13,19). Surgical intervention is required to repair these detachments, but the resulting visual acuity may be impaired. In patients undergoing surgical repair of a retinal detachment due to CMV retinitis, continued treatment of the CMV retinitis is essential to prevent relapse of the retinitis and subsequent redetachment.

VII. CONCLUSION

In conclusion, untreated CMV retinitis is a progressive, destructive, and blinding ocular disorder. Because it is a frequent infection in patients with

AIDS, it greatly adds to the morbidity of this disease. Ganciclovir is an effective treatment for CMV retinitis; it can arrest the progression of the disease and preserve visual acuity. While relapse does occur in patients treated with ganciclovir and kept on maintenance therapy, this relapse appears to represent a failure of the immune system and often responds to a second course of induction therapy.

REFERENCES

1. Jabs DA, Green WR, Fox R, Polk BF, Bartlett JG. Ocular manifestations of acquired immune deficiency syndrome. Ophthalmology 1989; 96:1092-1099.
2. Murray HW, Knox DL, Green WR, Susel RM. Cytomegalovirus retinitis in adults. Am J Med 1977; 63:574-584.
3. Pollard RB, Egbert PR, Gallagher JG, Merigan TC. Cytomegalovirus retinitis in immunosuppressed hosts. I. Natural history and effects of treatment with adenine arabinoside. Ann Intern Med 1980; 93:655-664.
4. Egbert PR, Pollard RB, Gallagher JG, Merigan TC. Cytomegalovirus retinitis in immunosuppressed hosts. II. Ocular manifestations. Ann Intern Med 1980; 93:664-670.
5. Fiala M, Chatterjee SN, Carson S, Poolsawat S, Heiner DC, Saxon A, Guze LB. Cytomegalovirus retinitis secondary to chronic viremia in phagocytic leukocytes. Am J Ophthalmol 1977; 84:567-573.
6. Holland GN, Pepose JS, Pettit TH, Gottlieb MS, Yee RD, Foos RY. Acquired immune deficiency syndrome. Ocular manifestations. Ophthalmology 1983; 90:859-873.
7. Rosenberg PR, Uliss AE, Friedland GH, Harris CA, Small CB, Klein RS. Acquired immunodeficiency syndrome. Ophthalmology 1983; 90:874-878.
8. Palestine AG, Rodrigues MM, Macher AM, Chan CC, Lane HC, Fauci AS, Masur H, Longo D, Reichert CM, Steis R, Rook AH, Nussenblatt RB. Ophthalmic involvement in acquired immunodeficiency syndrome. Ophthalmology 1984; 91:1092-1099.
9. Freeman WR, Lerner CW, Mines JA, Lash RS, Nadel AJ, Starr MB, Tapper ML. A prospective study of the ophthalmologic findings in the acquired immune deficiency syndrome. Am J Ophthalmol 1984; 97:133-142.
10. Newsome DA, Green WR, Miller ED, Kiessling LA, Morgan B, Jabs DA, Polk BF. Microvascular aspects of acquired immune deficiency syndrome retinopathy. Am J Ophthalmol 1984; 98:590-601.
11. Pepose JS, Holland GN, Nestor MS, Cochran AJ, Foos RY. Acquired immune deficiency syndrome. Pathogenic mechanisms of ocular disease. Ophthalmology 1985; 92:472-484.
12. Jacobson MA, O'Donnell JJ, Porteous D, Brodie HR, Feigal D, Mills J. Retinal and gastrointestinal disease due to cytomegalovirus in patients with the acquired immune deficiency syndrome: Prevalence, natural history, and response to ganciclovir therapy. Quar J Med 1988; 67:473-486.
13. Jabs DA, Enger C, Bartlett JG. Cytomegalovirus retinitis and acquired immunodeficiency syndrome. Arch Opthalmol 1989; 107:75-80.

14. Henderly DE, Freeman WR, Smith RE, Causey D, Rao NA. Cytomegalovirus retinitis as the initial manifestation of the acquired immune deficiency syndrome. Am J Ophthalmol 1987; 103:316-320.
15. Holland GN, Sison RF, Jatulis DE, Haslop MG, Sakamoto MJ, Wheeler NC, The UCLA CMV Retinopathy Study Group. Survival of patients with acquired immune deficiency syndrome after development of cytomegalovirus retinopathy. Ophthalmology 1990; 97:204-211.
16. Hoechst H, Dieterich D, Bozzette S, Reichman RC, Connor JD, Leibes L, Sonke RL, Spector SA, Valentine F, Pettinelli C, Richman DD. Toxicity of combined ganciclovir and zidovudine for cytomegalovirus disease associated with AIDS. Ann Intern Med 1990; 113:111-117.
17. Henderly DE, Freeman WR, Causey DM, Rao NA. Cytomegalovirus retinitis and response to therapy with ganciclovir. Ophthalmology 1987; 94:425-434.
18. Orellana J, Teich SA, Friedman AH, Lerebours F, Winterkorn J, Mildvan D. Combined short- and long-term therapy for the treatment of cytomegalovirus retinitis using ganciclovir (BW B759U). Ophthalmology 1987; 94:831-838.
19. Gross JG, Bozzette SA, Mathews WC, Spector SA, Abramson IS, McCutchan JA, Mendez T, Munguia D, Freeman WR. Longitudinal study of cytomegalovirus retinitis in acquired immune deficiency syndrome. Ophthalmology 1990; 97:681-686.
20. Holland GN, Buhles WC, Mastre B, Kaplan HJ, UCLA CMV Retinopathy Study Group. A controlled retrospective study of ganciclovir treatment for cytomegalovirus retinopathy. Use of a standardized system for the assessment of disease outcome. Arch Ophthalmol 1989; 107:1759-1766.
21. D'Amico DJ, Sholnik PR, Koslof BR, Pimhsten P, Hirsch MS, Schooley RT. Resolution of cytomegalovirus retinitis with zidovudine therapy. Arch Ophthalmol 1988; 106:1168-1169.
22. Guyer DR, Jabs DA, Brant AM, Beschorner WE, Green WR. Regression of cytomegalovirus retinitis with zidovudine. A clinicopathologic correlation. Arch Ophthalmol 1989; 107:868 874.
23. Pepose JS, Newman C, Bach MC, Quinn TC, Ambinder RF, Holland GN, Hodstrom PS, Frey HM, Foos RY. Pathologic features of cytomegalovirus retinopathy after treatment with the antiviral agent ganciclovir. Ophthalmology 1987; 94:414-424.
24. Palestine AG, Stevens G, Lane HC, Masur H, Fujikawa LS, Nussenblatt RB, Rook AH, Manischewitz J, Baird B, Megill M, Quinnan G, Gelmann E, Fauci AS. Treatment of cytomegalovirus retinitis with dihydroxy propoxymethyl guanine. Am J Ophthalmol 1986; 101:95-101.
25. Collaborative DHPG Treatment Study Group. Treatment of serious cytomegalovirus infections with 9-(1,3-dihydroxy-2-propoxymethyl)guanine in patients with AIDS and other immunodeficiencies. N Engl J Med 1986; 314:801-805.
26. Holland GN, Sidikaro Y, Kreiger AE, Hardy D, Sakamoto MJ, Frenkel LM, Winston DJ, Gottlieb MS, Bryson YJ, Champlin RE, Ho WG, Winters RE, Wolfe PR, Cherry JD. Treatment of cytomegalovirus retinopathy with ganciclovir. Ophthalmology 1987; 94:815-823.
27. Jabs DA, Newman C, de Bustros S, Polk BF. Treatment of cytomegalovirus retinitis with ganciclovir. Ophthalmology 1987; 94:824-830.

28. Laskin OL, Cederberg DM, Mills J, Eron LJ, Mildvan D, Spector SA. Ganciclovir for the treatment and suppression of serious infections caused by cytomegalovirus. Am J Med 1987; 83:201.
29. Jacobson MA, O'Donnell JJ, Brodie HR, Wofsy C, Mills J. Randomized prospective trial of ganciclovir maintenance therapy for cytomegalovirus retinitis. J Med Virology 1988; 25:339-349.
30. Jabs DA. CMV retinitis and AIDS. Ganciclovir treatment results. Testimony before the FDA advisory committee meeting, May 22, 1989.
31. Erice A, Chou S, Biron KK, Stanat SC, Balfour HH, Jordan MC. Progressive disease due to ganciclovir-resistant cytomegalovirus in immunocompromised patients. N Engl J Med 1989; 320:291-293.

7

Intravitreal Ganciclovir Therapy for Cytomegalovirus Retinopathy

M.-H. Heinemann
*Cornell University Medical College
and Memorial Sloan-Kettering Cancer Center
New York, New York*

I. INTRODUCTION AND RATIONALE

Cytomegalovirus (CMV) infection of the retina has emerged as the most common ocular opportunistic infection complicating the acquired immunodeficiency syndrome (AIDS). While the prevalence of CMV retinitis among AIDS patients is not known, many investigators believe that up to 25% of patients with AIDS will develop this infection at some time during the course of their illness (1). The retinal necrosis caused by CMV is inexorably progressive and will result in profound loss of vision and eventual blindness if left untreated. It is fortunate, therefore, that antiviral agents have become available that can, in most cases, arrest the progression of the retinitis and transform areas of full-thickness retinal necrosis into chorioretinal scar tissue.

Standard therapy for CMV retinitis currently involves systemic therapy with intravenously administered ganciclovir sodium, a congener of the nucleoside acyclocir. Ganciclovir has been shown to be an effective therapy for CMV retinitis with a very high initial response rate (2-4). Long-term maintenance therapy is required, however, to prevent progression or recrudescence of the retinitis, and a significant number of patients will develop areas of reactivation despite maintenance therapy with ganciclovir (1,3). Systemic therapy with GCV is frequently complicated by myelosuppression and neutropenia that often require attenuation or discontinuation of treatment (4). Drug-induced neutropenia is most common at the end of induction therapy (5 mg/kg q 12 hr), and the incidence of granulocytopenia tends to increase with the duration of therapy. Granulocytopenia is the most common precipitating factor in the attenuation or discontinuation of systemic ganciclovir therapy, accounting for 65% of interruptions or terminations of treatment (3). While treatment with intravenously administered ganciclovir can usually be resumed once the granulocyte count has risen, such intermittent treatment commonly leads to reactivation of retinitis, resulting in additional retinal necrosis and further impairment of vision in many cases. Although it has been demonstrated that ganciclovir can be concurrently administered with zidovudine (AZT) (500 mg per day), drug-induced myelosuppression often requires that the doses of one or both drugs be reduced or that administration of one or both be discontinued.

An alternative to systemic ganciclovir therapy for the treatment of CMV retinitis is the use of intravenously administered foscarnet. Preliminary data suggest that intravenously administered foscarnet is roughly comparable to ganciclovir in arresting the progression of retinitis; however, it too has significant systemic toxicity (especially nephrotoxicity), and maintenance therapy often has to be discontinued or the maintenance dosage of drug reduced (5). Reactivation of retinitis while on maintenance foscarnet therapy has been described, but it is not known if these phenomena are more less common than with ganciclovir maintenance therapy.

Regardless of which antiviral agent is used, long-term intravenous therapy via indwelling venous catheters carries with it a significant risk of complications. These include the perioperative and operative risks of implantation of catheters and catheter-associated sepsis. Immunocompromised patients with indwelling catheters are particularly vulnerable to a wide variety of opportunistic systemic infections. In addition, many of the patients under therapy for CMV retinitis have significant reductions in visual acuity and peripheral field and thus have difficulty with catheter hygiene and drug preparation and administration. Recent improvements in the design of these catheters have reduced the frequency of catheter-associated infections but the long-term use of these devices remains hazardous.

In view of the high morbidity associated with systemic antiviral therapy and the high reactivation rate among patients while on full or attenuated doses of maintenance therapy, the use of intravitreally administered ganciclovir was put forward as an alternative therapeutic strategy. Limited clinical experience has suggested that intravitreally administered ganciclovir may be effective in treating sight-threatening CMV retinitis in those patients who for one reason or another are intolerant of systemic antiviral therapy (Figures

1 and 2). The use of intravitreal ganciclovir has also been proposed as adjunctive therapy for patients who can receive only attenuated doses of systemic ganciclovir or foscarnet.

Henry, Cantrill, and co-workers (6) were the first to treat a patient with intravitreal ganciclovir. Their report suggested that serial intravitreal injections were well tolerated by the patient and were effective in arresting the progression of the retinitis. In addition, pharmacokinetic data collected from the patient indicated no significant systemic absorption of ganciclovir, and that twice-weekly injections of 200 μg provided intraocular concentrations of ganciclovir above the ID_{50} of CMV. In a subsequent study, Ussery and associates (7) reported that 11 of 14 eyes treated with intravitreal injections of ganciclovir demonstrated suppression of retinitis after intermittent, short-term therapy.

The safety and efficacy of long-term intravitreal ganciclovir were evaluated in a series of 10 patients by Cantrill and associates (8) and in a series of seven patients by the author (9). These studies indicated that long-term

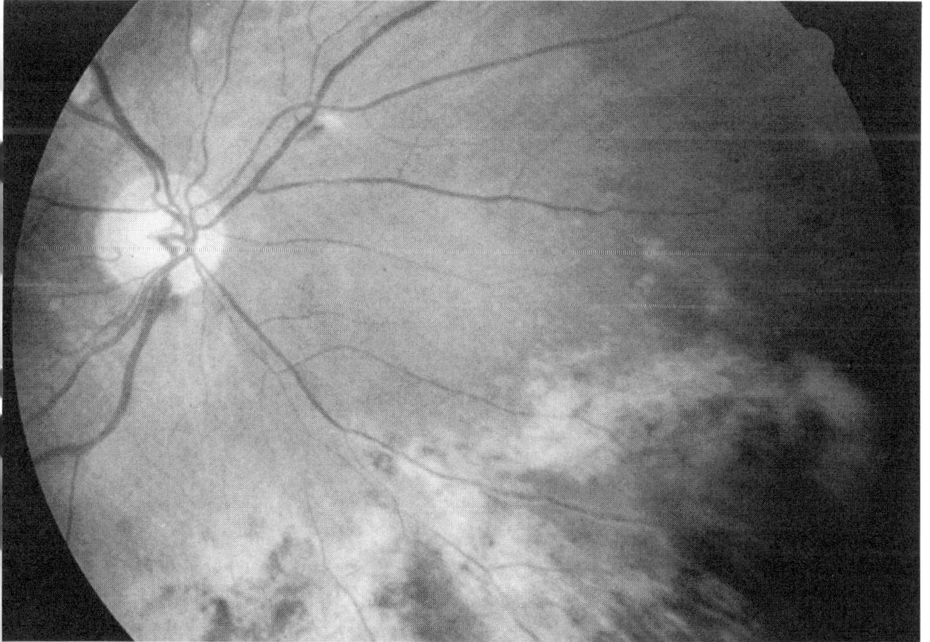

Figure 1 Fundus photograph of eye with large area of active, necrotizing retinitis before treatment with intravitreal ganciclovir.

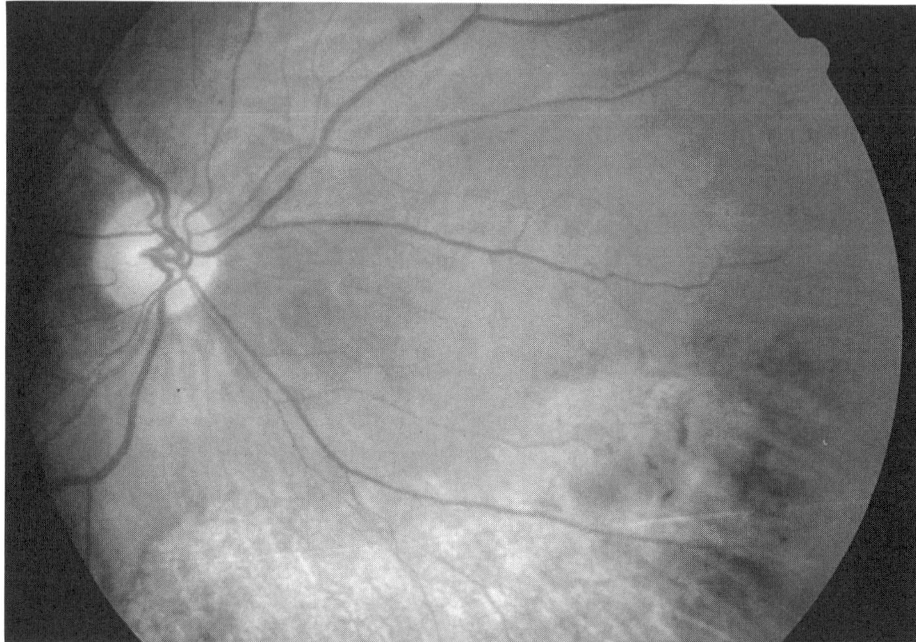

Figure 2 The same retina as in Figure 1 after an induction course of 6 weeks of intravitreal treatment. The retina has become atrophic, chorioretinal scarring has begun, and there is little or no retinal opacification. The retinitis has not progressed as compared with the pretreatment photograph.

therapy—up to 58 weeks of treatment—was, for the most part, well tolerated, and, at least during the initial phases of treatment, effective in suppressing the retinitis and improving or stabilizing visual acuity. On the basis of these initial observations, a prospective, multicenter clinical trial was initiated by the AIDS Clinical Trials Group at the National Institute of Allergy and Infectious Diseases to determine the safety and efficacy of intravitreal ganciclovir therapy in AIDS patients with active CMV retinitis who are intolerant of systemic therapy because of neutropenia.

II. PHARMACOLOGICAL AND TOXICITY DATA

Limited data exist on the pharmacokinetics and toxicity of intravitreally administered ganciclovir. Pulido and associates (10) performed acute toxicity studies in rabbits who had received injections of 10, 20, 40, 80, 100, 200, and 400 μg of ganciclovir. The retinas of animals receiving 40 and 400 μg, as well as those of control animals receiving injections of normal saline, were studied electrophysiologically before treatment and 7 days postoperatively. No electroretinographic abnormalities were detected. Histologic study of treated eyes failed to disclose any abnormalities. More extensive toxicologic studies have been performed by Syntex Laboratories (11). In these studies no drug-related abnormalities were detected either ophthalmoscopically or histologically in eyes of rabbits treated up to three times weekly with doses of ganciclovir up to 400 μg per injection.

In the report by Henry and co-workers (6), the elimination half-life of intravitreal ganciclovir from vitreous humor was estimated at over 13 hours. Analyses of vitreous concentrations of ganciclovir in patients treated by means of intravitreal injection suggest that the ID_{50} for CMV is maintained for more than 60 hours after a single 200-μg dose. These conclusions should be qualified, as concentrations of ganciclovir necessary to inhibit replication of human CMV may be as high as 10 mg/L (11). The limited pharmacokinetic data suggest that such levels may be difficult to achieve in human, inflamed eyes (as opposed to smaller, uninflamed rabbit eyes), and as a result weekly or even twice-weekly injections as given during long-term treatment regimens may be insufficient to control viral replication.

In patients in the literature who have been treated on a long-term basis, there has been no evidence of toxicity from repeated intravitreal injections, but it should be emphasized that adverse reactions to injection or drug toxicity may be difficult to evaluate clinically in eyes that are extensively damaged by necrotizing retinitis (8,9,12). Many patients reported mild discomfort after injections. Conjunctival scarring and episcleral and scleral inflammatory changes were evident in patients who had undergone multiple injections. Some patients developed low-grade, short-term vitreal inflammatory changes, manifested by intravitreal cellular infiltrate and mild clouding of the vitreous. The status of the lens was not compromised in any treated patient. The most serious complications reported were two cases of *Staphylococcus epidermidis* endophthalmitis, which both responded to prompt vitreous surgery and systemic and intracameral antibiotic therapy (8,9). A retinal detachment attributable to injection occurred in the series reported by Ussery and associates (7).

III. INDICATIONS FOR INTRAVITREAL GANCICLOVIR THERAPY

Indications for intravitreal ganciclovir therapy have yet to be defined, but patients with active, sight-threatening CMV retinitis (retinitis within 3000 μm of the fovea and/or 1500 μm of the optic nerve) who are intolerant of systemic therapy are among those most likely to benefit from this mode of therapy. Because CMV retinitis is a manifestation of systemic viral infection, and because the development of retinitis in a previously uninvolved eye in patients not treated with systemic therapy is common, intravitreal therapy should not be initiated in patients with CMV retinitis if systemic therapy can be given (1,12). Systemic therapy may include systemically administered ganciclovir or foscarnet, or combination therapy such as systemic ganciclovir and granulocyte-macrophage colony-stimulating factor, which can mitigate the neutropenic effects of therapy with ganciclovir alone. It remains to be seen whether intravitreally administered ganciclovir may be of value as adjunctive therapy to low-dose systemic ganciclovir therapy or whether "booster" doses of intravitreal drug may be of benefit in patients who manifest progression of retinitis while on maximal systemic therapy (reinduction dose) and who cannot tolerate other systemic antiviral agents.

Certain exclusion criteria do exist for intravitreal therapy. Patients who are markedly thrombocytopenic (platelet count $<25,000/\text{mm}^3$) are at high risk of developing intraocular hemorrhage during or after the injection procedure. Patients who have external ocular infections (e.g., conjunctivitis or blepharitis) should not undergo intraocular injection. Opacification of the ocular media such as that caused by vitreous hemorrhage, dense cataract, or corneal opacity makes difficult visualization of the posterior ocular structures—retina, optic nerve, and central retinal artery—and as a result intraocular injections cannot be safely performed nor the effects of treatment adequately evaluated.

IV. TECHNIQUE OF DRUG ADMINISTRATION

Clinical experience to date suggests that a 200-μg dose of ganciclovir in an injection volume of 0.1 ml can be safely injected through the pars plana into the vitreous compartment. Ganciclovir is reconstituted with 0.9% sodium chloride free of preservatives and serially diluted to yield a solution with concentration of 2 mg/ml. A small volume is filtered through a 22-μm filter, and 0.1 ml of this solution is used for injection.

To minimize the chance of infection the eye is copiously irrigated with sterile saline after application of topical anesthetics and placement of a self-retaining eyelid speculum. Agents such as proparacaine or 4% cocaine may be used. Pretreatment with topical antibiotics such as gentamicin 1 day before treatment may also be considered. Injections may safely be made over the pars plana (3.5 to 4.0 mm from the corneascleral limbus) (Figure 3). Injections are administered with a tuberculin syringe fitted with 30-gauge, 1/2-inch needles.

Following injection, indirect ophthalmoscopy should be performed to check for patency of the central retinal artery because transient elevations of intraocular pressure are common following intraocular injections.

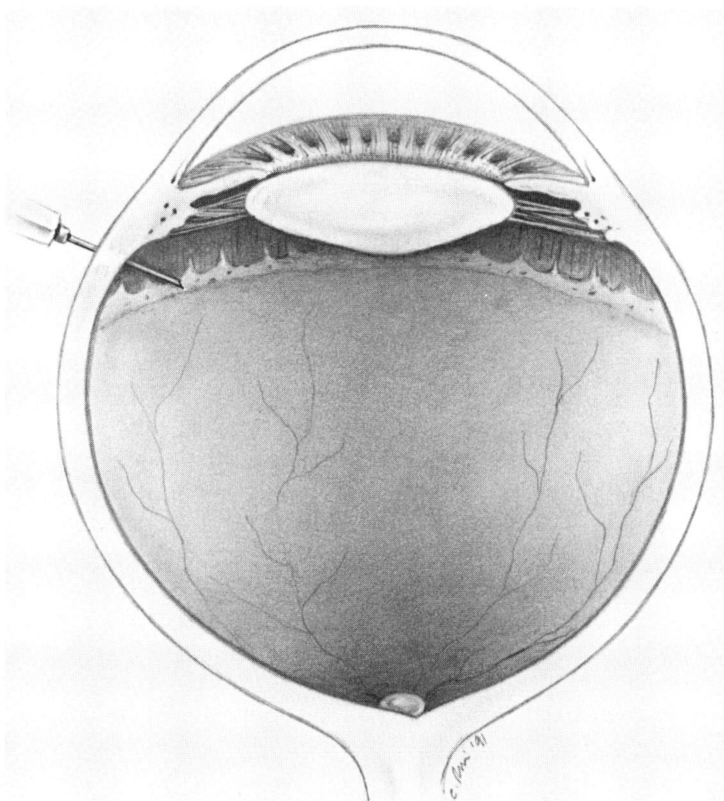

Figure 3 Schematic representation of ocular anatomy illustrating injection site through the pars plana. Injections are most conveniently made in the infero- and supcrotemporal quadrants of the eye, roughly 3.5 to 4.0 mm from the corneoscleral limbus.

The optimal treatment regimen for administration of intravitreal ganciclovir is not known. Initial clinical reports suggest that an initial induction period of twice-weekly injections for 2 to 3 weeks followed by weekly injections is effective in most cases (7-9).

V. COMPLICATIONS OF INTRAVITREAL THERAPY

In general, intraocular injections, when carefully performed, can be given repeatedly over extended periods of time without seriously compromising the eye. Reported complications of intravitreal ganciclovir therapy have been few. The most serious among them are bacterial endophthalmitis and retinal detachment. For practical considerations, most patients treated with intravitreal injections will be treated in an outpatient clinical facility, where the risk of contamination is great. Sterilization of the conjunctiva, irrigation of the injection site, careful injection technique, and preparation of injection solutions by the pharmacy will all reduce—but not eliminate—the risk of infection associated with the procedure. Timely recognition of endophthalmitis, should it develop, is critical. Prompt initiation of antibiotic therapy and vitrectomy can, in most cases, treat the infection, even in immunocompromised patients.

Eyes with CMV retinitis, both active and inactive, are particularly vulnerable to developing retinal detachments, especially if they have received antiviral therapy (13). CMV causes full-thickness retinal necrosis, and retinal break formation, which can lead to retinal detachment, is very common. While injection through the pars plana will not cause retinal detachment directly, several factors associated with the injection procedure may contribute to development of detachments. Despite the use of sharp, small-bore (30-gauge) needles, the globe is deformed and the pars plana and vitreous base violated during injections. Repeated injections may unfavorably alter the vitreous and cause vitreoretinal traction that may result in detachment, especially in eyes with large areas of necrotic and atrophic retina. Nevertheless, retinal detachment attributable to intravitreal injections in patients with CMV retinitis is rare.

VI. SUMMARY

The treatment of cytomegalovirus retinitis in patients with AIDS remains a major therapeutic challenge for ophthalmologists and internists despite the rapid development of antiviral therapies. The nature of the disease, an inexorably progressive process leading to profound visual impairment, coupled with the difficulties of administering highly toxic medications have conspired to make treatment difficult. Intravitreal treatment of CMV retinitis may have a place in the management of disorder, although indications for this method of treatment remain to be clarified. For patients intolerant of systemic therapy with ganciclovir or foscarnet, or combination therapies such as ganciclovir and GM-CSF, intravitreal therapy may be the only treatment available to patients with sight-threatening disease. The role of intravitreal therapy is, however, limited by several factors. These include the fact that CMV retinitis is a manifestation of systemic disease and, if they are not treated systemically, patients are at risk for developing retinitis in the other eye or other organ infection such as colitis and pneumonitis. It remains to be determined if intravitreal therapy is safe. While initial studies indicate that intravitreal therapy is a safe and effective salvage therapy for CMV retinitis, complications, while unusual, may be severe and vision-threatening. Finally, although intravitreal therapy is technically simple, it can psychologically and physically trying for patients to undergo an indefinite series of injections. However, when systemic treatment options are no longer available to the patient, intravitreal therapy may be the only alternative to progressive visual loss leading to blindness.

REFERENCES

1. Jabs DA, Enger C, Bartlett JG. Cytomegalovirus retinitis and acquired immunodeficiency syndrome. Arch Ophthalmol 1989; 107:75-80.
2. Holland GN, Sidikaro Y, Krieger AE, Hardy D, Sakamoto MJ, Frenkel LM, Winston DJ, Gottlieb MS, Bryon YJ, Champlin RE. Treatment of cytomegalovirus retinopathy with ganciclovir. Ophthalmology 1987; 94:815-823.
3. Jabs DA, Newman C, DeBustros S, Polk BF. Treatment of cytomegalovirus retinitis with ganciclovir. Ophthalmology 1987; 94:824-830.
4. Collaborative DHPG Study Group. Treatment of serious cytomegalovirus infections with 9-(1,3-dihydroxy-2-propoxymethyl) guanine in patients with AIDS and other immunodeficiencies. N Engl J Med 1986; 314:801-806.
5. Lehoang P, Girard B, Robinet M. Foscarnet in the treatment of cytomegalovirus retinitis in acquired immune deficiency syndrome. Ophthalmology 1989; 96:865-873.
6. Henry K, Cantrill H, Fletcher C, Chinnock BJ, Balfour HH. Use of intravitreal ganciclovir (dihydroxy propoxymethyl guanine) for cytomegalovirus retinitis in a patient with AIDS. Am J Ophthalmol 1987; 103:17-23.
7. Ussery FM, Gibson SR, Conklin RH, Piot DF, Stool EW, Conklin AJ. Intravitreal ganciclovir in the treatment of AIDS-associated cytomegalovirus retinopathy. Ophthalmology 1988; 95:640-647.
8. Cantrill HL, Henry K, Melroe NH, Knobloch WH, Ramsay RC, Balfour HH. Treatment of cytomegalovirus retinitis with intravitreal ganciclovir. Ophthalmology 1989; 96:376-374.
9. Heinemann MH. Long-term intravitreal ganciclovir therapy for cytomegalovirus retinopathy. Arch Ophthalmol 1989; 107:1767-1772.
10. Pulido J, Peyman GA, Lesar T, Vernot J. Intravitreal toxicity of hydroacyclovir (BW-B759U): a new antiviral agent. Arch Ophthalmol 1985; 104:840-841.
11. Syntex Institute of Clinical Medicine Study Manual #1257. Syntex Research, Palo Alto, California, 1986.
12. Freeman WR. Intraocular antiviral therapy. Arch Ophthalmol 1989; 107:1737-1739.
13. Pepose JS, Newman C, Bach MC, Quion TC, Ambinder RF, Holland GN, Hodstrom PS, Frey HM, Foos RY. Pathologic features of cytomegalovirus after treatment with the antiviral agent ganciclovir. Ophthalmology 1987; 94:414-424.

8

Monitoring AIDS-Related Cytomegalovirus Retinitis

Paul R. Montague and Thomas A. Weingeist
University of Iowa
Iowa City, Iowa

I. INTRODUCTION

Indirect ophthalmoscopy is the easiest way of screening, diagnosing, and following the clinical course of cytomegalovirus (CMV) retinitis related to the acquired immunodeficiency syndrome (AIDS). In fact, there is no more readily available way of visualizing the peripheral retina and thereby detecting the early signs of this vision-threatening infection before it becomes symptomatic. Unfortunately, the technique is not suitable for determining the efficacy of drug therapy because there is no objective way of documenting the findings of the examiner. Fundus photography provides the most accurate and the only objective means of monitoring retinitis suitable for evaluating drug therapy, but fundus photography also has its shortcomings. With fundus photography it is not possible to easily document changes between the equator of the globe and the ora serrata, where the peripheral retina ends. Optimal results are also dependent on effective pupillary dilation, clear ocular media, cooperation from the patient, and a skilled ophthalmic photographer. Ideally, clinical trials attempting to establish the efficacy of drug therapy for AIDS-related CMV retinitis should include both fundus photography and indirect ophthalmoscopy.

To date there have been no publications of a clinical trial in which serial fundus photography was properly utilized to document either the natural history of CMV retinitis or the efficacy of drug therapy in individuals with AIDS. To ensure appropriate documentation of the posterior ocular fundus during the course of drug studies, we have designed a photographic protocol that would enable masked readers to objectively grade photographs. This chapter is intended to serve as a guide for future investigators interested in studying the effects of pharmaceutical agents on the retina.

II. OPHTHALMOSCOPIC APPEARANCE OF AIDS-RELATED CMV RETINITIS

The opthalmoscopic appearance of a white necrotizing retinitis with an advancing edge is distinctive of CMV retinitis, especially when observed in an

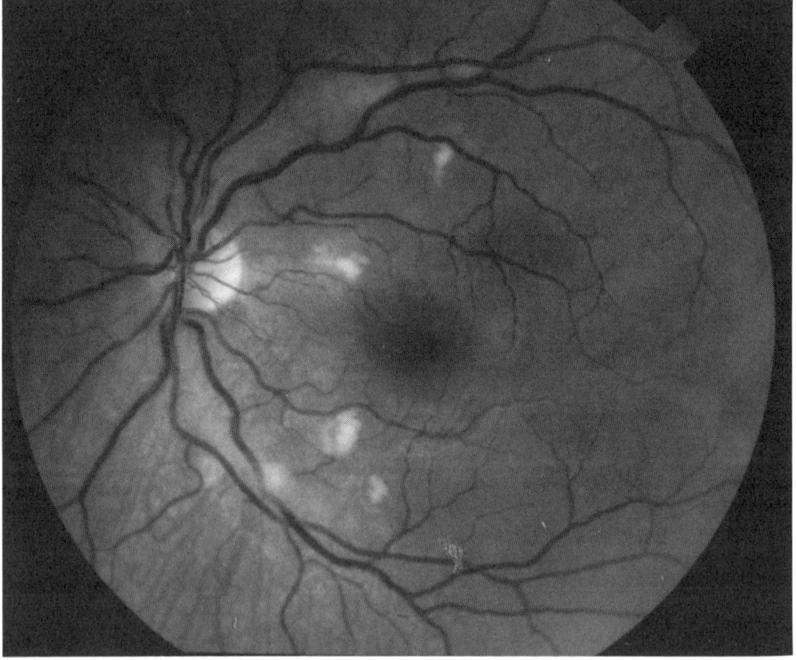

(a)

Figure 1 (a) The early onset of CMV retinitis characterized by a small white retinal lesion may be difficult to distinguish from a cotton-wool spot associated with HIV retinitis. (b, c) Serial fundus photography conclusively demonstrates that some of the earlier lesions were due to CMV retinitis while others were cotton-wool spots.

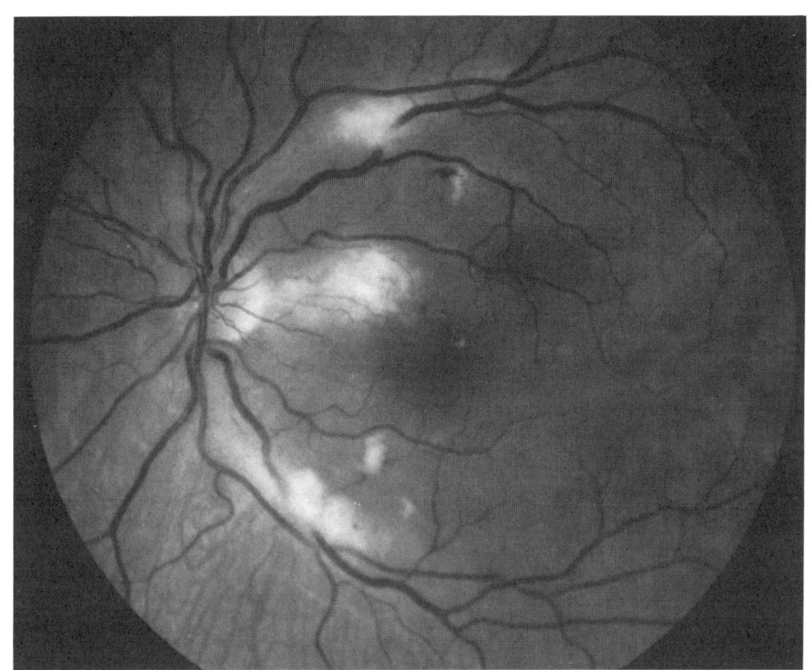

(b)

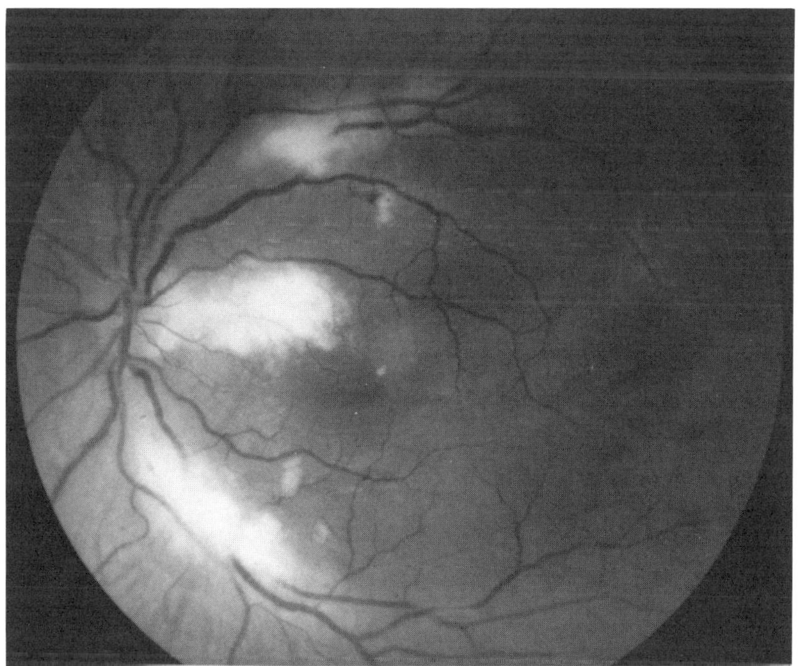

(c)

immunocompromised individual. Initially, retinal lesions may appear as either scattered white dots or white granular patches without any characteristic regional predilection. The early clinical lesions may be difficult to distinguish from cotton-wool spots (Figure 1). As the disease evolves, vascular sheathing, retinal exudates, and retinal hemorrhages commonly occur. If untreated, CMV infection results in full-thickness necrosis of the retina. The destruction of the retina is usually so extensive and the immune system so compromised that the underlying pigment epithelium is unable to produce the characteristic pigmentary changes seen with healing *Toxoplasma gondii* lesions and other infectious diseases occurring in individuals with a normal immune response. Other ocular manifestations of CMV infection include swelling of the optic disc and rhegmatogenous retinal detachment.

Three forms of CMV retinitis have been described in patients with AIDS. The "fulminant" form is characterized by dense retinal whitening, retinal

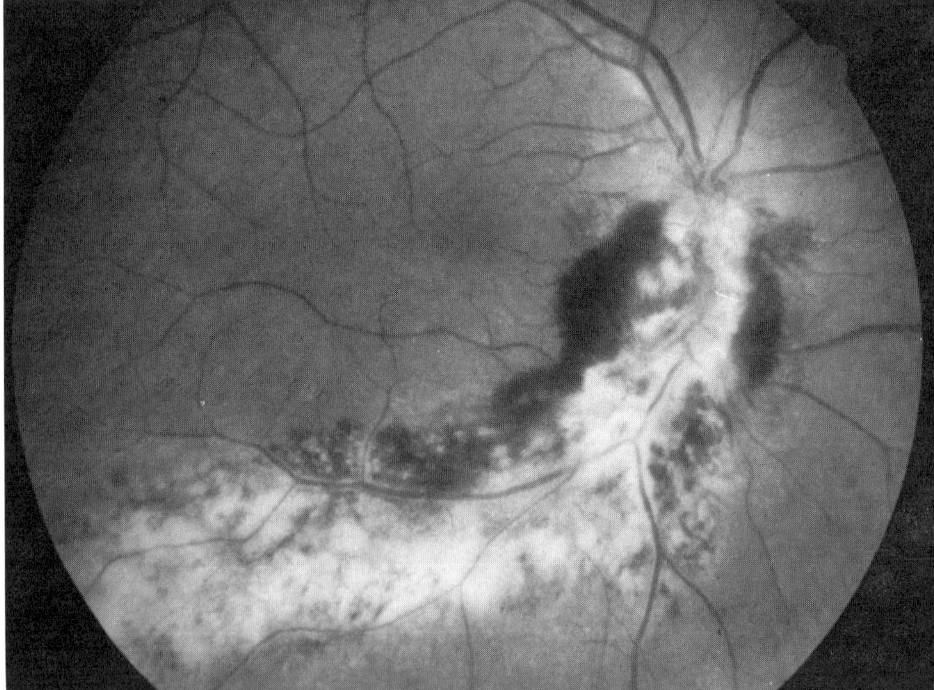

Figure 2 Fulminant form of CMV retinitis. The ophthalmoscopic appearance of these white necrotic retinal lesions with hemorrhage has been described as resembling pizza or scrambled eggs with catsup.

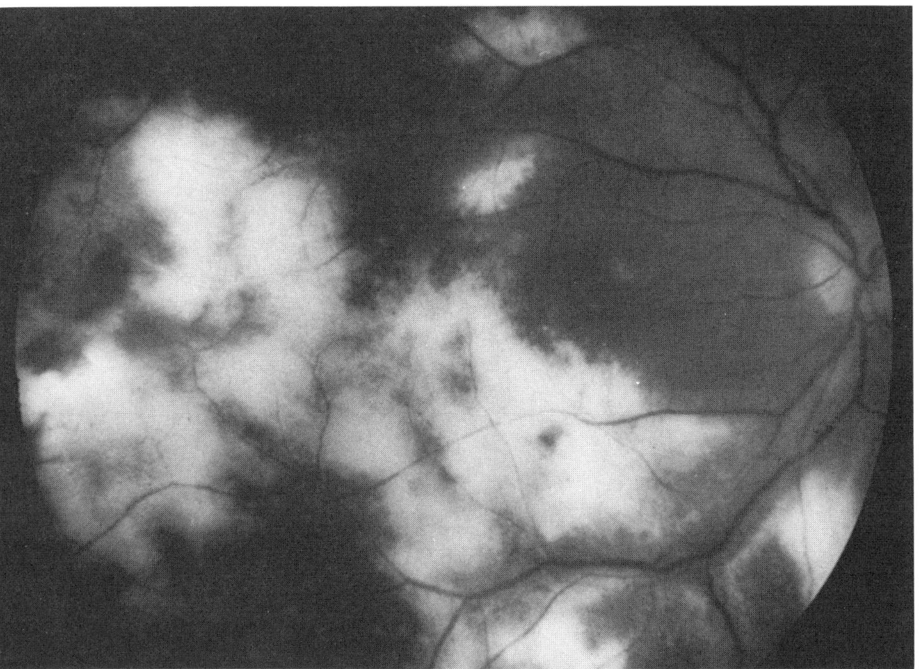

Figure 3 Granular form of CMV retinitis. Ophthalmoscopically these lesions appear drier and are less often associated with retinal hemorrhage.

hemorrhages, and inflammatory vascular sheathing. Lesions are usually found adjacent to major retinal vessels (Figure 2). The "granular" form is usually not associated with hemorrhage or vasculitis. Lesions frequently have a central area of retinal atrophy and gliotic scarring, possibly indicating that the lesions are relatively longstanding with slow centrifugal spread (1-6) (Figure 3). A third and relatively uncommon form may occur in association with "frosted-branch angiitis," so named because of its distinctive appearance (7) (Figure 4). The factors leading to these different forms are unknown. Granular lesions may be more common in the peripheral retina.

III. "HEALED" CMV RETINITIS

If medical intervention results in resolution of the CMV infection, the chalky white lesions appear to break up and the necrotic retina becomes translucent. As the process continues, the remaining retinal elements become transparent. The underlying retinal pigment epithelium and choroid develop a brown, fine

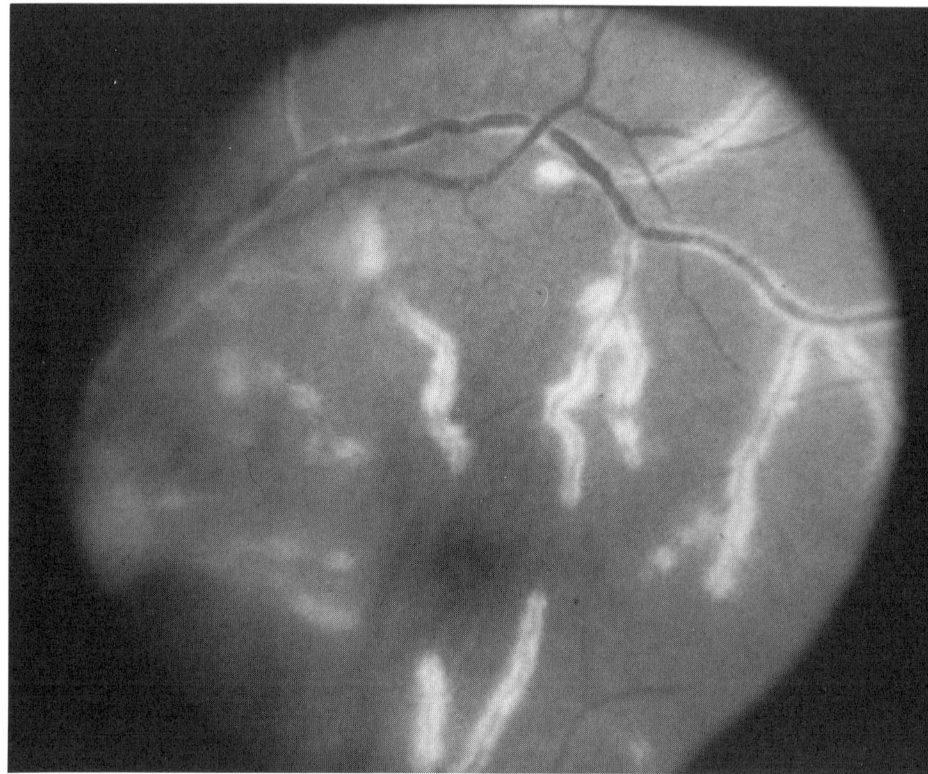

Figure 4 Frosted retinal periphlebitis may occur as an uncommon manifestation of AIDS-related CMV retinitis. This distinctive ophthalmoscopic picture may also arise from other viral infections that are not associated with AIDS. (Courtesy of Warren M. Sobol, M.D.)

granular appearance, and the choroidal vessels become increasingly prominent due to baring of the sclera and the generalized loss of pigmentation from the retinal pigment epithelium and choroid. At this stage the CMV retinitis is said to have healed or undergone regression (8) (Figure 5).

IV. REACTIVATION OF CMV RETINITIS

In patients with AIDS-related CMV retinitis, withdrawal of antiviral therapy usually results in reactivation of CMV retinitis. These recurrences, or "breakthroughs," are characterized by advancement of the borders of lesions

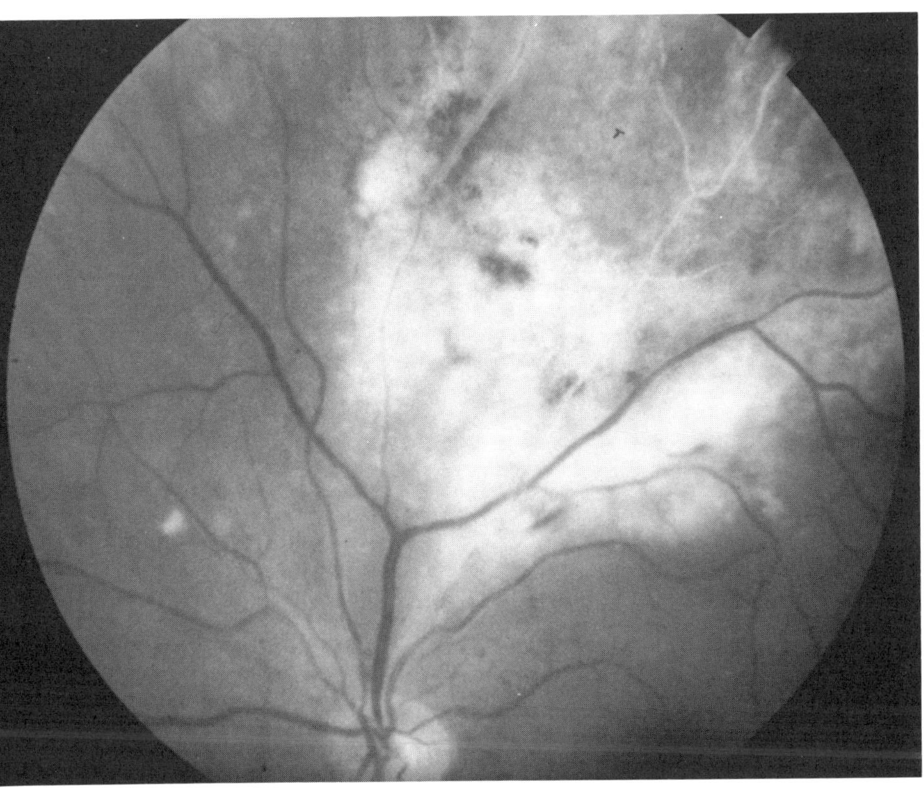

(a)

Figure 5 (a) Baseline photograph of CMV retinitis demonstrating retinal opacification and hemorrhage. (b) Follow-up photograph approximately 3 months after ganciclovir therapy. Note the reduction in retinal opacification, the granular pigmentary changes, and the baring of the underlying choroidal vessels characteristic of "healed" CMV retinitis.

and the development of new isolated areas of retinal involvement. The creeping advancement of lesions resembles the spreading of a brushfire (Figure 6). Failure of the margins of lesions to expand appears to be the most sensitive indication that CMV retinitis is responding to therapy. It should be remembered that new lesions can develop only within viable retina. Recurrences most often arise along the "healed" margins of lesions rather than within the center of lesions that have been devastated by the virus.

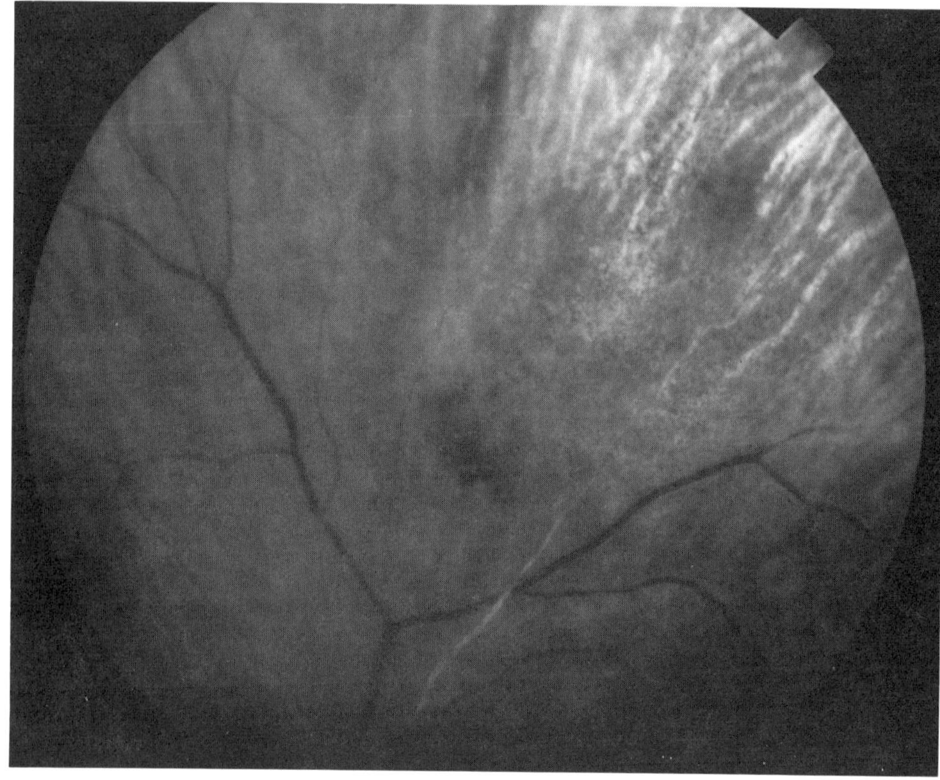

(b)   Figure 5 *continued*

V. INDIRECT OPHTHALMOSCOPY

Indirect ophthalmoscopy should be performed routinely to diagnose and monitor cytomegalovirus retinitis and other HIV-related retinal diseases. Subretinal, intraretinal, and preretinal hemorrhages; cotton-wool spots; retinal edema; retinal atrophy; intraretinal whitening; and perivascular sheathing are among the most common findings in CMV retinitis. In these patients, the ocular media usually remain relatively clear and free of inflammatory cells, compared with individuals who are able to mount a normal inflammatory reaction. Evaluation of the peripheral retina is essential because CMV retinitis often occurs anterior to the equator, beyond the limits of direct ophthalmoscopy and before patients develop visual symptoms.

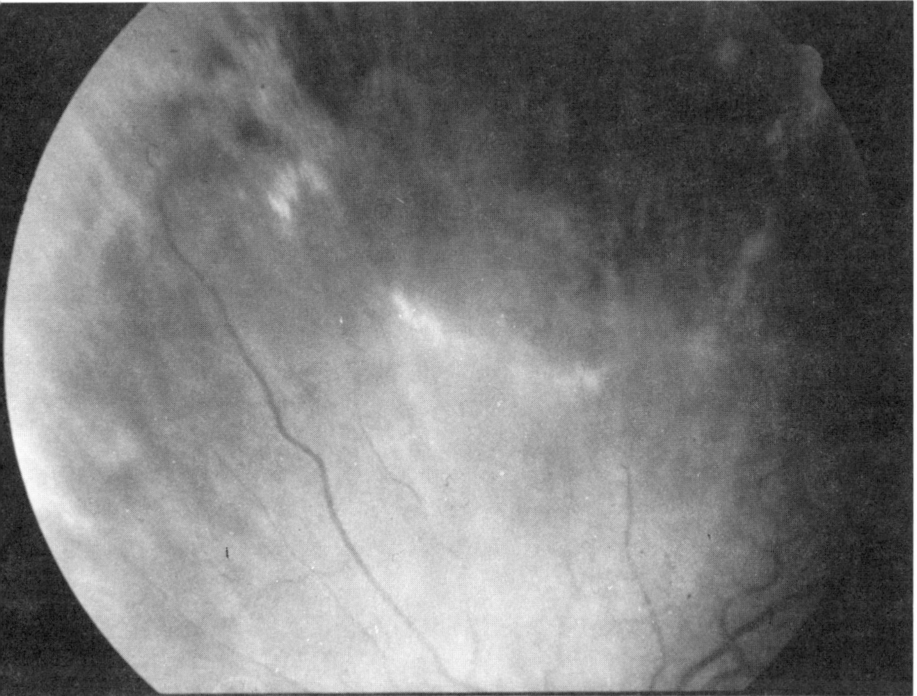

Figure 6   Recurrences of CMV retinitis are characterized by the development of new lesions or an advancing border from a "healed" lesion, which resembles the spreading of a brushfire.

Due to the extensive retinal involvement that commonly occurs, and the relatively small changes that might constitute progression of retinal disease, indirect ophthalmoscopy is not an adequate means of monitoring AIDS-related retinitis when evaluating drug therapy.

VI. OCULAR FUNDUS PHOTOGRAPHY

Fundus photography, when performed according to a repeatable protocol, provides accurate documentation of most of the posterior retina that can be used to determine remission or progression of ocular infection while providing a permanent record for unbiased analysis.

Fundus cameras may be classified into three categories, according to the area of the retina that can be documented in a single photograph. Normal-angle cameras photograph between 30 and 40 degrees of the ocular fundus, which is almost exactly the area delineated by the major vascular arcades or macula. Wide-angle cameras photograph between 45 and 60 degrees of the fundus. Ultrawide-angle cameras cover areas greater than 60 degrees.

As the angle of view of a fundus camera increases, the magnification of the image on the film decreases, and the size of the pupil required for photography increases. The wide-angle (45-60-degree) cameras provide the optimal compromise. Using nine 60-degree fields (Figure 7), the majority of the posterior retina can be documented. Similar coverage with a 30-degree camera would require over 30 photographs, making the photographic session intolerable for the patient and identification of peripheral fields during the evaluation process extremely difficult, if not impossible.

Generally, a 4.5-mm pupil is required for wide-angle photography of the posterior pole. Wider dilation is necessary for photography of the periphery.

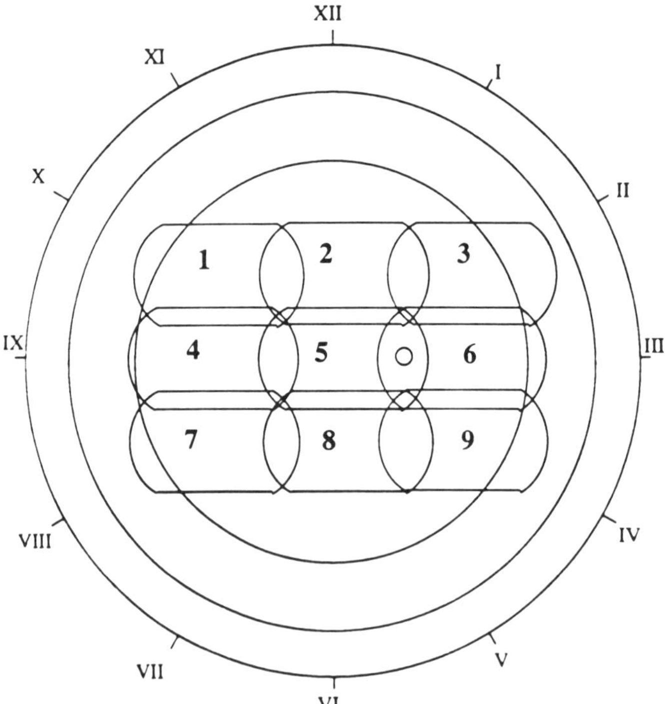

Figure 7 Schematic diagram of nine standard photographic fields of the posterior ocular fundus attainable with a 60-degree camera.

Peripheral fundus photographs taken through inadequately dilated pupils have a blue-black shadow at the edge. If increased dilation cannot be obtained, manipulation of the fundus camera to shift the shadow and using two or more photographs for the same field may provide an adequate view. The already difficult task of photographing the peripheral retina is further complicated by the inability of debilitated patients to tolerate lengthy sessions at the fundus camera.

VII. FLUORESCEIN ANGIOGRAPHY

At the present time, fluorescein angiography fails to provide any additional insight into the efficacy of drug therapy. In addition, it places an unnecessary burden on patients and increased hazard on medical personnel. Fluorescein angiography is occasionally of value when studying unusual ophthalmoscopic observations or documenting previously unpublished findings that present a diagnostic challenge (*Pneumocystis carinii* choroiditis) (9).

VIII. PHOTOGRAPHIC EVALUATION OF AIDS-RELATED CMV RETINITIS

Subtle changes in the ophthalmoscopic appearance of CMV retinitis are often difficult to detect except by carefully documented serial fundus photography. As new areas of retina become involved, the retina becomes less transparent. Progressive involvement by CMV infection leads to full-thickness retinal necrosis and opacification.

The complexity of evaluating changes in the ocular fundus is compounded by the fact that multiple lesions must be assessed and hemorrhages often obscure the retina.

Evaluation of patients with AIDS-related retinitis is facilitated by dividing the ocular fundus into three zones (8) (Figure 8). Zone 1 includes the macula, optic disc, and peripapillary area. The macula is located within the temporal vascular arcades, an area within 3000 μm, or two disc diameters, of the center of the fovea. The peripapillary area is arbitrarily defined. It extends 1500 μm, or one disc diameter, from the optic disc margin. CMV retinal involvement of zone 1 is immediately threatening to central vision and therefore requires urgent treatment. Zone 2 is located between the equator of the globe and the border of zone 1. Zone 3 is the part of the fundus anterior to the equator. Involvement of zones 2 and 3 do not affect visual acuity immediately. However, without treatment, CMV retinitis progresses relentlessly and eventually leads to blindness either from damage to the macula and optic disc within zone 1 or from retinal tears in zones 2 and 3 that result in retinal detachment.

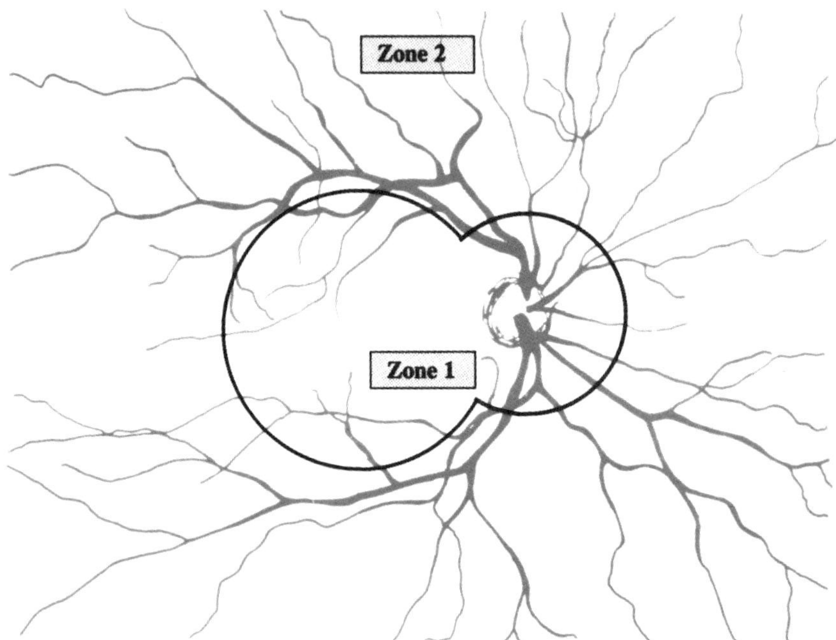

Figure 8   The ocular fundus divided into three zones. Zone 1: macula, optic disc, and peripapillary area. Zone 2: between anterior border of zone 1 and equator. Zone 3 (not shown): equator to ora serrata, the anteriormost border of the retina.

IX. PHOTOGRAPHIC PROCEDURE

Mapping of zones 1 and 2 can be accomplished with sufficient detail for evaluation of AIDS-related retinitis with nine 60-degree photographic fields. The central field is centered on the papillomacular bundle, midway between the fovea and optic disc, encompassing all of zone 1. The other eight fields surround the central field, overlapping their neighbors by about 25% of the picture area (Figure 7).

In order to facilitate wide-angle photography of the periphery, the pupil should be dilated to at least 4.5 mm with topical sympathomimetic and parasympatholytic agents such as Cyclogyl and Neo-Synephrine. Some wide-angle fundus cameras may require wider dilation, depending on their optical design. Adequate dilation has been achieved when shadow-free photographs of all nine fields can be obtained.

X. PHOTOGRAPHIC FINDINGS AND GRADING SCHEME

Side-by-side comparisons of current visit to baseline for each photographic field will reveal changes in the size, location, and intensity of each lesion.

The presence of new lesions or the expansion of the borders of old lesions (greater than a certain number of microns) constitutes *failure* of therapy. *Stabilization* occurs if there are no new lesions and no changes have occurred in old lesions. *Improvement* occurs if there is reduction in intensity of retinal whitening, there are no new lesions, and the borders of *all* lesions have not advanced (8).

Many factors must be taken into consideration in establishing a grading system. Among the most important are how to deal with hemorrhage, which may obscure boundaries of lesions, and determining the minimal lesion size that will constitute CMV retinitis.

Overlying hemorrhage that obscures the boundaries of CMV lesions presents a grading problem. Since the exact border across the hemorrhage is unknown, areas of hemorrhage on either the baseline or the follow-up visit should be ignored during analysis of the margins of CMV retinitis.

The parameters used to grade "improvement," "stabilization," and "progression" or "failure" are arbitrary. Progression of 1500 μm or more may be tolerable in zones 2 and 3, but would be unacceptable within zone 1.

In order to avoid difficulty in distinguishing between cotton-wool spots and small CMV lesions, it is essential to define the exact minimum size a small white retinal lesion must be before designating it. CMV white retinal lesions usually must be 500 μm in length or greater, or one-quarter disc area in size, before they can be reliably distinguished from cotton-wool spots (Figure 1).

XI. CONCLUSION

Monitoring AIDS-related CMV retinitis can best be achieved by using a combination of indirect ophthalmoscopy and wide-angle fundus photography. Careful photographic documentation of the posterior ocular fundus permits objective evaluation by masked graders of the efficacy of drug therapy. In the future, drug studies are likely to be facilitated by computer-assisted analysis of fundus photographs.

ACKNOWLEDGMENT

This work was supported in part by an unrestricted grant from Research to Prevent Blindness, New York.

REFERENCES

1. Holland GN, Pepose JS, Pettit TH, Gottlieb MS, Yee RD, Foos RY. Acquired immune deficiency syndrome: ocular manifestations. Ophthalmology 1983; 90: 859-873.

2. Freeman WR, Lerner CW, Mines JA, Lash RS, Nadel AJ, Starr MB, Tapper ML. A prospective study of ophthalmologic findings in the acquired immune deficiency syndrome. Am J Ophthalmol 1984; 97:133-142.
3. Friedman AH. The retinal lesions of the acquired immune deficiency syndrome. Trans Am Ophthalmol Soc 1984; 82:447-491.
4. Palestine AG, Rodrigues MM, Macher AM, Chan C-C, Lane HC, Fauci AS, Masur H, Longo D, Reichert CM, Steis R, Rook AH, Nussenblatt RB. Ophthalmic involvement in acquired immunodeficiency syndrome. Ophthalmology 1984; 91:1092-1099.
5. Pepose JS, Holland GN, Nestor MS, Cochran AJ, Foos RY. Acquired immune deficiency syndrome: pathogenic mechanisms of ocular disease. Ophthalmology 1985; 92:472-484.
6. Jabs DA, Enger C, Bartlett JG. Cytomegalovirus retinitis and acquired immunodeficiency syndrome. Arch Ophthalmol 1989; 107:75-80.
7. Kleiner RC, Kaplan HJ, Shakin JL, Yannuzzi LA, Crosswell HH, McLean WC. Acute frosted retinal periphlebitis. Am J Ophthalmol 1988; 106:27-34.
8. Holland GN, Buhles WC, Mastre B, Kaplan HJ. Controlled retrospective study of ganciclovir treatment for cytomegalovirus retinopathy. Am J Ophthalmol 1989; 107:1759-1766.
9. Sneed SR, Blodi CF, Berger BB, Speights JW, Folk JC, Weingeist TA. *Pneumocystis carinii* choroiditis in patients receiving inhaled pentamadine (letter). N Engl J Med 1990; 322:936-937.

9

Ganciclovir Treatment of Cytomegalovirus Gastrointestinal Disease in Patients with AIDS

Douglas T. Dieterich
New York University School of Medicine
New York, New York

I. INTRODUCTION

Cytomegalovirus (CMV) infection of the gastrointestinal tract has been described in the literature at least since 1925 (1). Since the development of the use of immunosuppressive drugs in organ transplants and the occurrence of human immunodeficiency virus (HIV) infection, it has taken on a much greater significance. CMV has also been found in the gastrointestinal tract of geriatric patients and in patients with inflammatory bowel disease (2-4). Diagnosing CMV in the gastrointestinal tract now is even more important because there is effective therapy available to treat it.

In 1981, when the HIV epidemic was just beginning, I saw my first patient with CMV colitis: a 35-year-old homosexual man who was admitted to Bellevue Hospital in New York City with diarrhea, dehydration, and cachexia. All stool tests were negative several times, and after replacement of fluids and electrolytes he was referred to the gastroenterology department. He was suspected of having what was called at the time "gay-related immunodeficiency," or GRID. A colonoscopy revealed a patchy colitis and a very large cavernous rectosigmoid ulcer. The pathology department reported that the biopsies indicated "intracytoplasmic amebiasis," the theory being that the immune defect was allowing the ameba to become intracytoplasmic. Intravenous metronidazole had no effect, and two more biopsies had the same result. The patient died, and the autopsy revealed intracytoplasmic inclusion bodies in the brain, retina, lung, liver, colon, and, of course, the rectum. These were diagnostic of cytomegalovirus infection throughout the body. The pathologists now know what inclusion bodies look like but in 1981 CMV disease of the rectum was so uncommon that many pathologists failed to consider the diagnosis.

This case points out several important points in the care of HIV-infected patients. We were correctly biopsying the sites of suspected lesions. However, we did not immediately recognize the pathogen that was present all along. CMV is now found in up to 90% of autopsies of HIV-infected patients (5,6). It is a major cause of illness among transplant recipients and with acquired immunodeficiency syndrome (AIDS) patients and has a significant effect on survival in both groups. This chapter discusses the diagnosis and therapy of CMV infection of the GI tract in AIDS patients.

II. NATURAL HISTORY AND SCOPE OF CMV GASTROINTESTINAL DISEASE

A. Incidence of Gastrointestinal Disease in AIDS Patients

Very little has been written about the overall incidence of CMV in the gastrointestinal tract of AIDS patients. However, it is clear that AIDS patients suffer from an enormous amount of gastrointestinal disease. Anthony et al. (7), in a study of 100 patients with AIDS, prospectively found that 80% of the homosexual men and 58% of the intravenous drug users suffered from diarrhea. Lane et al. (8) reported that 60% of 85 AIDS patients suffered gastrointestinal symptoms. Heise et al. (9) found 98 of 200 HIV-infected patients suffering gastrointestinal symptoms. In France, Girard et al. (10) found that 62% of a group of AIDS patients reported diarrhea. There is little doubt that symptoms in both the upper and lower gastrointestinal tracts afflict AIDS patients in high numbers, approximating 60 to 80%.

In four autopsy studies of AIDS patients published in the 1980s (5,11-13), the gastrointestinal tract was involved 88, 58, 60 and 50% of the time, respectively. The metaanalysis of these data yields a cumulative number of 46 of 74, or 62%. The overall incidence of CMV from any site on autopsy in those four studies was 74 of 91, or 81%.

How much of this gastrointestinal disease is caused by CMV is a difficult question. Through 1987 there were 22 reported cases of CMV gastrointestinal involvement in the literature (14-20). Since then it has become clear that CMV is a significant pathogen (21), and several articles have appeared about treatment (22,23). The literature about incidence is still confusing, but I will summarize it briefly (see also Table 1). Francis et al. (24) studied 190 consecutive endoscopic biopsies from AIDS patients. Eighteen of 190 (8.9%) had CMV. Ten of 129 (7.7%) of HIV-positive patients compared with eight of 61 (13%) of the patients with AIDS had CMV on biopsy, which is consistent with the fact that CMV is usually a late disease in HIV infection, usually presenting in patients with fewer than 100 cells. Rene et al. (25) in an autopsy study in 1988 found gastrointestinal CMV in seven of 24 (29%). Cosnes et al. (26) found two of 45 (4.4%), Stamm and Grant (27) two of 28 (7%), Heise et al. (9) 28 of 98 (29%), Boylston et al. (28) 21 of 279 (7.5%), Masur et al. (29) one of eight (12.5%), Buhles et al. (30) 42 of 314 (13.3%), the DHPG Collaborative Study Group (31) eight of 26 (31%), and Dieterich et al. (32) 101 of 193 (52%). Metaanalysis of these data reveals that 188 of 1205, or 15.6% of patients with gastrointestinal symptoms have CMV infection of the gastrointestinal tract. In a 1988 study, Smith et al. (33) looked closely at 20 patients with AIDS and diarrhea. One or more etiologies was found in 17 (85%). CMV was found in nine (45%).

Two series, as yet unpublished, that have somewhat larger numbers of patients may shed some light on incidence. Through October 1988, Syntex had data on 5678 cases of CMV infection for which ganciclovir was dispensed (Table 2). The non-AIDS cases were primarily transplant patients: 222 (3.9%)

Table 1 Incidence in AIDS Patients of Gastrointestinal Disease Caused by CMV

Author (Ref.)	No. of patients	GI disease	Percentage
Francis et al. (24)	190	18	8.9
Rene et al. (25)	24	7	29.8
Cosnes et al. (26)	45	2	4.4
Stamm and Grant (27)	28	2	7.0
Heise et al. (9)	98	28	29.0
Boylston et al. (28)	279	21	7.5
Masur et al. (29)	8	1	12.5
Buhles et al. (30)	314	42	13.3
DHPG Collab Grp. (31)	26	8	31.0
Dieterich et al. (32)	193	101	52.0
Subtotal	1205	188	15.6
Syntex (unpub.)	5678	804	14.1
Dieterich (unpub.)	683	128	19.0
Total	7566	1068	14.0

Table 2 Breakdown of Gastrointestinal Disease in 5678
CMV-Infected Patients (Syntex Database 1985-1988)

	No. of patients	Percentage
Non-AIDS		
Upper GI	222	3.9
Lower GI	99	1.7
Liver	274	4.8
Subtotal	595	10.4
AIDS		
Upper GI	376	6.6
Lower GI	395	6.9
Liver	33	0.6
Subtotal	804	14.1
Total gastrointestinal CMV	1399	24.6
Total CMV	5678	100%

had upper GI disease, 99 (1.7%) had lower GI disease, and 274 (4.8%) had
CMV hepatitis. The overall incidence of gastrointestinal CMV in this group
was 10.4%. In contrast, the AIDS patients had a much higher incidence of
upper and lower GI disease: 376 (6.6%) and 395 (6.9%), respectively. AIDS
patients had a much lower incidence of CMV hepatitis 33 (0.6%) than did
the transplant patients. Overall, then, 14.1% of the CMV infections in AIDS
patients were gastrointestinal.

In an unpublished series at New York University, 683 endoscopies were
performed on AIDS patients from 1981 through 1988. Of those, 128 (19%)
had a positive biopsy for CMV. The available data therefore seem to suggest
an incidence of around 15% for gastrointestinal CMV, although I believe it
will be higher when more patients have more endoscopic biopsies.

B. Diagnosis of Gastrointestinal CMV

Metaanalysis of data is fraught with hazards, not the least of which is dif-
fering methodology and investigator bias. Finding CMV on gastrointestinal
biopsies is not easy. It requires assiduous biopsying of multiple sites even if
they appear endoscopically or radiologically normal. Not all groups do this,
and not all pathologists painstakingly look for CMV inclusions under the
microscope.

The investigators of the two series with the highest incidences of CMV, Heise et al. (9) and Dieterich et al. (32), are gastroenterologists who have an interest in the disease and search for it diligently. Our technique is to screen every patients several times for pathogens in the stool. If negative, colonoscopy and/or upper endoscopy is performed. Even in a normal colon, 10-12 biopsies are taken from right, transverse, and sigmoid colon, similar to the technique described for screening for dysplasia in ulcerative colitis. During the upper endoscopy, biopsies are taken from the distal duodenum/jejenum, antrum, and esophagus in a similar manner, endoscopic appearance notwithstanding. In a recent abstract, Rene et al. (34) statistically examined 229 AIDS patients for predictive factors for intestinal infection. They found that 102 of 229, or 44.5%, had infections. The two factors that most strongly correlated with gastrointestinal infection ($p < 0.001$) were diarrhea and extraintestinal CMV.

I firmly believe that endoscopic biopsy in AIDS patients with gastrointestinal symptoms will yield a high percentage of treatable CMV disease. In addition, if the first biopsy is negative and clinical suspicion is high, there are two options. The most logical one is to rebiopsy. The other is to treat empirically with ganciclovir. The second option must be weighed very carefully in view of the potential risks of ganciclovir therapy and the question of whether to use maintenance therapy. I would not recommend it unless at least two endoscopic biopsies are negative. The etiology of ulcers and other gastrointestinal lesions may be not CMV but primary HIV lesions of the esophagus or colon (35,36), or other diseases such as herpes or torulopsis globrata, and this must be kept in mind when deciding on therapy.

III. MANIFESTATIONS AND SITES OF DISEASE

Cytomegalovirus can and does infect the entire gastrointestinal tract from the mouth to the rectum, including the liver, biliary tree, and pancreas (37). Unlike transplant patients, who suffer more CMV hepatitis and upper gastrointestinal disease, AIDS patients seem to have more colitis. The distribution seems to be quite different in the two immunocompromised states.

A. Oropharynx

Oropharyngeal ulcers are not common manifestations of cytomegalovirus infection, but they do occur. Many of these ulcers do not have CMV in biopsies and may be idiopathic or caused by HSV or HIV. The ulcers caused by herpes simplex generally respond to acyclovir and if severe may require parenteral administration. Several investigators have used either local or systemic steroids (38) in CMV-negative oral ulcers with good success. The rare ulcer caused by CMV can be treated with ganciclovir, usually successfully.

B. Esophagus

Esophageal disease in HIV-infected patients is a controversial topic. There are only a few references about CMV or other causes of esophageal disease in AIDS patients. In general, most physicians who treat AIDS patients will treat odynophagia medically, at first with antifungal agents. By far the most common cause of odynophagia and dysphagia is *Candida esophagitis*. If it is present in the oropharynx, then treatment with ketoconazole, fluconazole, and/or clotrimazole troches is usually the first step. If there is no thrush or if the odynophagia persists, then upper endoscopy is the procedure of choice. Barium swallow, while reportedly diagnostic, is a poor substitute for an endoscopic biopsy. It is estimated that more than half of all esophageal disease seen by endoscopy in HIV patients would not be seen on x-ray (see Figures 1-4).

When an esophageal ulcer or severe esophagitis is found, what are the odds that it will be CMV? Only two studies shed any light on this matter at all. Connolly et al. (39) studied 154 patients, 10 (6.4%) of whom had esophageal ulcers. Four of these 10, or 40%, had CMV. Gould et al. (40) looked at 180 patients. Twenty had esophageal biopsies: 10 of the 20 (50%) had Candida and four (20%) had CMV. Grippon et al. (41) described a giant esophageal ulcer caused by CMV. In our series at New York University (32), 22 of 193 (11.4%) patients with AIDS and CMV infections treated with ganciclovir had upper gastrointestinal disease. The Syntex group indicated that 6.6% of their AIDS patients had upper gastrointestinal disease. Overall, it seems that about 20 to 40% of esophageal ulcers are definitely caused by CMV. If these biopsies are repeated, then the yield of CMV is increased considerably.

What is the etiology if CMV is not involved? Kotler et al. (36) have described HIV particles in situ studies of CMV-negative biopsies. Indeed Rabenek et al. (42) have described acute HIV infection presenting with painful esophageal ulcers. It stands to reason that if the acute infection can cause ulceration, then it can recur. These chronic ulcers may be treated with AZT, diet, and perhaps systemic or locally injected steroids (38). If they persist, they should be biopsied at least four separate times before CMV is ruled out, and in problematic cases empiric ganciclovir is not entirely out of line. A rare cause (I have seen only two in over 100 cases) of esophageal ulceration is herpes simplex. Biopsy of that lesion, which is usually more diffuse with multiple smaller ulcers, is diagnostic.

C. Stomach

CMV gastritis without esophageal disease is rarely reported. However, there is in the literature one case of an antral mass caused by CMV (43) and several

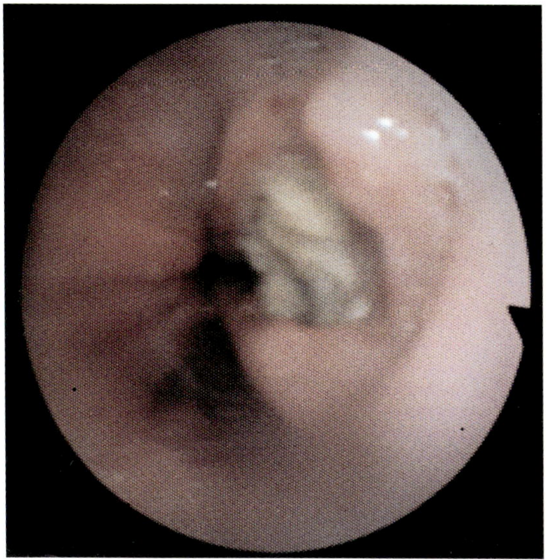

Figure 1   Cytomegalovirus esophageal ulcer.

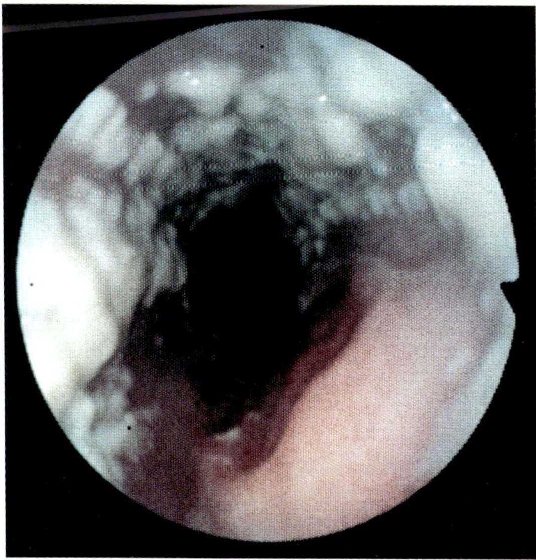

Figure 2   Cytomegalovirus esophageal ulcer opposite *Candida* esophagitis.

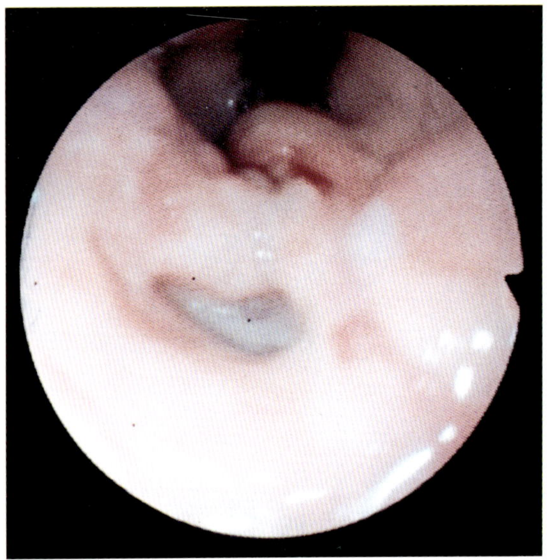

Figure 3 Cytomegalovirus esophageal ulcer in an esophageal lymphoma.

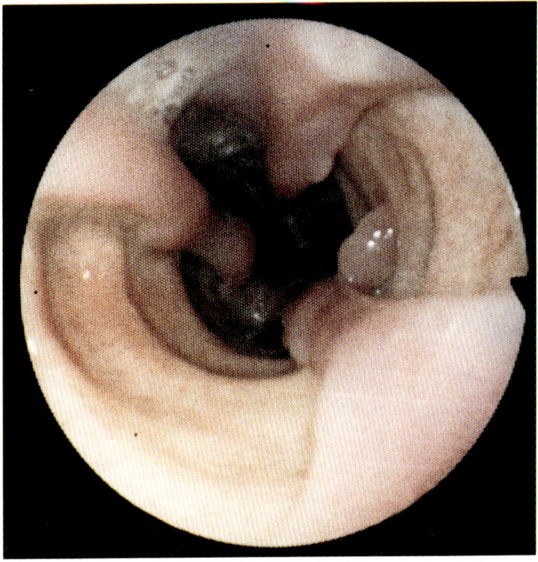

Figure 4 "Primary HIV" esophageal ulcer, no cytomegalovirus identified.

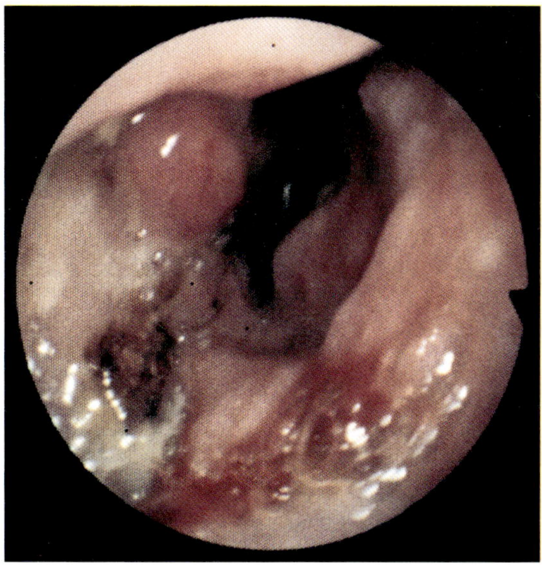

Figure 5 Duodenal lymphoma with cytomegalovirus on biopsy.

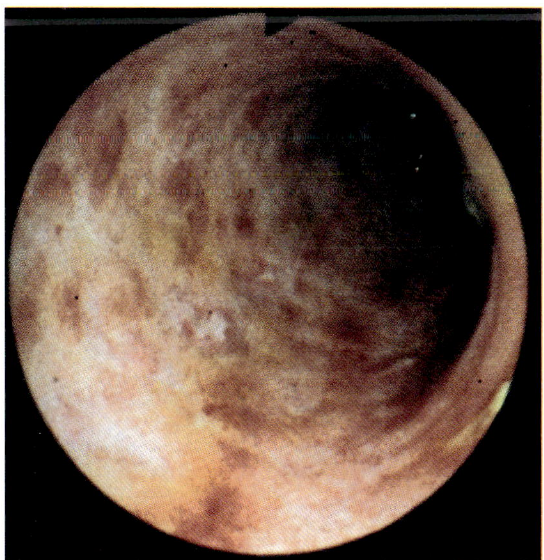

Figure 6 Cytomegalovirus colitis, patchy erythema.

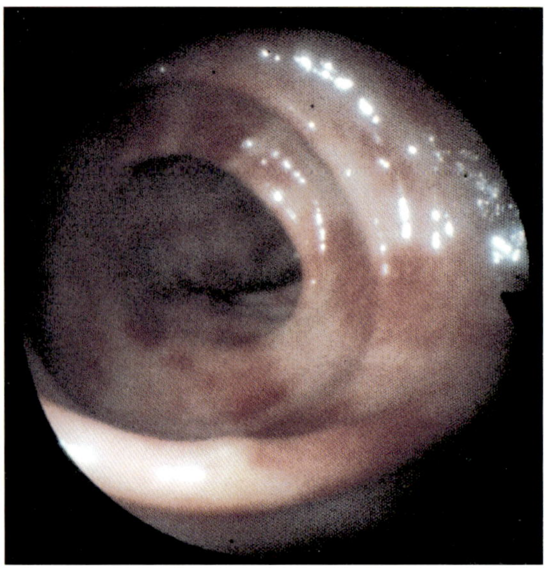

Figure 7 Cytomegalovirus colitis, patient R.F.

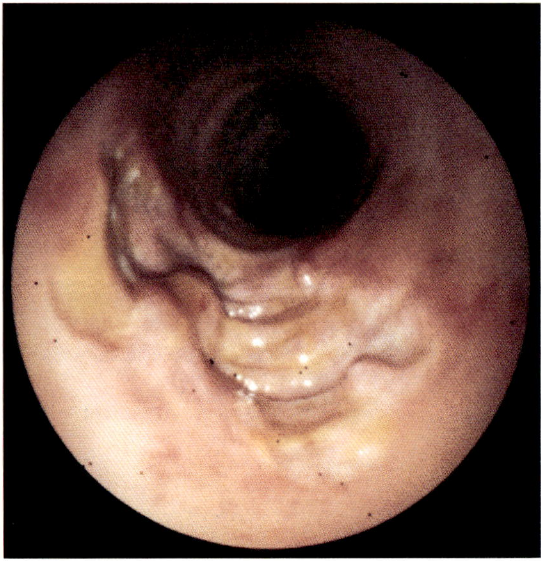

Figure 8 Deep cytomegalovirus ulcers in patient R.F. 18 months into therapy with ganciclovir.

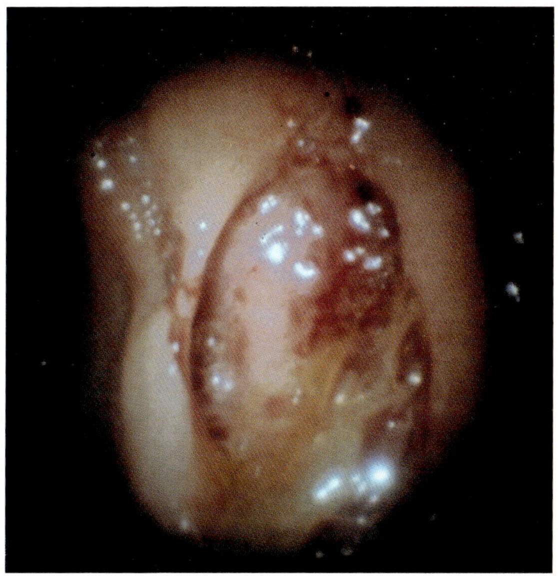

Figure 9 Large deep cecal ulcer caused by cytomegalovirus.

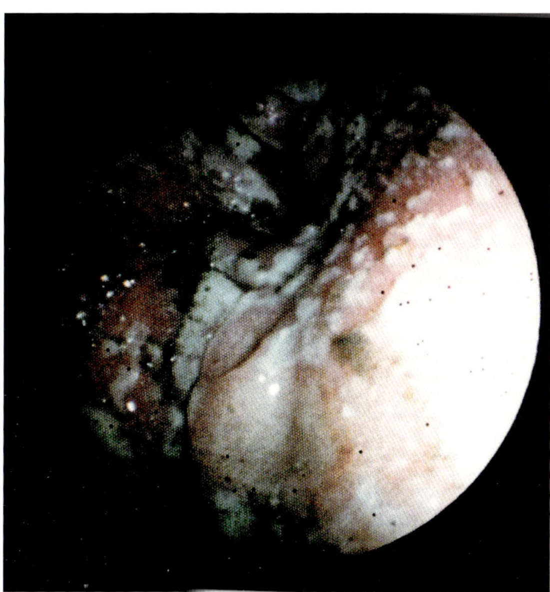

Figure 10 Cytomegalovirus rectal ulcer (center) surrounded by candidiasis.

of esophageal and gastric involvement (44-46). In my experience, a normal-appearing stomach will often yield CMV inclusion bodies on biopsy. Occasionally, Kaposi's sarcoma lesions in the stomach when biopsied will show CMV. In addition, I have seen three patients who underwent gallium scan for a fever of undetermined origin with significant uptake in the stomach. Upon biopsy, all three had CMV gastritis and fever, which resolved when treated with ganciclovir.

In summary, CMV does involve the stomach with both ulcers and gastritis, but less commonly than it does the esophagus. In the stomach and small bowel, CMV is also found with such neoplasms as lymphomas and Kaposi's sarcoma. This is especially important in light of therapy. Therefore, it is doubly vital to take multiple biopsies of any suspicious ulcer or lesion as well as of normal-appearing intervening areas.

D. Small Bowel

Cytomegalovirus is also a cause of enteritis in AIDS patients. This can present in three different ways. Diffuse enteritis caused by CMV usually produces fever, abdominal pain, and sometimes diarrhea. Malabsorption is variable in these patients, but the so-called wasting syndrome is common. This may be due less to actual small intestinal damage than to the hypermetabolic catabolic state produced by the actue infection. There is some evidence that this wasting can be reversed by treatment with ganciclovir (47). Biopsy from the distal duodenum or jejunum is usually positive. The second way is CMV infection along with small bowel lymphoma, which is much less common. This is an important combination because both diseases are treatable, but if one is missed the prognosis is much poorer. Finally, CMV infection of the ileum causcs ulcers and, not infrequently, perforation (48). CMV is responsible for more than 30% of surgery performed in AIDS patients (see Section IV). When an AIDS patient presents to the emergency room with free air under the diaphragm, a perforated ileal ulcer caused by CMV is the most likely diagnosis (see Figure 5).

Kotler et al. (47) have correlated survival with wasting and shown that it can be reversed with ganciclovir therapy of the CMV. In addition, Dieterich et al. (32) noted a survival advantage for maintenance treatment of CMV infections without regard to their site of presentation.

E. Liver and the Biliary Tree

CMV also infects the biliary tree. It has been implicated as a major cause of acalculous cholecystitis leading to surgery in AIDS patients (49-51). Not infrequently, CMV in the biliary tree is also associated with cryptosporidiosis and they are found together on biopsy or autopsy (52). Dowsett et al. (53) described sclerosing cholangitis in AIDS patients. Two of four (50%) had CMV infections of the biliary tree. In addition, Jacobson et al. (54) described a series of 36 patients with CMV, 12 (33%) of whom had cholestatic liver chemistries.

Hepatitis caused by CMV is a much more common infection in transplant patients than in patients with AIDS. In the Syntex database, 4.8% of the non-AIDS patients had hepatitis while only 0.6% of the AIDS patients did. This is a large series of 5678 patients treated compassionately with ganciclovir nationwide. The diagnosis is made on liver biopsy. The characteristic enzyme picture is of elevated alkaline phosphatase and GGTP, with mild elevation of ALT and AST. Fever and sometimes right-upper-quadrant tenderness along with malaise and fatigue are the symptoms. It is somewhat surprising that this infection is not encountered more often in AIDS patients. This may be because many of the transplant-related infections are primary infections and the AIDS-related ones are reactivations.

F. Colon and Rectum

The colon is the gastrointestinal organ most often affected by CMV infection. In our series of 69 patients with gastrointestinal CMV, 46 (67%) had colitis (22). All the original reports from the early literature (e.g., Ref. 1) mention the colon as the infected organ. The reason for this is not clear; however, the magnitude and importance of the problem are enormous. If 70% of AIDS patients sometimes experience diarrhea in their clinical course, and in some series (32,33) the incidence of CMV involved in that diarrhea is 50%, then 35% of all the AIDS patients in the United States will have CMV of the GI tract, primarily colitis. The usual presentation is that of an AIDS patient with fewer than 100 T cells who has diarrhea with mutliple negative stool tests. Some investigators say three—others say six—negative stool tests should be done before endoscopic biopsy of the jejunum and colon is performed. The diarrhea may be intermittent or constant, watery or bloody. It may or may not be accompanied by tenesmus. There is no characteristic pattern. Some patients have no discernible diarrhea. Occasionally during a fever investigation, gallium scans will be positive for parts of the colon and, upon colonoscopic biopsy, CMV colitis found. The bottom line, though, is that after a number of stool examinations, colonoscopy and biopsy is the procedure of choice (Figures 6-8).

Is sigmoidoscopy and biopsy adequate, or is colonoscopy necessary? In 44 patients with CMV colitis at New York University (55), 19 had biopsies evaluable for location of disease. Only eight of 19 (42%) had positive biopsies from the rectum or sigmoid when the biopsies were positive from the transverse and right colon. Clearly, the answer is that colonoscopy is the procedure of choice. I recommend colonoscopy with 10-12 biopsies taken at random intervals throughout the colon. It is especially noteworthy that 11 of 44 (25%) of these patients had normal-appearing colonic mucosa endo-

Table 3 Surgery in AIDS Patients: Etiology

Author (Ref.)	CMV found	No. of patients	Percentage
Wilson et al. (57)	11	36	31
Wexner et al. (58)	7	14	50
Dorfler et al. (59)	3	3	100
Ferguson (60)	2	14	14
Robinson et al. (61)	3	21	14
DeRiso et al. (62)	1	1	100
Burke et al. (63)	1	1	100
Frank and Raicht (48)	2	2	100
Total	30	92	33

scopically. Even if the mucosa appears normal, multiple random biopsies should be taken.

The appearance of CMV colitis is quite variable. Sometimes, as just stated, it appears totally normal. It can look only mildly friable or have patchy erythema. The entire colon may be affected by pancolitis with ulcers, or only local areas (usually the cecum) may be inflamed (Figures 6-8). Large ulcers may be present, especially in the end stage (Figure 9), throughout the colon from the cecum to the rectum and continuing outside to the anus. These large rectal ulcers can be cavernous when viewed endoscopically (Figure 10). the patchy appearance with hemorrhagic areas corresponds to the vascular improvement on pathology (56).

IV. SURGERY

The importance of CMV in the surgery of patients with AIDS cannot be overestimated. There are nine reports in the literature of surgery in AIDS patients and the causes for surgery. Wilson et al. (57) noted 11 of 36 (31%), Wexner et al. (58) seven of 14 (50%), Dorfler et al. (59) three of three (100%), Ferguson (60) two of 14 (14%), Robinson et al. (61) three of 21 (14%), Frank and Raicht (48) two of two (100%) (see Table 3). There are three individual case reports of CMV necessitating surgery (62,63). Metaanalysis of these data yields 30 of 92, or 33% of surgery in AIDS patients caused by CMV. Whenever surgery is contemplated in an AIDS patient, then, CMV should be considered a prime suspect.

V. PATHOLOGY

Like the endoscopic appearance, the pathological appearance of CMV is diverse. Occasionally, the colonic crypts are well preserved and there is little inflammation, but there are numerous cells with typical CMV inclusions present. These are described by Waisman et al. (56) as "enlarged": "The viral inclusion body is most prominent in the nucleus and is surrounded by a clear halo, but the cytoplasm is also abnormal and slightly agranular." Some centers will do immunoperoxidase staining and CMV DNA in situ probing. This will increase slightly the yield of CMV diagnoses. However, a good pathologist with assiduous searching under H & E staining can do almost as well. Rotterdam et al. (64) and this author have reported on a system for classifying the grade of CMV infection on biopsy. This will help to quantify CMV infection for evaluative purposes, especially in studies of treatment of gastrointestinal CMV. This system is suitable for CMV disease in both the upper and lower gastrointestinal tracts.

In the esophagus, CMV produces deep ulcers with inclusion bodies found in mesenchymal cells and not epithelial cells (65). This is in sharp contrast to herpes infections, which preferentially infect squamous epithelial cells (56).

VI. TREATMENT

The treatment for CMV gastrointestinal disease is the same as that for CMV retinitis, with some modifications: ganciclovir 5 mg/kg IV BID for 14 days and then maintenance treatment with 6 mg/kg IV daily. Is it necessary to treat CMV gastrointestinal disease? The answer is an unequivocal yes. The only data we can bring to bear on the situation are some natural history data (65). In that series, all 11 patients with gastrointestinal disease before ganciclovir treatment were quite ill. The median time to progression was 1 month. The median time to death was 2 months. That is a very poor prognosis. In comparison, in our first paper (22), we noted a clinical response rate of 75% improved and 23% stabilized. The median time to relapse was 9 weeks after the end of therapy, and the median survival was 6 months.

An expanded version of this first group of results (23) confirmed the original results. To date, these are the only two published series of results in the gastrointestinal tract. The original report (31) described eight gastrointestinal cases, seven of which responded to ganciclovir therapy. The data from the compassionate use of ganciclovir are clear; the drug can induce a remission 75 to 85% of the time. Many investigators use maintenance therapy, but there are no hard data to support it. The median time to relapse in our study was 9 weeks. Some patients went as long as 1 year before relapsing; others relapsed quite quickly or developed retinitis. I use maintenance therapy in all the gastrointestinal patients I treat, partly because it can delay the onset of relapse and partly because I am convinced that it prolongs survival (32).

The use of ganciclovir for the treatment of CMV gastroenteritis in transplant patients was recently reported (67). This study was a randomized, double-blind, placebo-controlled study in a group of bone marrow transplant patients. The results indicated that, although ganciclovir sterilized the viral cultures, there was no difference in symptoms between the two groups and no endoscopic difference. This seems to be a different disease than it is in AIDS patients. Although 81% of the patients in this study had diarrhea, only two of 37 patients had sigmoidoscopy and none had colonoscopy. This indicates a clear difference in the two groups of patients and their diagnostic examinations. In addition, the immune status of transplant patients generally improves as time passes after the actual procedure, while AIDS patients' immunity inexorably declines. In this group of transplant patients, evaluated in this way, ganciclovir was not better than supportive care.

Fortunately, in 1986 we also began a double-blind, placebo-controlled study of CMV colitis in AIDS patients (68). The code has just been broken on this study, and the results show a significant benefit for ganciclovir treatment (68). This study enrolled 62 patients in four medical centers. All patients underwent colonoscopy before and after a 14-day course of ganciclovir 5 g/kg IV twice daily. A highly significant reduction of CMV cultures from colon and urine was noted ($p < 0.001$). A clear trend without statistical significance was that the placebo patients lost an average of 3 pounds in 14 days while the ganciclovir patients maintained their weight. Development of extracolonic CMV disease was more common in the placebo group [seven of 23 (30%)] than in the ganciclovir group [three of 28 (11%)]. That difference was statistically significant ($p = 0.026$). Finally, 20 of 32 (63%) ganciclovir patients and only 11 of 30 (33%) of placebo patients had reductions in colonoscopy score and successful completion of the study. This study indicates that ganciclovir is effective therapy for CMV colitis in AIDS patients.

What about other drugs for the treatment of CMV in the gastrointestinal tract? There is only one report published to date of foscarnet's use in the gastrointestinal tract (69). It only reports on five patients, and the results were not encouraging. However, several investigators have been using foscarnet in the gastrointestinal tract, and their results—unpublished as yet (B. Gazzard, personal communication, 1990)—have been generally comparable to those of ganciclovir. I have used foscarnet in 11 patients with relapsed CMV disease and have gotten seven partial or complete responses in patients who have relapsed on ganciclovir.

VII. CONCLUSIONS

From this review of the literature, several points should stand out. Cytomegalovirus is a significant cause of disease in the gastrointestinal tract of

AIDS patients; it may be responsible for as much as half of all diarrhea and a third of all esophageal disease. It is reponsible for a third of all surgeries in AIDS patients and causes significant mortality in that group. On the positive side, CMV can be treated effectively with ganciclovir and possibly with foscarnet. If side effects such as neutropenia develop, GM-CSF may be helpful (Chapter 13). I would recommend both immediate induction therapy and then maintenance therapy with ganciclovir for all AIDS patients with biopsy-proven CMV gastrointestinal disease. If relapse occurs and cannot be treated with reinduction or is due to a resistant virus, then I would recommend trying foscarnet. If neutropenia is the only problem, a concurrent trial of GM-CSF is warranted. In virtually all cases, however, ganciclovir will be adequate therapy for CMV gastrointestinal disease.

REFERENCES

1. Von Glahn WC, Pappenheimer AM. Intranuclear inclusions in visceral disease. Am J Pathol 1925; 5:445-465.
2. Freeman HJ, Shnitka TK, Piercey JRA, Weinstein WM. Cytomegalovirus infection of the gastrointestinal tract in a patient with late onset immunodeficiency syndrome. Gastroenterology 1977; 73:1397-403.
3. Cooper HS, Raffensperger EC, Jonas L. Cytomegalovirus inclusions in patients with ulcerative colitis and toxic dilatation requiring colonic resection. Gastroenterology 1977; 72:1253-1256.
4. Sidi S, Graham JH, Razvi SA, Banks PA. Cytomegalovirus infection of the colon associated with ulcerative colitis. Arch Surg 1979; 114:857-859.
5. Reichert CM, O'Leary TJ, Levens DL, Simrell CR, Macher AM. Autopsy pathology in the acquired immune deficiency syndrome. Am J Pathol 1983; 112:357-382.
6. Kronawitter U, Goebel D, Zieta CH, Zoller W, Eder M. Clinical versus post mortem findings in patients with HV infection. Programs and Abstracts IV International Conference on AIDS, Stockholm, 1988.
7. Anthony MA, Brandt LJ, Klein RS, Bernstein LH. Infectious diarrhea in patients with AIDS. Dig Dis Sci 1988; 33:1141-1146.
8. Lane GP, Lucas CR, Smallwood RA. The gastrointestinal and hepatic manifestations of the acquired immunodeficiency syndrome. Med J Australia 1989; 150:139-43.
9. Heise W, Mostertz P, Anastch K, Akorde J, Page M. Gastrointestinal findings in HIV infection. Clinical aspects, microbiological findings and endoscopic picture. Deutsche Medizinische Wochenschrift 1988; 113:1588-1593.
10. Girard PM, March C, Maslo C, Rene P, Leport J, Matheron S, Michon C, Coulaud JP, Saimot AB. Digestive manifestations in acquired immunodeficiency disease. Annales de Medecine Interne (Paris) 1987; 138:411-415.
11. Guarda LA, Luna MA, Smith JL. AIDS: Post mortem findings. Am J Clin Pathol 1984; 81:549-557.

12. Neidt GW, Schmela RA. AIDS: Clinicopathologic study of 56 autopsies. Arch Pathol Lab Med 1985; 109:727-765.

13. Mobley K, Rotterdam HZ, Lerner CW. Autopsy findings in AIDS. Pathol Ann 1985; 20:45-65.

14. Gertler SL, Pressman J, Price P, Brozinsky S, Miyai K. Gastrointestinal cytomegalovirus infection in a homosexual man with severe acquired immunodeficiency syndrome. Gastroenterology 1983; 85:1403-1406.

15. Guttman D, Raymond A, Gelb A. Virus-associated colitis in homosexual men: two case reports. Am J Gastroenterol 1983; 78:167-169.

16. Frank D, Raicht RF. Intestinal perforation associated with cytomegalovirus infection in patients with acquired immune deficiency syndrome. Am J Gastroenterol 1984; 79:201-205.

17. Meiselman MS, Cello JP, Margetten W. Cytomegalovirus colitis. Report of the clinical, endoscopic and pathologic findings in two patients with the acquired immune deficiency syndrome. Gastroenterology 1985; 88:171-175.

18. St. Onge G, Ezahler GH. Giant esophageal ulcer associated with cytomegalovirus. Gastroenterology 1982; 83:127-130.

19. Knapp AB, Horst DA, Eliopoulos G, Gramm H, Gaber LW, Falchuk KR. Falchuk ZM, Trey C. Widespread cytomegalovirus gastroenterocolitis in a patient with acquired immunodeficiency syndrome. Gastroenterology 1982; 85:1399-1402.

20. Balthazar EJ, Megibow AJ, Fazzini E, Opulencia JF, Engel I. Cytomegalovirus colitis: radiographic findings in 11 patients. Radiology 1985; 155:585-589.

21. Dieterich DT. Cytomegalovirus: A new gastrointestinal pathogen in immunocompromised patients (editorial). Am J Gastroenterol 1987; 82:764-765.

22. Chachoua A, Dieterich DT, Krasinski K, Greene J, Laubenstein L, Wernz J, Buhles W, Koretz S. 9-(1,3-dihydroxy-2-propoxymethyl)guanine (ganciclovir) in the treatment of cytomegalovirus gastrointestinal disease with the acquired immunodeficiency syndrome. Ann Intern Med 1987; 107:133-137.

23. Dieterich DT, Chachoua A, Lafleur F, Worrell C. Ganciclovir treatment of gastrointestinal infections caused by cytomegalovirus in patients with AIDS. Rev Infect Dis 1988; 10(suppl 3).

24. Francis ND, Boylston AW, Roberts AH, Parkin JM, Pinching AJ. J Clin Pathol 1989; 42:1055-1064.

25. Rene E, Marche C, Chevalier T, Rouzioux C, Regnier B, Saimot AG, Negesse Y, Matheron S, Leport C, Wolff B. Cytomegalovirus colitis in patients with acquired immunodeficiency syndrome. Dig Dis Sci 1988; 33:741-750.

26. Cosnes J, Darmoni SJ, Evard D, Le Quintret Y. Value of digestive endoscopic examination in acquired immunodeficiency syndrome (45 cases). Annales of Gastroenterologie et d'Hepatologie (Paris) 1986; 22:123-128.

27. Stamm B, Grant JW. Biopsy pathology of the gastrointestinal tract in human immunodeficiency virus associated disease: a 5 year experience in Zurich. Histopathology 1988; 13:531-540.

28. Boylston AW, Cook HT, Francis ND, Goldin RD. Biopsy pathology of acquired immune deficiency syndrome (AIDS). J Clin Pathol 1987; 40:1-8.

29. Masur J, Lane HC, Palestine A, Smith PD, Manischewitz J, Stevens G, Fujidawa I, Macher AM, Nussenlatt R, Baird B. Effect of 9-(1,3-dihydroxy-2-prop-

oxymethyl)guanine on serious cytomegalovirus disease in eight immunosuppressed homosexual men. Ann Intern Med 1986; 104:41-44.

30. Buhles WC, Mastre BJ, Tinker AJ, Strand V, Koretz SH. Ganciclovir treatment of life- or sight-threatening cytomegalovirus infection: experience in 314 immunocompromised patients. Rev Infect Dis 1988; 10(suppl 3):s495-506.

31. DHPG Collaborative Study Group. Treatment of serious cytomegalovirus infections with 9-(1,3-dihydroxy-2-propoxymethyl)guanine in patients with AIDS and other immunodeficiencies. N Engl J Med 1986; 314:801-805.

32. Dieterich DT, Dugan M, Blank K, Chachoua A. Ganciclovir (DHPG) treatment of cytomegalovirus infections in 183 AIDS patients. IV International Conference on AIDS, Stockholm, 1988, abstract 7193.

33. Smith PD, Lane HC, Gill VJ, Manischewitz JF, Quinnan GV, Fauci AS, Masur H. Intestinal infections in patients with the acquired immunodeficiency syndrome. Ann Intern Med 1988; 108:328-334.

34. Rene E, Verdon R, Roze C, Vallot T, Matheron S, Leport C, Marche C, Ruszniewski P. Intestinal infections during AIDS: Who should be investigated? Gastroenterology 1990; 98:A471.

35. Kotler DP, Reka S. Modulation of HIV production by rectal mucosa in vitro. Gastroenterology 1990; 98:A457.

36. Kotler DP, Wilson CS, Haroutiounian G, Fox CH. Detection of human immunodeficiency virus-1 by 35S-RNA in situ hybridization in solitary esophageal ulcers in two patients with the acquired immune deficiency syndrome. Am J Gastroenterol 1989; 84:313-317.

37. Joe I, Ansher AP, Gordin PM. Severe pancreatitis in an AIDS patient in association with cytomegalovirus infection. South Med J 1989; 82:1444-1445.

38. Kotler DP, Reka S, Borcich A, Winkler WP. Corticosteroid therapy of idiopathic esophageal ulcers in AIDS. Gastrointes Endosc 1990; 36:191A.

39. Connolly GM, Hawkins D, Harcourt-Webster JN, Parsons PA, Husain OA, Gazzard BG. Oesophageal symptoms, their causes, treatment, and prognosis in patients with the acquired immunodeficiency syndrome. Gut 1989; 30:1033-1039.

40. Gould B, Kory WP, Raskin JB, Ibe MJ, Redlhammer DE. Esophageal biopsy findings in the acquired immunodeficiency syndrome (AIDS): clinicopathologic correlation in 20 patients. South Med J 1988; 81:1395-1396.

41. Grippon P, Baetz A, Peroy O, Rozenbaum W, Karkouche B, Bousquet O, Opolon P. Giant esophageal ulcer in a cytomegalovirus infection in a patient with the acquired immunodeficiency syndrome. Gastroenterol Clin Biol 1985; 9: 844-845.

42. Rabenek L, Popovic M, Garnter S, McLean DM, Mcleod WA, Read E, Wong KK, Boyko WJ. Acute HIV infection presenting with painful swallowing and esophageal ulcers. JAMA 1990; 263:2318-2322.

43. Alta G, Turnage R, Eckhauser FF, Agha I, Ross S. A submucosal antral mass caused by cytomegalovirus infection in a patient with acquired immunodeficiency syndrome. Am J Gastroenterol 1986; 81:714-717.

44. Freedman PG, Weiner BC, Balthazar EJ. Cytomegalovirus esophagogastritis in a patient with acquired immunodeficiency syndrome. Am J Gastroenterol 1985; 80:434-437.

45. Spiller RC, Lovell D, Silk DB. Adult acquired cytomegalovirus infection with gastric and duodenal ulceration. Gut 1988; 29:1109-1111.
46. Balthazar EJ, Megibow AJ, Hulnick DH. Cytomegalovirus esophagitis and gastritis in AIDS. Am J Roentgenol 1985; 144:1201-1204.
47. Kotler DP, Tierney AR, Altilio D, Wang J, Pierson RN. Body mass repletion during ganciclovir treatment of cytomegalovirus infections in patients with acquired immunodeficiency syndrome. Arch Intern Med 1989; 149:901-905.
48. Frank D, Raicht RF. Intestinal perforation associated with cytomegalovirus infection in patients with acquired immune deficiency syndrome. Am J Gastroenterol 1984; 79:201.
49. Aaron JS, Wynter CD, Kirton OC, Simko V. Cytomegalovirus associated with acalculous cholecystis in a patient with acquired immune deficiency syndrome. Am J Gastroenterol 1988; 83:879-881.
50. Ong PI, Ellis ME, Tweeedle DE, Gerguson G, Haboubi NY, Knox WF. Cytomegalovirus cholecystitis and colitis associated with the acquired immunodeficiency syndrome. J Infect 1989; 18:73-75.
51. Agha FP, Nostrant TT, Abrams GD, Mazanec M, Van Moll L, Gumucio JJ. Cytomegalovirus cholangitis in a homosexual man with acquired immunodeficiency syndrome. Am J Gastroenterol 1986; 81:1068-1072.
52. Blumberg RS, Kelsey P, Perrone T, Dickersin RI, Laquaglia M, Ferruci J. Cytomegalovirus and cryptosporidium associated acalculous gangrenous cholecystis. Am J Med 1984; 76:118-123.
53. Dowsett JP, Miller R, Davidson R, Vaira D, Polydorou A, Cairns FR, Weller IV. Sclerosing cholangitis in acquired immunodeficiency syndrome. Case reports and review of the literature. Scand J Gastroenterol 1988; 23:1267-1274.
54. Jacobson MA, Cello JP, Sanda MA. Cholestasis and disseminated cytomegalovirus disease in patients with the acquired immunodeficiency syndrome. Am J Med 1988; 84:218-224.
55. Dieterich DT, Rahmin M, Rotterdam H, Dolitsky D. Cytomegalovirus colitis in AIDS: Presentation in 33 patients. V International Conference on AIDS, Montreal, 1989, MBP116.
56. Waisman J, Rotterdam HZ, Neidt GN, Lewin K, Racz P. AIDS: An overview of the pathology. Pathol Res Pract 1987; 182:729-754.
57. Wilson SE, Robinson G, Williams RA, Stabile BF, Cone R, Sarfeh IJ, Miller DR, Pasaro E. Acquired immune deficiency syndrome (AIDS): Indications for abdominal surgery, pathology, and outcome. Ann Surg 1989; 210:428-433.
58. Wexner SD, Smithy WR, Trillo C, Hopkins BS, Dailey TH. Emergency colectomy for cytomegalovirus ileocolitis in patients with the acquired immune deficiency syndrome. Dis Colon Tectum 1988; 31:755-761.
59. Dorfler H, Eisenhut C, Geissler K, Remberger K, Goebel FD. Klin Wochenschr 1988; 66:69-74.
60. Ferguson CM. Surgical complications of acquired immune deficiency virus infection. Am Surg 1988; 54:4-9.
61. Robinson G, Wilson SP, Williams KA. Surgery in patients with acquired immune deficiency syndrome. Arch Surg 1987; 122:170-175.

62. DeRiso AJ, Kemeny MM, Torres RA, Oliver JM. Multiple jejunal perforations secondary to cytomegalovirus in a patient with acquired immune deficiency syndrome. Case report and review. Dig Dis Sci 1989; 34:623-629.
63. Burke G, Nichols I, Balogh K, Hammer S, Jensen W, Pomposelli P, Jenkins R. Perforation of the terminal ileum with cytomegalovirus vasculitis and Kaposi's sarcoma in a patient with acquired immunodeficiency syndrome. Surgery 1987; 102:540-545.
64. Rotterdam H, Yi-Jin She, Dieterich DT. Diagnosis and grading of CMV colitis: Comparison of H & E stains, DNA in-situ hybridization and immunoperoxidase stains for early and late antigens. V International Conference on AIDS, Montreal, 1989, MBP127.
65. Villar LA, Massanari RM, Mitros FA. Cytomegalovirus infection with acute erosive eosphagitis. Am J Med 1984; 76:924-928.
66. Strand V, Dieterich DT, Chachoua A, DHPG Collaborative Study Group. Natural history of untreated cytomegalovirus infections in AIDS patients. IV International Conference on AIDS, Stockholm, 1988, 7198.
67. Reed EC, Wolford JL, Kopecky KJ, Lilleby KE, Dandliker PS, Todaro JL, Mcdonald GB, Meyers JD. Ganciclovir for the treatment of cytomegalovirus gastroenteritis in bone marrow transplant patients. Ann Intern Med 1990; 112: 505-510.
68. Dieterich DT, Kotler D, Busch D, Crumpacker C, Mastre BJ, Dumond C, DeArmand B, Buhles W. Randomized, placebo-controlled study of ganciclovir treatment of cytomegalovirus colitis in AIDS patients. VI International Conference on AIDS, San Francisco, 1990, F894.
69. Weber JN, Thom S, Barrison I, Unwin R, Forster S, Jeffries DJ, Boyston A, Pinching AJ. Cytomegalovirus colitis and oesophageal ulceration in the context of AIDS: clinical manifestations and preliminary report of treatment with foscarnet. Gut 1987; 28:482-487.

10

Ganciclovir Treatment of Solid-Organ Transplant Recipients with Cytomegalovirus Disease

David R. Snydman
New England Medical Center
Boston, Massachusetts

I. INTRODUCTION

Cytomegalovirus (CMV) is the most significant viral pathogen affecting solid-organ transplantation (1). Among renal transplant recipients, 25% of patients with CMV pneumonia are likely to die from their pneumonia or from complications related to severe CMV disease (2). Furthermore, the mortality rate for ventilator-dependent patients with CMV pneumonia is 95% (3). Until recently, therapy of cytomegalovirus-associated disease with a variety of viral agents, such as adenine arabinoside, leukocyte interferon, or acyclovir, has been largely unsuccessful (4-6). However, the newly developed antiviral agent ganciclovir has been used with some success in the treatment of life-threatening or serious cytomegalovirus disease in solid-organ transplant recipients (7-21).

This review will summarize the state of our knowledge in the use of ganciclovir for the treatment of CMV-associated disease in solid-organ transplant recipients. Where possible, the contrast between treatment of patients with acquired immunodeficiency syndrome (AIDS) with ganciclovir and the treatment of solid-organ transplant recipients will be discussed.

It is important to note that there have been no randomized, controlled trials of the use of ganciclovir for the treatment of CMV disease in solid-organ transplant recipients. Furthermore, in analyzing all the published reports to date, there are clearly variations in these series regarding case definitions and the criteria for classification of clinical cure, or clinical improvement. Moreover, severity of illness at entry, ventilator dependence, rapidity of diagnosis, variability in dosage regimens, and the completeness of clinical and virologic follow-up vary greatly among many of the studies (7-24). Therefore, comparisons between the different groups of patients treated with ganciclovir are virtually impossible.

Despite the lack of prospective, randomized trials, there is some evidence that ganciclovir is beneficial in treating the CMV syndromes seen in transplantation. This review will attempt to summarize the largest studies to date in order to place ganciclovir use in the solid-organ transplant population in some perspective.

II. CMV PNEUMONIA

In general, treatment of CMV pneumonia in solid-organ transplant recipients has been successful in approximately two-thirds of all patients treated. Table 1 summarizes these reports.

Most reports of CMV pneumonia therapy with ganciclovir do not provide sufficient detail regarding serologic status of transplant recipients, relationship of initiation of ganciclovir treatment to day of disease onset, or disease severity to make meaningful statements about probability of cure. It is clear from the data in Table 1 that there is a wide diversity of clinical responses among the different series. Some investigators defined clinical improvement or response to therapy as stabilization of CMV infection with improved oxygenation and evidence of elimination of CMV. In two studies, cure was defined as a return to normal oxygenation and resolution of pneumonia off study drug. In those patients who were ventilator-dependent, cure was defined as removal of the need for ventilatory support.

Some of the differences in outcome noted in Table 1 may be ascribed to differences in severity of illness and timing of initiation of therapy in relation to disease onset. For example, in the reports by Snydman (10) and Metselaar and Weimar (17), both of which actually demonstrate the lowest survival rates, 15 of the 17 patients from the two series were ventilator-dependent, yet six of 15 (40%) survived. Previous studies have shown a 95% mortality among such patients (2). None of these patients relapsed, and all six survivors were cured of their CMV-associated pneumonia.

In the largest single series of CMV pneumonia in solid-organ transplant recipients, Keay et al. (8) demonstrated improvement in CMV pneumonia in

Table 1 Treatment of CMV Pneumonia in Solid-Organ Transplant Recipients with Ganciclovir

Author (Ref.)	Average daily dose (mg/kg/d)	Type of transplant (no. of patients)	Clinical outcome (%)	Virologic outcome (%)
Paya et al. (7)	NS[a]	Liver (2) Kidney (2)	Cure (100)	Cleared (75)
Keay et al. (8)	10	Heart (8) Heart-lung (6)	Improved (77)	Cleared (100)
Erice et al. (9)	7.5	Kidney (3)	Cure (67) Improved (33)	Cleared (100)
Snydman (10)	3	Kidney (12)	Cure (33) Improved (17)	Cleared (33)
Gudnason et al. (11)	7.5	Kidney (1) Liver (3)	Improved (100)	Cleared (75)
Stratta et al. (12)	10	Liver (15)	Cure (94)[b]	Cleared (NS[a])
Thomson and Jeffries (13)	5-11	Renal (12) Heart (6) Liver (6)	Improved (75)	Cleared (68)[c]
Harbison et al. (14)	7.5	Liver (4) Kidney (2)	Improved (67)	Cleared (50)
Watson et al. (15)	7.5	Heart (4)	Improved (100)	Cleared (100)
Salmella et al. (16)	10	Liver (4)	Improved (75)[d]	Cleared (100)
Metselaar and Weimar (17)	10	Renal (6)	Cure (67)	NS[a]
Dussaix and Wood (18)	10	Liver (2)	Cure (100)[d]	Cleared (100)
D'Allesandro et al. (19)	10	Liver (2)	Cure (100)	Cleared (100)
de Hemptinne et al. (20)	10	Liver (4)	Cure (75) Improved (25)	Cleared (75)
Mai et al. (21)	NS[a]	Liver (9) Kidney (3)	Cure (83)	Cleared (83)
Total		116	79%	80%

[a]Not stated.
[b]Overall response rate for series was 94%; response of patients with pneumonia not stated explicitly; some patients received unselected immune globulin.
[c]68% of total series had virologic response; virologic response in pneumonia not stated explicitly.
[d]All patients received CMV hyperimmune globulin.

77% of heart and heart-lung transplant recipients with CMV pneumonia. In general, most other studies demonstrate both a clinical and virologic response approaching 75 to 80% among solid-organ transplant recipients with CMV pneumonia.

Generally, relapses of CMV pneumonia do not occur following successful ganciclovir therapy. However, Stratta et al. (12) have reported a 56% relapse rate among patients treated for CMV pneumonia. This is generally contrary to our own experience. We have only rarely seen relapses occur.

Information regarding timing of ganciclovir therapy with respect to disease onset and outcome is generally lacking. Hecht et al. (22), in prospectively followed renal transplant patients at risk for primary CMV disease, did provide evidence suggesting that early initiation of therapy may be associated with an improved clinical outcome.

From these studies, there is surely suggestive evidence of both a clinical and virologic response to ganciclovir therapy of CMV pneumonia among solid-organ transplant recipients. There are no obvious differences in response rates among the different types of solid-organ transplant recipients. These data stand in marked contrast to ganciclovir therapy of CMV pneumonia in bone marrow transplantation (23). The differences may be due to immunopathological differences in the CMV pneumonic process in marrow transplantation versus that in solid-organ transplantation. However, caution should be exercised in overinterpreting the "improvement" category. Some of these patients died with progressive respiratory failure or superinfection but lacked evidence of CMV at autopsy.

III. CMV HEPATITIS

Although CMV hepatitis may occur in any solid-organ transplant setting, cytomegalovirus-associated hepatitis occurs most frequently in the liver transplant recipient (24). In liver transplantation, the occurrence of CMV hepatitis in the transplanted organ has been a cause for concern; however, many cases resolve spontaneously without the need for specific anti-CMV therapy (24).

Ganciclovir has been used in a number of patients to treat CMV hepatitis, primarily in those patients who have undergone liver transplantation. Table 2 lists the response rates in a number of published series. Generally, the response rates for patients with CMV hepatitis as the major manifestation of CMV disease are slightly greater than those seen with CMV pneumonia. This difference may reflect the less serious nature of CMV disease seen in CMV hepatitis compared to patients who develop CMV pneumonia. The virologic response rates are generally quite similar to those seen in CMV pneumonia.

Relapses of treated CMV hepatitis are generally uncommon. However, Stratta and colleagues (12) demonstrated a 10% rate of relapse in those with CMV hepatitis as their only manifestation of CMV disease. However, this relapse rate was significantly less frequent than the rate of relapse in patients with disseminated disease or multiorgan involvement.

Table 2 Treatment of CMV Hepatitis in Solid-Organ Transplant Recipients with Ganciclovir

Author (Ref.)	Average daily dose (mg/kg/d)	Type of transplant (no. of patients)	Clinical outcome (%)	Virologic outcome (%)
Paya et al. (7)	NS	Liver (5) Kidney (1)	Improved (85)	Cleared (67)
Gudnadson et al. (11)		Liver (2)	Improved (50)	Cleared (50)
Erice et al. (9)		Liver (1)	Improved (100)	Cleared (100)
D'Allesandro et al. (19)	10	Liver (2)	Cured (100)	Cleared (100)
de Hemptinne et al. (20)	10	Liver (4)	Cured (100)	Cleared (100)
Thomson and Jeffries (13)	5-11	Liver (1) Renal (2)	Improved (100)	Cleared (68)
Harbison et al. (14)	7.5	Liver (7)	Improved (42)	Cleared (56)
Salmella et al. (16)	10	Liver (3)	Improved (100)	Cleared (100)
Barkholt et al. (25)	7.5	Liver (5)	Improved (60)[b]	NS[a]
Metselaar and Weimar (17)	5	Renal (2)	Improved (100)	NS[a]
Stratta et al. (12)	10	Liver (34)	Improved (94)[c]	NS[a]
Total		69	84%	75%

[a]Not stated.
[b]Three patients received immune globulin.
[c]Some patients received immune globulin.

IV. CMV RETINITIS

CMV retinitis generally occurs as a late complication in solid-organ transplantation (26). The initial response rate to treatment with ganciclovir is generally excellent. Table 3 lists the few series exclusive of AIDS in which solid-organ transplant patients with CMV retinitis have been reported. Indi-

Table 3 Outcome of Cytomegalovirus-Associated Retinitis in Solid-Organ Transplant Recipients Treated with Ganciclovir

Author (Ref.)	No. of patients	Clinical response rate (%)	Virologic response (%)	Relapse rate (%)
Snydman (10)	4	100	100	75
Keay et al. (8)	3	67	NS[a]	67
Thomson and Jeffries (13)	4	100	NS[a]	NS[a]
Total	11	91	100	56

[a]Not stated.

vidual cases from several other reports are not included in this table. The initial response rate to ganciclovir therapy in CMV retinitis is over 90%. However, relapses are common and retreatment or maintenance therapy may be necessary. In our experience, lifelong maintenance therapy is generally not necessary. If a patient relapses after induction therapy, I generally retreat with a full course, and follow with maintenance treatment. However, in the transplant recipient receiving a stable immunosuppressive regimen, a gradual tapering and withdrawal of ganciclovir therapy may be possible. This stands in marked contrast to patients with AIDS, who require lifelong therapy (27).

V. ADVERSE EFFECTS

In the solid-organ transplant recipient, the most common adverse effect of treating CMV disease with ganciclovir is neutropenia (Table 4). Since all the studies conducted to date have been open-label, compassionate-use, one cannot differentiate the occurrence of adverse events from some manifestations of the underlying disease being treated or the concomitant medications being employed in these patients. Other frequently occurring adverse events have included thrombocytopenia; central nervous system toxicity, including coma, hallucinations, and seizures; and renal insufficiency. Many other adverse events, including fever, abnormal liver function tests, rash, and hemolysis, have been reported, but their relationship to the use of ganciclovir has been unclear, especially in view of the large number of concomitant medications used in many of these patients (13).

Generally the dose-limiting adverse events are neutropenia and thrombocytopenia. Dosage reduction or interruption may be necessary to prevent life-threatening toxicity. The marrow aplasia is generally temporary, although we have seen an occasional patient in whom aplasia has lasted 2 months or more.

Table 4 Frequency of Adverse Events Reported in Solid-Organ Transplant Recipients Treated with Ganciclovir

Adverse event	No. of events ($n = 122$) (%)
Neutropenia	37 (30)
Thrombocytopenia	6 (5)
Central nervous system	8 (7)
Renal	4 (3)

Resistance of cytomegalovirus to ganciclovir, which has been reported in bone marrow transplantation patients and patients with AIDS receiving long-term maintenance ganciclovir therapy for retinitis, has not been reported in solid-organ transplant recipients (28). Clearly, such isolates may be pathogenic and surveillance for such occurrences will be necessary.

VI. DOSING

The virtually total renal clearance of ganciclovir makes it necessary to adjust dosage in renal insufficiency (29). This may be particularly problematic in patients with changing renal function, such as those individuals undergoing therapy for renal allograft rejection. Dosage must be modified considerably (see Chapter 4), according to established nomograms. Unfortunately, determinations of ganciclovir levels are not generally available. Therefore, dosage adjustment must be empiric. Supplemental doses are necessary during hemodialysis and hemofiltration (29).

VII. FUTURE CONSIDERATIONS

A. Prophylaxis

Despite the lack of randomized, controlled clinical trials of the use of ganciclovir in solid-organ transplant recipients who develop CMV disease, there are a number of examples in which the drug has been shown to be beneficial in treating CMV disease of the lung, liver, retina, and gastrointestinal tract. The impression that early therapy may be beneficial or that "prophylaxis" of CMV disease in high-risk individuals, such as those receiving OKT3, may be useful has recently led a number of transplant centers to employ early institution of therapy in such patients (12,18). Controlled trials of ganciclovir prophylaxis are currently underway in bone marrow and heart transplant recipients. Over the next few years, it is likely that the greatest use of this antiviral agent will be prophylactic in order to avoid the immunopathological events that complicate the development of CMV infection (30).

B. Combination with Immune Globulin

An additional consideration in the use of ganciclovir has been combined therapy with immune globulin for therapy of CMV pneumonia. Experimental evidence in animal models suggests that there is synergy between ganciclovir and immune globulin in treating established CMV infection (31). Although no evidence exists in solid-organ transplant recipients, there are a number of studies that support the use of large doses of immune globulin with ganciclovir in the therapy of CMV pneumonia in bone marrow transplant recipients (32-34). Despite the lack of information in solid-organ transplant patients, the use of such a combination has become common in some centers (12,18). Controlled trials using these different approaches are surely warranted to substantiate the cost-effectiveness of such an approach.

REFERENCES

1. Ho M. Cytomegalovirus. Biology and infection. In Greenough WB III, Merigan TC (Eds), Current Topics in Infectious Disease, New York, Plenum, 1982.
2. Peterson PK, Balfour HH Jr, Marker SC, Fryd DS, Howard RJ, Simmons RL. Cytomegalovirus disease in renal allograft recipients: a prospective study of the clinical features, risk factors and impact on renal transplantation. Medicine (Baltimore) 1980; 59:283-300.
3. Simmons RL, Matas AJ, Rattazzi LC, Balfour HH Jr, Howard RJ, Najarian JS. Clinical characteristics of the lethal cytomegalovirus infection following renal transplantation. Surgery 1977; 82:537-546.
4. Wade JC, Hintz M, McGuffin RW, Springmeyer SC, Connor JD, Meyers JD. Treatment of cytomegalovirus pneumonia with high-dose acyclovir. Am J Med 1982; 73(suppl 1A):249-256.
5. Meyers JD, McGuffin RW, Bryson YJ, Cantell K, Thomas ED. Treatment of cytomegalovirus pneumonia after marrow transplant with combined vidarabine and human leukocyte interferon. J Infect Dis 1982; 146:80-84.
6. Shepp DH, Newton BA, Meyers JD. Intravenous lymphoblastoid interferon and acyclovir for treatment of cytomegaloviral pneumonia. J Infect Dis 1984; 150:776-777.
7. Paya CV, Hermans PE, Smith TF, et al. Efficacy of ganciclovir in liver and kidney transplant recipients with severe cytomegalovirus infection. Transplant 1988; 46:229-234.
8. Keay S, Petersen E, Icenogle, et al. Ganciclovir treatment of serious cytomegalovirus infection in heart and heart-lung transplant recipients. Rev Infect Dis 1988; 10(S3):S563-S572.
9. Erice A, Jordan MC, Chace BA, et al. Ganciclovir treatment of cytomegalovirus disease in transplant recipients and other immunosuppressed hosts. JAMA 1987; 257:3082-3087.
10. Snydman DR. Ganciclovir therapy for cytomegalovirus disease associated with renal transplants. Rev Infect Dis 1988; 10(S3):S554-S560.
11. Gudnason T, Belani KK, Balfour HH Jr. Ganciclovir treatment of cytomegalovirus disease in immunocompromised children. Pediatr Infect Dis 1989; 8:836-840.
12. Stratta RJ, Shaefer MS, Markin RS, et al. Clinical patterns of cytomegalovirus disease after liver transplantation. Arch Surg 1989; 124:1443-1450.
13. Thomson MH, Jeffries DJ. Ganciclovir therapy in iatrogenically immunosuppressed patients with cytomegalovirus disease. J Antimicrob Chemother 1989; 23(SE):61-70.

14. Harbison MA, DeGirolami PC, Jenkins RL, Hammer SM. Ganciclovir therapy of severe cytomegalovirus infections in solid-organ transplant recipients. Transplant 1988; 46:82-88.

15. Watson FS, O'Connell JB, Amber IJ, et al. Treatment of cytomegalovirus pneumonia in heart transplant recipients with 9-(1,3-dihydroxy-2-propoxymethyl)guanine (DHPG). J Heart Transplant 1988; 7:102-105.

16. Salmella K, Hockerstedt K, Lautenschlager I, et al. Ganciclovir in the treatment of severe cytomegalovirus disease in liver transplant patients. Transplant Proc 1990; 22:238-240.

17. Metselaar HJ, Weimar W. Cytomegalovirus infection and renal transplantattion. J Antimicrob Chemother 1989; 23(suppl E):37-47.

18. Dussaix E, Wood C. Cytomegalovirus infection in pediatric liver transplant recipients. Transplantation 1989; 48:272-274.

19. D'Alessandro AM, Pirsch JD, Stratta RJ, et al. Successful treatment of severe cytomegalovirus infections with ganciclovir and CMV hyperimmune globulin in liver transplant recipients. Transplant Proc 1989; 21:3560-3561.

20. De Hemptinne B, Lamy ME, Sahzzoni M, et al. Successful treatment of cytomegalovirus disease with 9-(1,3-dihydroxy-2-propoxymethyl)guanine. Transplant Proc 1988; 20(S1):652-655.

21. Mai M, Nery J, Sutker W, et al. DHPG (gancyclovir) (SIC) improves survival in CMV pneumonia. Transplant Proc 1989; 21:2263-2265.

22. Hecht DW, Snydman DR, Crumpacker CS, et al. Ganciclovir for treatment of renal transplant-associated primary cytomegalovirus pneumonia. J Infect Dis 1988; 157:187-190.

23. Reed EC, Dandliker PS, Meyers JD. Treatment of cytomegalovirus pneumonia with 9-[2-hydroxy-1-(hydroxymethyl)ethoxymethyl]guanine in the treatment of cytomegalovirus pneumonia. Ann Intern Med 1986; 105:214-215.

24. Paya CV, Hermans PE, Weisner RH, et al. Cytomegalovirus hepatitis in liver transplantation: Prospective analysis of 93 consecutive orthotopic liver transplantations. J Infect Dis 1989; 160:752-758.

25. Barkholt LM, Ericzon BG, Ehrnst A, et al. Cytomegalovirus infections in liver transplant patients: incidence and outcome. Transplant Proc 1990; 22:235-237.

26. Pollard RB, Egbert PR, Gallagher JG, Merigan TC. Cytomegalovirus retinitis in immunosuppressed hosts. I. Natural history and effects of treatment with adenine arabinoside. Ann Intern Med 1980; 93:655.

27. Mills J, Jacobson MA, O'Donnell JJ, et al. Treatment of cytomegalovirus retinitis in patients with AIDS. Rev Infect Dis 1988; 10(S3):S522-S527.

28. Erice A, Chou S, Biron KK, et al. Progressive disease due to ganciclovir-resistant cytomegalovirus in immunocompromised patients. N Engl J Med 1989; 320:289-293.

29. Somadossi JP, Bevan R, Ling T, et al. Clinical pharmacokinetics of ganciclovir in patients with normal and impaired renal function. Rev Infect Dis 1988; 10(S3):S506-S514.

30. Grundy JE. Virologic and pathogenetic aspects of cytomegalovirus infection. Rev Infect Dis 1990; 12(S7):S711-S719.

31. Rubin RH, Lynch P, Pasternak MS, et al. Combined antibody and ganciclovir treatment of murine cytomegalovirus-infected normal and immunosuppressed BALB/c mice. Antimicrob Agents Chemother 1989; 33:1975-1979.
32. Reed EC, Bowden RA, Dandliker PS, et al. Treatment of cytomegalovirus pneumonia in marrow transplant patients with ganciclovir and intravenous cytomegalovirus immunoglobulin. Ann Intern Med 1988; 109:783-788.
33. Emanual D, Cunningham I, Jules-Elysee K, et al. Cytomegalovirus pneumonia after marrow transplantation successfully treated with the combination of ganciclovir and high dose intravenous immune globulin. Ann Intern Med 1988; 109: 777-782.
34. Schmidt GM, Kovacs A, Zaia JA, et al. Ganciclovir/immunoglobulin combination therapy for the treatment of human cytomegalovirus-associated interstitial pneumonia in bone marrow allograft recipients. Transplantation 1988; 46:905-907.

11

Ganciclovir Treatment of Bone Marrow Transplant Recipients with Cytomegalovirus Disease

John A. Zaia and Gerhard M. Schmidt
City of Hope National Medical Center
Duarte, California

I. INTRODUCTION

A. Comparison of Bone Marrow Transplantation and Solid-Organ Transplantation

With the development of bone marrow transplantation (BMT) in the late 1970's, a major complication of the procedure was severe cytomegalovirus (CMV) infection (1,2). This was of particular note because the most serious syndrome, CMV-associated interstitial pneumonia (CMV-IP), occurred in 15-25% of all BMT recipients and was nearly always fatal. At that time, CMV-IP was well recognized as an important problem of other immuno-suppressed populations and as one of the most severe manifestations of CMV infection (3). Nevertheless, life-threatening CMV infection was less frequent in these other immunodeficient groups, and, clearly, the spectrum of clinical disease appeared different in BMT from that seen in solid-organ transplantation. In renal transplantation, in fact, although the rate of infection with CMV was as high as in BMT recipients, the high prevalence of asymptomatic infection initially obscured the specific clinical syndrome attributable to CMV (4). Eventually, it was recognized that reactivation of CMV occurred both in the recipient and in the organ itself, accounting for the spectrum of clinical syndromes (5,6). Many studies have reported fever, leukopenia, thrombocytopenia, mononucleosis, hepatitis, and pneumonitis during the 2-3 months after transplantation (6). Late, after renal transplantation, CMV-associated retinitis occurs in a small percentage of recipients. With the use of more intensive immunosuppression, and the development of heart, heart-lung, and liver transplantation, the heterogeneity of CMV-associated diseases continues to be expanded (7).

Similar to solid-organ transplantation, the CMV-associated syndromes occurring after BMT include marrow-suppressive events such as leukopenia and thrombocytopenia, enteritis, and hepatitis (8). However, the most consistent life-threatening event associated with CMV infection noted after BMT was CMV-IP. The initial observations described by Meyers et al. (2) indicated that 26% of allogeneic BMT recipients developed CMV-IP, with a mortality of nearly 100%. Thus, CMV-IP became the leading infectious problem after marrow transplantation, and the use of a variety of antiviral strategies, including ganciclovir (GCV), in this population will be reviewed in this chapter.

B. Heterogeneity of CMV-Associated Disease

As with the different transplantation groups, there is a wide variation in the spectrum of CMV-associated disease observed in various populations, including both normal and immunodeficient persons (9). It is important to appreciate this heterogeneity for what it tells us about the mechanisms of disease. In normal individuals, CMV infection occurs in young infants and in adolescent persons. During these primary infections, disease is rare and, when it occurs, is more frequently seen in the adolescent and the young adult. It is not known why some persons with primary CMV infection develop severe disease and others have only mild disease, but, presumably, this is related to host variation in immune response to virus (9).

In AIDS patients and in neonates, CMV infection can be progressive and relatively unchecked for many weeks with relatively little symptomology (10,11). Nevertheless, in this group of patients, the central nervous system (CNS) complications, and particularly the retinitis, demonstrate the neurotropism of this virus. The virus itself is capable of producing tissue damage, and, as described below (see Section II), this is a direct consequence of virus infection. However, the neurotropic aspects of CMV infection are much less commonly observed in solid-organ transplantation and, despite the severity of other manifestations of CMV, are almost never seen in the marrow transplant recipient. CMV retinitis is a late complication of infection, and it is possible that this difference in the CMV disease spectrum between the AIDS patient and the BMT recipient is due to the fact that, in the past, CMV infection was fatal in a subgroup of marrow recipients, thus removing the possibility of late complications.

The principal difference in disease seen in CMV infection in transplantation recipients, compared to groups in which CNS complications are common, is the predominance of mononucleosislike symptoms (compare Refs. 6-11). The cardinal features of CMV infection in the transplant recipient are fever, neutropenia, thrombocytopenia, and malaise. These signs and symptoms, of course, occur during CNS syndromes and during enteritis and hepatitis in all involved patients, but they are more frequently seen without other organ-specific involvement. This has suggested an aspect of disease pathogenesis that is separate from the organ-tropic features of disease. Furthermore, because these symptoms have been associated with immunological abnormalities characteristic of transplant populations, such as host versus graft disease or graft versus host disease (GVHD), the possibility has been raised that the disease complex associated with CMV in certain situations is due not so much to the virus as to the host response to the infection (12,13). If this is true, then the approach to treatment, and especially to the development of antiviral therapy, must take into consideration this aspect of disease pathogenesis. It is important to understand that chemotherapy directed to inhibition of virus replication will be effective in treating disease only when the syndrome is a direct effect of continuing virus replication. If the virus-associated disease complex is due to nonviral factors, then antiviral therapy is more likely to be successful when used prophylactically and, unless used early, will fail to treat existing disease. The management of CMV infection in the BMT recipient illustrates this point, as will be discussed below (see Section IV) and underlines the importance of clearly separating the viral and nonviral components of disease pathogenesis in planning treatment strategy.

II. PATHOGENESIS OF CMV DISEASE AFTER MARROW TRANSPLANTATION

A. Direct Effect of Virus in Pathogenesis

The mechanism of disease pathogenesis must explain the clinical syndromes that can be associated either with prolonged and continuous expression of infectious virus or with minimal amounts of CMV but no less serious infection. The pathogenesis of CMV-associated diseases is only beginning to be understood, and, at a molecular level, we are nowhere near an explanation of the relatively complex events that accompany CMV infection and may be relevant to disease occurrence. Nevertheless, by combining clinical and laboratory observations, it is possible to develop a hypothesis for CMV pathogenesis.

In simplest terms, it appears that there are disease syndromes that occur because of persistent virus infection, and there are other syndromes that occur because the host is reacting to that infection. It is well recognized that there may be chronic and persistent viral shedding following either primary or re-activated CMV infection, and that this can be associated with asymptomatic infection or with frank disease (9). For reasons not yet known, asymptomatic infection occurs in the great majority of all persons who are infected with CMV, and this includes marrow transplant recipients (13). The mechanism by which asymptomatic CMV infection results in resolution of infection is unknown. It is inferred from observations of more severe disease in immuno-deficient populations that the immune response to CMV leads to a resolution of infection. In fact, it is possible that resolution of infection is really only an equilibrium between continuous high and low levels of virus reactivation. It is recognized that the presence of cytotoxic lymphocyte function is pro-tective from CMV-IP after BMT (14), but the role of humoral and cellular factors contributing to resolution of infection remains poorly characterized. The possibility exists, then, that we never actually resolve the primary infec-tion or, if we do, that reactivation occurs readily in response to physiological changes in the host.

In addition, the host with CMV infection is potentially altered by a relatively large genetic load of viral DNA, which could play a role in pathogenesis. CMV contains more than 200 gene sequences, and these could be in a rela-tive state of activation at most times. The important question to be asked is whether this new and persistently active genetic information can contribute to disease. Looked at from this level, then, an additional complexity must be considered in appreciating CMV pathogenesis. It is possible that when pathogenetic mechanisms are known in more detail for the herpesviruses, this will be far different from conventional schemes of pathogenesis for other clinical infectious disease (9).

We can begin to address this issue by asking which clinical syndromes are determined by persistent CMV infection. Two clinical settings of profound immunoincompetence—that of the fetus and that of the person with advanced AIDS—can be associated with severe CMV infection, and the infection often involves tissue of neuronal origin or of gastrointestinal origin (10,11). The resultant clinical syndromes appear to be determined by the cytopathic ef-fects of the virus. It appears, in fact, based on the asymptomatic aspect of infection in most individuals, that the degree to which host immune func-tion is altered plays a role in the level of persistence of CMV infection, and in the face of unbridled virus replication certain organs are targeted for disease (see Figure 1). Thus, in congenital infections and in AIDS, the target organs are the brain, nervous tissue such as the retina and the adrenal gland, and gut tissue. As noted above, except for the liver, these organs are usually not involved in CMV syndromes in normal persons and are relatively infre-quent in immunosuppressed groups considering the high frequency of infec-tion. The fact that inhibition of CMV infection with appropriate antiviral

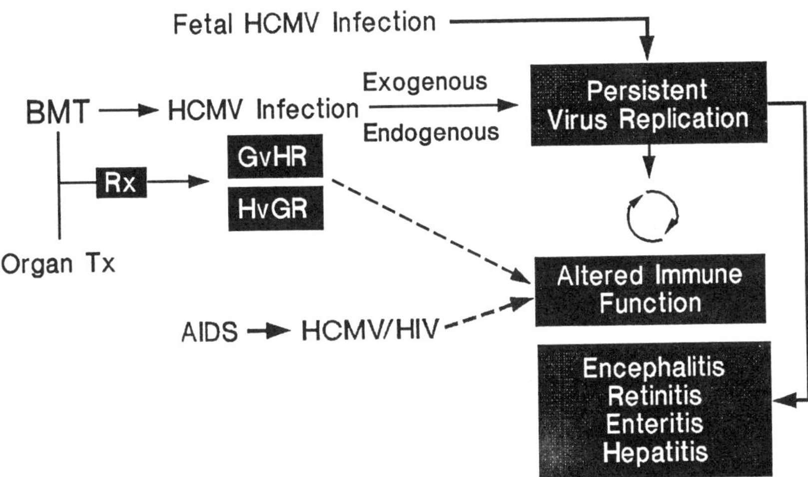

Figure 1 Virus-determined syndromes of CMV infection. The level of persistent virus replication determines the amount of direct CMV cytopathology, and this directly influences the development of disease in tissues of central nervous system and gut origin. Persistence of CMV infection, in turn, is regulated by the degree of altered immune function and, with profound disturbances of function, this can result in encephalitis, retinitis, adrenalitis, enteritis, and hepatitis. In AIDS patients, both human immunodeficiency virus type 1 (HIV) and CMV influence the level of altered immune function. In transplant (Tx) recipients of bone marrow (BMT) or solid organs, therapy (Rx) of graft versus host reaction (GvHR) or of host versus graft reaction (HvGR) leads to the immune function alteration. In fetal CMV infection, unbridled virus replication leads directly to CNS and gut disease.

agents such as GCV can be therapeutic in syndromes such as retinitis and enteritis in AIDS patients is evidence that persistence of virus infection is the driving force in these diseases (15,16).

Why are retinitis, enteritis, and hepatitis less frequently observed after marrow transplantation than are the syndromes of fever, mononucleosis, and pneumonitis? In the simplified model of pathogenesis shown in Figure 1, it is presumed that these diseases do not develop directly from persistent virus replication. CMV infection is necessary, but other events are occurring that are more important for pathogenesis. If this is true, then these syndromes should not respond to antiviral therapy, and, in fact, it has been well shown (see Section IV below) that antiviral agents usually fail to treat CMV-associated diseases in this population. For example, both CMV-IP and CMV-associated enteritis after BMT have failed to respond to GCV therapy (17, 18). Yet, as noted, these diseases are usually associated with persistent virus infection, and virus replication was promptly inhibited by the GCV therapy (15,16). Thus, it appears that CMV-IP and CMV enteritis are different diseases in the marrow recipient compared to the AIDS patient.

B. Effect of Nonviral Factors on Pathogenesis

The implication of this is that there is a host component that contributes to disease, and inhibition of virus replication, while efficacious in managing disease produced by virus-induced cytopathology, will have little impact on diseases derived from the host-contributed pathogenetic elements (19). This, in fact, is well recognized in other herpes viral syndromes such as herpes simplex virus (HSV)-induced mucocutaneous disease. Acyclovir (ACV) therapy can inhibit HSV replication in reactivation disease very effectively, and yet ACV therapy results in no significant alteration of disease severity when used more than 24 hours after symptoms of virus reactivation occur. In fact, ACV treatment of recurrent HSV mucocutaenous disease is effective only when used very early after virus reactivation (20).

The effect of persistent CMV infection on host functions is illustrated in Figure 2. In this schema, the alterations in host immune function, determined in part by the CMV infection and in part by the direct or indirect effects of GVHD, in conjunction with cellular effects of CMV infection, result in a level of immune reactivity that leads to CMV-IP. It is clearly recognized that the expression of CMV-encoded products can result in protein-specific immune activation (21). There is evidence, as noted above, that immune reactivity resulting in cytotoxic lymphocyte function is protective after BMT (14).

The question that is unresolved at this time is how immune activation can result in organ-specific pathology such as CMV-IP. It is well known from the past decade of clinical investigation that there are immunological disturbances associated with CMV infection (22), and it is thought that this abnormality is based at the macrophage level (23-25). It is recognized, for example, that interleukin-1 (IL-1) and IL-2 are abnormal after CMV infection (26,27), and the implication is that CMV infection results in a disturbed regulation of the immune system.

Recently, Dudding et al. (28) have reported that CMV-infected macrophages, previously primed with phorbol ester, have an altered ability to produce IL-1β and tumor necrosis factor-α (TNFα). This further suggests that CMV infection is associated with a metabolic derangement of cells that impairs their ability to produce or to respond to mediators of the immune response. There is, as yet, no evidence that cytokine abnormalities or growth factor disturbances are important in CMV-associated disease. Nevertheless, it is recognized that CMV infection is associated with enhanced susceptibility

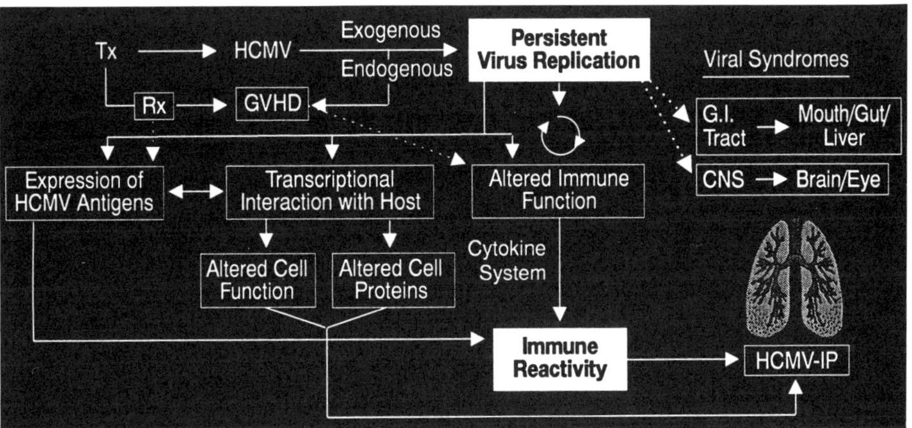

Figure 2 Pathogenesis of CMV-associated syndromes in marrow transplant recipients. Following marrow transplantation (Tx), CMV infection occurs from exogenous or endogenous sources, leading to persistent virus replication. This results in expression of viral antigens, transcriptional interaction with host cells, and alteration in immune function. In addition, the treatment (Rx) of graft versus host disease (GVHD) and the interaction of CMV and GVHD contribute to the state of altered immune function. In this hypothesis, the direct and indirect effects of CMV infection result in increased immune reactivity that is mediated by disturbances in the regulation of the cytokine system and causes CMV-associated interstitial pneumonia (CMV-IP). Viral syndromes derived directly from virus replication bypass this complex pathway, producing diseases of the gastrointestinal (G.I.) tract and the central nervous system (CNS).

to other infections (29), indicating that host resistance factors are functionally altered. It can be hypothesized that humoral mediators of immunological function are abnormally controlled after CMV infection, and these will eventually be shown to mediate specific disease syndromes, such as CMV-IP. There already are reports that describe the putative role of TNFα in busulfan-induced pneumonitis (30) and of other cytokines in pulmonary inflammation (31). It is not unlikely that abnormal regulation of these cellular growth factors important to normal immune function will explain some of the pathological processes seen during CMV infection, and that it could even account for the organ-specific aspects of these syndromes.

C. Effects of CMV Infection of Cellular Function

Before we can appreciate how CMV infection results in altered immunity, we must further explore the effect of CMV infection on cellular functions that could contribute to disease. It has been known for many years that CMV alters host cell DNA synthesis (32), and the specific cellular effects of this alteration are only beginning to be understood. The CMV genome encodes sequences with molecular mimicry involving the HLA system (33,34), and it has been reported that CMV affects the level of HLA expression (21). However, there has been no definitive evidence that virus-induced alteration of the major histocompatibility system disrupts normal immune function. Similarly, selective cellular proteins are either down- or up-regulated during CMV infection. For example, fibronectin-specific RNA is down-regulated immediately after infection, without concomitant alteration in β-actin messenger RNA (35), and the physiological effects of specific down-regulation of an immunologically significant protein such as this are unknown. It is likely that other proteins necessary for optimal host function will be found to be altered by CMV infection.

We are only beginning to understand how macromolecular events are mediated at the subcellular level, but clearly CMV affects signal transduction systems in such a way that it can be inferred that these might be important in pathogenesis. The second-messenger systems, in which phosphokinase-C activation pathways and calcium-mediated activation pathways mediate signal transduction from membrane interactions with specific ligands (36), have been shown by Albrecht and co-workers to be involved in CMV infection (37). Alteration of these pathways can inhibit CMV replication in vitro, and it has been suggested that these effects could be important in explaining certain chromosomal abnormalities associated with CMV infection in vitro (38).

In regard to clinical disease, it can be hypothesized further that the virus, in acting as a ligand and interrupting these same pathways, basically creates a pathological disturbance of this cellular biostat (9). We would hypothesize that for CMV-associated disease in marrow transplant recipients, the common vehicle for determining symptomatic consequences of CMV infection is immune dysfunction. What we are asked to understand, in terms of pathogenesis, is how one can get from persistent CMV infection to a specific or nonspecific functional disturbance, such as altered immune regulation, and from there to a specific clinical syndrome. A T-cell immunodeficiency has been reported in which there is a defect in signal transduction (39), and therefore it is not difficult to imagine that second-messenger alterations by CMV infection could have effects on the immune system. In this regard, it has been observed that the promotor-regulatory region of the major immediate-early gene of CMV contains functional response elements that are similar to those of certain cytokines (40,41).

Boldogh et al. (42) have reported that CMV infection up-regulates the transcription of proto-oncogenes and that this is mediated by a membrane transduction phenomenon. This suggests that CMV, merely acting as a ligand, can influence cellular proliferation and gene transcription. Such cellular perturbations undoubtedly extend to other areas of transcriptional regulation that could have profound clinical importance. For example, Duncombe et al. (43) have reported that there is increased production of interferon gamma and of TNFα by peripheral blood mononuclear cells from marrow transplant recipients when these cells are cocultured with marrow fibroblasts infected with CMV. Although there is no clear connection between TNFα and clinical disease, TNFα has been associated with graft rejection and with GVHD, events related to CMV infection (44-46). Similarly, CMV infection of bone marrow cells has been reported to alter the ability of these cells to respond to growth factors in vitro, and it is possible that the marrow failure observed in the spectrum of CMV-associated disease after BMT is a result of virus-induced physiological derangements (47). This would explain why the use of antiviral chemotherapy could have either no effect or only a delayed effect on clinical disease, and development of better therapy will require more complete understanding of the precise pathogenetic events during CMV infection. Thus, basic research observations are beginning to be linked to the clinical understanding of symptomology, and hopefully this will lead to more successful prevention and treatment of this disease.

III. CMV-ASSOCIATED SYNDROMES AFTER BMT

A. Nonspecific CMV Syndromes

As mentioned already, in most marrow transplant recipients CMV infection is not associated with significant clinical signs and symptoms; however, few accurate incidence rates of fever, neutropenia, thrombocytopenia, and malaise are available for CMV infection after BMT. The incidence of CMV infection varies with recipient and donor CMV-serologic status, but except for the seronegative recipient of a seronegative marrow donor, the incidence of infection is in the range of 70-80% (48). In a prospective study of 127 allogeneic BMT recipients at City of Hope, the occurrence of fever was shown to correlate with the presence of positive blood cultures, as illustrated in Figure 3 (13). Unlike solid-organ transplantation, there are no prospective studies that describe the occurrence of other nonspecific signs of CMV infection after BMT, and the description of similar clinical syndromes of arthalgia, malaise, and wasting associated with CMV infection in solid-organ transplant recipients (5-7) provides the basis for linking such events to CMV after BMT.

B. CMV-Associated Pneumonitis

The syndrome of CMV-IP is defined as a pulmonary disease having roentgenographic evidence of interstitial changes, evidence of CMV infection in

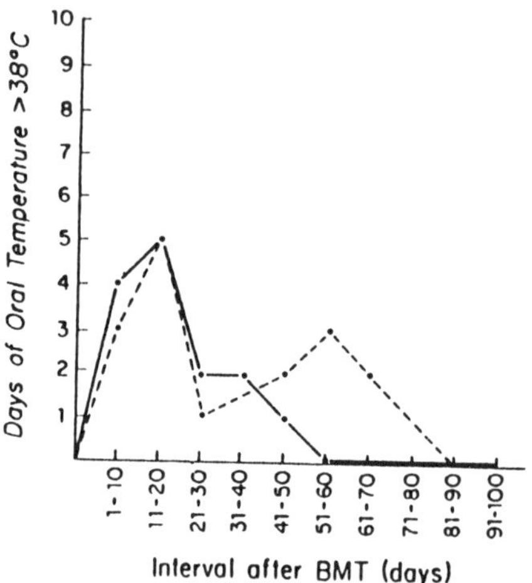

Figure 3 Time of occurrence of fever after bone marrow transplantation (BMT) in patients followed prospectively for CMV infection of blood. The mean number of days of oral temperature $<38\,°C$ is compared at intervals after BMT for patients (n = 59) with no positive CMV blood cultures and at least five negative cultures for CMV (solid line) and for patients (n = 48) with at least three positive CMV blood cultures (dashed line). (Adapted from Ref. 12.)

the lower respiratory tract, and the absence of other microbiological agents or histopathology that would explain the syndrome. Among the risks for developing this disease, the first and foremost is the occurrence of CMV infection, and the second major risk for CMV-IP is the development of GVHD (48). All other risk factors, such as age, conditioning regimen, and disease status, appear to be derivatives of these two predisposing elements in the pathophysiology. In 559 BMT recipients reviewed by Meyers et al. (2), CMV infection occurred in 60% of those with GVHD but in only 42% of those with no GVHD. More important, the incidence of CMV-IP was higher in those with GVHD whether during primary or recurrent infection. Disease occurs in greatest number in allogeneic marrow recipients who are CMV-seropositive prior to BMT. CMV-IP is much less frequent in autologous BMT (49,50) and is rarely seen after syngeneic marrow transplantation (51). The incidence of CMV-IP in allogenic BMT varies from 15-30% and has periods of relatively high or low incidence, and the mortality associated with this disease in the pre-GCV era was 80-100% (see Table 1, Section IV). The occurrence of CMV-IP does not appear to be declining, and in a 2-year period at City of Hope just prior to the use of GCV prophylaxis, 40 (25%) patients of 160 total transplant recipients developed CMV-IP. The incidence is un-

Table 1 Experience with Antiviral Agents for the Treatment of CMV-IP in BMT

Agent	Reference	Survival (%)
Interferon (IFN)	55	0
Acyclovir	58	14
Vidarabine/IFN	56	14
Acyclovir/IFN	57	23
	62	13
Foscarnet	63	0
Ganciclovir	64	10
	65	45
	66	22
	67	38
Ganciclovir/steroids	68	17
IGIV[a]	69	50
	70	21

[a]Intravenous immune globulin.

doubtedly related to selective factors such as a conditioning regimen and to unknown host factors, and this is assumed to play a role in producing variation in incidence from center to center.

The syndrome itself usually presents during the second or third months after BMT, with a median time of onset ranging from 52 to 62 days posttransplantation (1,2,8). The disease presents with cough and tachypnea and progresses to hypoxemia over 4-7 days. Prior to GCV-based treatment regimens, the course of disease was of two types: a more fulminant disease lasting < 14 days and a slower disease process that lasted ≥14 days (12). From the standpoint of patient management, peripheral cultures for CMV such as from urine and the throat do not predict for subsequent CMV-IP, but presence of CMV in blood is a predictor for this disease (52). At the City of Hope, the time from first evidence of CMV infection in blood to death in the more fulminant CMV-IP was 8 ± 15 days, and in the longer disease course for CMV-IP it was 28 ± 15 days (12). Because blood-culture results cannot routinely be reported in time for early treatment of CMV, we have utilized bronchoalveolar lavage (BAL) on day +35 post-BMT for determination of risk for CMV-IP and prophylactic treatment (see Section V).

The differential diagnosis of IP in the marrow recipient includes infection, recurrent leukemia, radiation/chemotherapy-related lung toxicity, and ideopathic IP. The types of infection associated with IP in this setting include other respiratory viruses, chlamydia, mycoplasma, *Legionella pneumophila*, *Mycobacterium tuberculosis*, and *Pneumocystis carinii*.

C. CMV-Associated Enteritis

CMV infection has been shown to produce severe gastrointestinal tract disease in immunodeficient persons, particularly those with AIDS (11). However, in marrow transplant recipients the exact incidence of CMV infection in the gut is not known. Hepatitis is undoubtedly the most frequent such infection, but because CMV infection is often concomitant with GVHD, liver transminase elevations are usually attributed to the latter. Ulceration of the gastrointestinal tract associated with CMV ranges from the esophagus (52) to the stomach, the small bowel, and the colon. The spectrum of disease due to CMV enteritis will vary based on the location of the lesions and on the overall severity of the CMV-associated syndrome, but, as reported by Reed et al. (18), this includes fever (33%), anorexia (81%), dysphagia (11%), nausea and vomiting (86%), upper (48%) and lower (8%) abdominal pain, diarrhea (81%), and intestinal hemorrhage (30%). In a controlled study evaluating GCV therapy, there was improvement or resolution of disease in approximately one-third of placebo recipients and stable disease in half of this group, but GCV failed to produce a change in symptoms despite a significant reduction in virus excretion (18). As noted above (see Section II), this suggests that the symptoms of CMV enteritis are likely not to be related to virus replication, and improvement in treatment will not require improved antiviral agents but, rather, a better understanding of this disease.

D. CMV-Associated Marrow Suppression

CMV-associated marrow suppression is an important but inadequately described clinical feature of CMV infection of marrow recipients (8). Suppression of graft function in association with CMV infection usually involves leukopenia but can be associated with thrombocytopenia and graft failure. Because of the association of CMV with solid-organ graft rejection, the effect of CMV infection on marrow engrafment has been explored in autologous BMT. Verdonck et al. (53) noted that CMV-seropositive recipients had delayed platelet recovery compared to seronegative recipients. Wingard et al. (49) have reported that platelet recovery is significantly slower in CMV-seropositive autologous BMT recipients with active CMV infection compared to a similar group without active CMV infection (49). However, in a description of 159 autologous marrow recipients, Reusser et al. (50) noted no effect of CMV infection on leukocyte or platelet recovery post-BMT. Nevertheless, there remain uncontrolled reports of marrow recovery during GCV treatment of CMV-associated graft failure (54).

IV. TREATMENT OF CMV-IP

A. Experience with Antiviral Agents

For the past decade, there have been many attempts to treat CMV-IP with available antiviral agents, and a summary of the treatment results of CMV-IP in the setting of allogeneic bone marrow transplantation is shown in Table 1. Nevertheless, when these agents were used either alone or in combination, the survival rates for CMV-IP in marrow recipients remained 0-23%, a result no different from those of the historic controls. Leukocyte-derived interferon (IFN) given at 2×10^4 to 6.4×10^5 units/kg per day, was used in eight marrow recipients with CMV-IP by Meyers et al. (55). All eight patients died of pneumonia, and virus was present in lung tissue from seven autopsy cultures. IFN was subsequently evaluated in combination with either vidarabine (araA) or acyclovir (ACV) (56,57). Using approximately the same IFN doses as above and araA doses ranging from 2.5-15 mg/kg per day, the survival remained poor, and there was significant marrow- and neurotoxicity (56). Acyclovir, when used alone to treat CMV-IP at doses as high as 1000 mg/M^2 per dose, has resulted in no improved survival but was associated with an antiviral effect (58). There has been evidence reported that, when combined in vitro with IFN, the concentration of ACV required to inhibit CMV is significantly reduced (59,60). ACV was used in combination with leukocyte-derived IFN in 13 marrow recipients with CMV-IP, and this resulted in a 23% survival rate, no consistent antiviral effect, and marked marrow and CNS toxicity (61). Subsequently, a purified form of lymphoblast-derived IFN was used in combination with ACV with similar poor results (62). Foscarnet, a pyrophosphate analog with activity against CMV and with effectiveness for treatment of CMV retinitis, has been used to treat CMV-IP in marrow recipients. When used at 9-20 mg/kg as a loading dose, followed by continuous infusion of 0.078-0.14 mg/kg per minute, there were no survivors among nine patients with CMV-IP (63).

Similarly, GCV, despite effectiveness in treating a variety of CMV-associated syndromes in immunosuppressed persons, has minimal effectiveness in treating CMV-IP in marrow transplant recipients. In the first published report of GCV therapy for CMV-IP by Shepp et al. (64), GCV was used at a total dose of 7.5-15 mg/kg per day in 10 persons, with survival in only one patient. Despite this high mortality, GCV treatment produced a prompt antiviral effect with suppression of CMV in blood, urine, and respiratory secretions in those who received at least 10 days of therapy (64). Erice et al. (65) reported that GCV used at 7.5 mg/kg per day for CMV-IP was associated with a 45% survival rate. In a study reported by Winston et al. (66), GCV used at a dose of 10 mg/kg per day resulted in a survival rate of 22% in nine marrow recipients with CMV-IP. In a multicenter study reported by Crumpacker et al. (67), eight of 21 (38%) GCV-treated marrow recipients survived CMV-IP. In this group, there was heterogeneity in terms of time of onset of CMV-IP, with approximately one-half of the group developing CMV-IP after day 80 post-BMT compared with the subjects in the study of Shepp et al. (64), all of whom developed CMV-IP prior to day 80. This suggests that either the disease itself was different or that the subject-to-subject variation in these two groups of patients resulted in varied outcomes. It is possible, as implied here, that GCV is more effective in persons late after BMT. GCV treatment has been reported to be effective in renal transplant recipients with CMV-IP, and it is not unlikely that marrow transplant recipients who develop late CMV-IP are better candidates for GCV therapy.

B. Experience with Antiviral Agents and/or Immune Globulin

The nearly uniform negative results of treatment of CMV-IP with antiviral approaches is strong evidence that the virus alone does not account for disease (see Section II above). Because of the possibility that CMV-IP could be caused by both CMV infection and the host response to infection, it was suggested that antiviral therapy be combined with immune response modification (12). The initial attempt to effect this combined treatment was reported by Reed et al. (68), who described the use of GCV and methylprednisolone in six marrow recipients with CMV-IP. In this study, GCV was given at a dose of 7.5 mg/kg per day, and steroid was given at 16 mg/kg per day for 1 week and then tapered over 14 days. Only one of six patients survived, and severe marrow and renal toxicity was observed in five patients. Clearly, this regimen produced no improvement.

The use of an intravenous immune globulin (IGIV), selected for high antibody to CMV (CMV-IGIV), has been evaluated for treatment of CMV-IP, with mixed results. In the initial study of Blacklock et al. (69), nine of 18 marrow recipients survived CMV-IP, some of whom were on mechanical ventilation due to their disease. This finding has not been confirmed, and a study by Reed et al. (70), in which 14 marrow recipients with CMV-IP were treated, failed to demonstrate a therapeutic effect with CMV-IGIV. In this latter study, a different preparation of IGIV and a different transplantation preparative regimen was used, and it remains possible that differences between these two studies are due to these uncontrolled factors.

These studies set the stage for regimens that combined GCV and IGIV (GCV/IVIG) for the treatment of CMV-IP. Animal studies at this same time deserve note because they provided additional observations relevant to the combination of GCV and immune globulin. In a mouse model of CMV-IP, Shanley and Pesanti (71) reported that GCV, while decreasing the amount of murine CMV infection in mouse lung, failed to prevent interstitial pneumonia. However, Wilson et al. (72) demonstrated that the combination of GCV and mouse immune serum would protect from a lethal challenge with MCMV. In this study neither GCV nor immune serum alone provided protection.

In 1987, the experiences of two BMT centers were reported, and these preliminary results suggested that the combined use of GCV and IGIV improved outcome of CMV-IP (73,74). Subsequently, several centers have published results using this type of therapeutic method (17,75,76). The comparison of results with these treatment regimens are shown in Table 2. In the study from the Fred Hutchinson Cancer Research Center, two IGIV products

Table 2 Treatment of CMV-IP with GCV/IGIV in Marrow Transplant Recipients

Center	Patient total	Survival (%)		Time of follow-up
		6 weeks	6 months	
FHCRC[a]	50[b]	25 (50)	16 (32)	9 months
	13[c]	5 (38)	5 (38)	5 months
MSKCC[d]	20[d]	14 (70)	6 (30)	24 months
COH[e]	40	32 (80)	15 (38)	18 months

[a]Data from the Fred Hutchinson Cancer Research Center; updated information courtesy of R. Bowden.
[b]Both groups of FHCRC patients received GCV at 2.5 mg/kg every 8 hours for 14 days and then at 5 mg/kg daily for 14 days. This group of patients received CMV IGIV (Cutter Laboratories) 400 mg/kg on days 1, 2, and 7 of treatment followed by 200 mg/kg on days 14 and 21.
[c]In addition to GCV, these patients received IGIV (Cutter Laboratories) 500 mg/kg every other day for nine doses.
[d]Data from the Memorial Sloan-Kettering Cancer Center, courtesy of D. Emanuel. Patients received GCV at 2.5 mg/kg every 8 hours for 14-20 days and then 5 mg/kg daily five times per week for 20 doses. IGIV (Baxter Healthcare) was given at 500 mg/kg every other day for 10 doses and then every 2 weeks for eight doses.
[e]These patients were treated with GCV at 5 mg/kg given twice daily for 21 days and then given daily five times per week until day 180 after transplantation or until significant immunosuppression was discontinued. IGIV (Baxter Healthcare) was given at 500 mg/kg every other day for 11 doses and then weekly until day 180 after transplantation.

have been used in conjunction with GCV (17). One product (CMV-IGIV) contained high-titer, CMV-specific antibody and was given at a dose of 400 mg/kg on days 1, 2, and 7, and then at half this dose on days 14 and 21. Of 50 patients in this group, 25 (50%) had at least a 6-week survival, and 16 patients (32%) were alive at 6 months, with a median follow-up of 9 months. In an additional group, patients were treated with a standard, commercially available IGIV containing a lower-titer CMV-specific antibody, and given at 500 mg/kg every other day for nine doses. Thirteen patients were entered into this group; five (38%) were alive at 6 weeks, and five (38%) were alive at 6 months, with a median follow-up of 5 months.

In results from Memorial Sloan-Kettering Cancer Center, 20 patients have received a regimen of IGIV consisting of 500 mg/kg every other day for 10 doses, and then every 2 weeks for eight doses (75). In this study, 14 (70%) of 20 patients were alive at 6 weeks, and 10 (30%) at 6 months, with a median follow-up of 24 months.

At the City of Hope, 40 patients have been treated with therapy that included antiviral induction treatment lasting 3 weeks, or until there is documented clearing of pulmonary CMV infection, followed by a maintenance treatment lasting until significant immunosuppressive medications were stopped (76). In this regimen, GCV was given at 10 mg/kg per day and IGIV at 500 mg/kg every other day for 21 days, at which time a repeat bronchoalveolar lavage (BAL) was performed, and if virus and cytology were negative for CMV, then the GCV was given at a dose of 5 mg/kg 5 days per week and IGIV at 500 mg/kg weekly until day +180 after BMT. With this treatment, 32 (80%) marrow recipients were alive 6 weeks after treatment was started, and 16 (40%) at the 6-month mark, with a median follow-up of 18 months.

This therapy was developed in pilot studies that were uncontrolled, but the survival rates were so different from the expected that further placebo-controlled studies in allogeneic BMT would have been unethical. A summary of the incidence of fatal IP at the City of Hope in the years 1980-1989 is shown in Figure 4. Before April 1985, no IGIV was used at City of Hope in BMT recipients, and from then on, different products were used sequentially. There was no significant difference in the incidence of CMV-IP during pilot studies using either conventional IGIV or CMV-antibody-enriched IGIV during 1985-1987. A significant difference in the incidence of fatal IP occurred, however, with the use of a GCV-plus-IGIV treatment regimen in 1987-1989 (23% vs. 3%; $p < 0.003$; see Figure 4). Admittedly, concomitant improvements in the management of marrow transplant recipients have occurred during this same time, and the incidence of fatal IP could have been influenced by these changes. But, conversely, marrow transplantation has been performed on increasingly more difficult patients during this same period, and this would tend to increase the risk for severe CMV-IP.

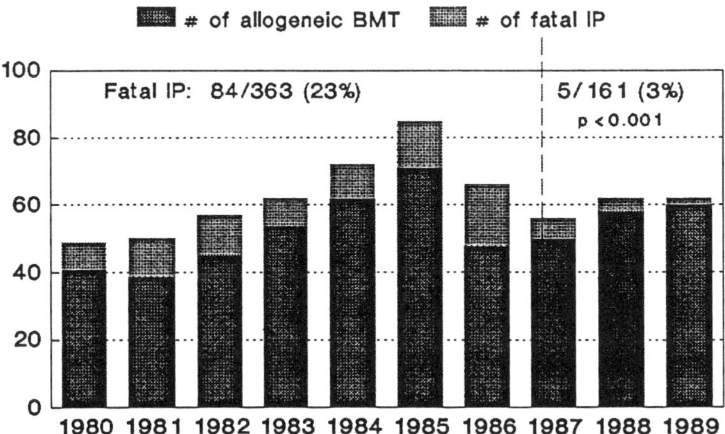

Figure 4 Incidence of fatal interstitial pneumonitis. The total number of bone marrow transplantations (BMT) and of cases of fatal interstitial pneumonitis (IP) occurring from 1980 to 1989 at City of Hope National Medical Center are shown. The vertical broken line indicates the beginning of therapy for cytomegalovirus-associated IP with ganciclovir and intravenous immune globulin.

It does not appear to be possible to clarify the issue regarding the effectiveness of GCV/IGIV for the management of CMV-IP in the BMT recipient with placebo-controlled treatment trials. We have attempted, instead, to analyze our current experience by determining whether CMV-IP remains a risk factor for survival in recently transplanted patients. In this analysis, we assume that CMV-IP should remain a risk factor associated with decreased long-term survival if the GCV/IGIV CMV-IP treatment regimen is not effective. A predictive model for survival has been developed at City of Hope and will be published in detail elsewhere (J. Nyland, personal communication). Briefly, in this model based on data from 72 recent BMT recipients, those with no subsequent IP who are transplanted in first complete remission of acute leukemia, or in first chronic phase of chronic lymphocytic leukemia, have a predicted survival on day 630 of 84% for those transplanted at age 15; this declines to 33% for those transplanted at age 45. Compared to this, patients transplanted with advanced leukemic disease and with subsequent IP will, in the group transplanted at age 15, have a 62% chance of being alive 630 days post-BMT, and this diminished to 4% for those transplanted at age 45. The significant factor in this model is age, and the occurrence of IP has no significant influence. This means that patients with and patients without IP have the same chance of long-term survival in our present BMT regimen, and this surprising result presumably is due to the ability to prevent death from CMV-IP by the initiation of GCV/IGIV treatment.

C. Details of Patient Management for CMV-IP

The treatment regimen for CMV-IP, adopted at many BMT centers in the United States, is similar to the regimen developed at City of Hope, and this is described in Table 3. The diagnosis of CMV-IP is established by BAL based on the occurrence of clinical symptoms, roentgenologic evidence of interstitial pneumonitis, histological or cultural evidence of CMV, and absence of other microbiological or histological explanation of IP. The most rapid and reliable diagnostic test for CMV in our experience has been centrifugal culture of BAL supernant fluid with stain 18 hours later for CMV immediate-early antigen (77). However, cytological evidence of CMV inclusion bodies in cells from BAL in the symptomatic patient is sufficient presumptive evidence for initiation of treatment. The dosage of GCV is 5 mg/kg IV given twice daily unless renal impairment is present (see Table 3). If the absolute neutrophil count is $<1000/mm^3$ for 2 consecutive days, the GCV should be stopped until the leukocyte count recovers. A repeat BAL is recommended

Table 3 Treatment Regimen for CMV-IP

Treatment phase[a]			
Ganciclovir	5 mg/kg	IV	q 12 h
IGIV	500 mg/kg	IV	QOD
Maintenance phase[b]			
Ganciclovir	5 mg/kg	IV	qd 5 days/week
IGIV	500 mg/kg	IV	q week
Dose adjustment[c]			

If neutrophils <1000 mm^3 for 2 consecutive days then discontinue ganciclovir until count recovers.

Renal impairment

Ganciclovir dose (mg/kg)	Dose interval	Serum creatinine
5	q 12 h	0.1-1.4
2.5	q 12 h	1.5-2.5
2.5	q 24 h	2.6-4.5
1.25	q 24 h	>4.5

[a]Treatment is recommended for at least 21 days *and* until clinical improvement and absence of CMV in repeat bronchoalveolar lavage.
[b]Maintenance therapy is recommended to continue until discontinuation of immunosuppressive therapy.
[c]The discontinuation of ganciclovir should also be based on the severity of CMV-IP and on whether the neutropenia is likely to be secondary to CMV infection.

at treatment day 21 to document that the initial antiviral therapy has been effective. We have not observed infectious (i.e., culture-positive) CMV in BAL after 21 days of therapy, but cytological evidence of CMV can be present. We continue induction-level therapy when histological evidence of infection persists. If infectious virus persists in respiratory secretions during therapy, use of another antiviral agent such as foscarnet should be considered.

It is useful to describe in a total of 40 patients the extended results observed at the City of Hope using this approach (76). The median onset of CMV-IP was day 52 post-BMT, with a range of 30-369 days. GCV induction treatment lasted a median of 21 days, with a range of 10-59 days, and GCV maintenance treatment was given for a median of 101 days, with a range of 10-180 days. Most patients responded within the initial 4-7 days of treatment with improvement in respiratory symptoms and signs, and roentgenographic improvement became apparent during the second and third week of therapy depending on disease severity (see Figure 5). Intensive monitoring of respiratory function

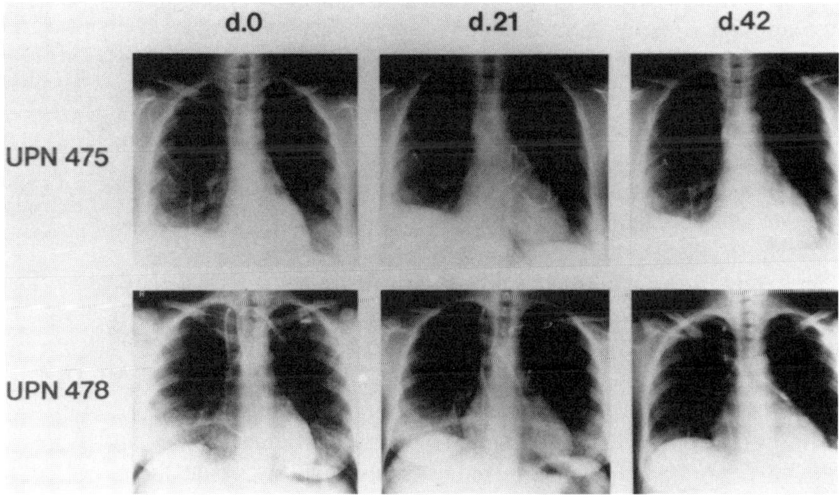

Figure 5 Course of treated human CMV-associated interstitial pneumonia. Two recipients of allogeneic bone marrow transplantation with unique patient numbers (UPN) 475 and 478 were treated with ganciclovir and intravenous immune globulin, as described in the text and in Table 3. Both patients responded to therapy with marked clinical improvement within 1 week. Chest reontgenograms are shown at the start of treatment (d.0), at the end of induction therapy (d.21), and after 21 days of maintenance therapy (d.42). (Adapted from Ref. 19.)

and early intervention for respiratory failure was provided to these patients. Nevertheless, of seven patients requiring mechanical ventilation, none survived the acute disease.

The main side effect was depression of white blood cells, with a pretreatment median of 5000/mm^3 and a nadir of 1200/mm^3. Other side effects included renal impairment, which never required dialysis, blurred vision, transient cortical blindness, and a severe rash with desquamation. Eight patients, or 20% of all patients treated, died within 42 days, and five of those patients died from CMV-IP.

The basis for the long-term maintenance therapy used here is the potential for recurrence of CMV infection and of CMV-IP. The City of Hope treatment regimen is given throughout the period of anti-GVHD therapy, and during this maintenance therapy with GCV-IGIV, we have not seen a case of CMV-IP. Although this treatment has resulted in an initial survival rate from CMV-IP of approximately 80%, this group of transplant recipients subsequently have had additional complications resulting in increased mortality. In total, 26 of the 40 patients treated here eventually died at a median of 152 days post-BMT, or 67 days following the event of interstitial pneumonia. In an attempt to determine the characteristics of those patients who responded to treatment compared to those who did not respond, a multivariant analysis of patient-related parameters was performed. There was no significant difference in outcome contributed by the stage of disease at time of transplantation. Fourteen of the 26 fatalities had been transplanted with advanced neoplastic disease, and 12 were in first clinical remission of acute leukemia or chronic phase of chronic lymphocytic leukemia. Fourteen patients had survived a disease that had a mortality rate of >90%, and they are now at a median of 606 days after bone marrow transplantation, or 531 days post-IP. Six of these 14 were transplanted in advanced disease, and eight were in first complete remission or in chronic phase of leukemia. The incidence of GVHD was not significantly different between those who survived and those who died. Overall, the causes of death in patients with CMV-IP were as follows: five patients died from CMV-IP, eight from GVHD, four from sepsis, four from relapsed leukemia, two with fungal pneumonia, one from veno-occlusive disease, and one with graft failure. In one patient, who died at an outside institution, the cause of death could not be established. Thus, a total of 15% of deaths were due to septic complications in this group of patients. We were concerned about the incidence of fungal sepsis in these patients, but analysis of fungal infections in patients on GCV/IGIV was not different from that in patients not receiving this regimen (data not shown).

D. Mechanism of Action of GCV/IGIV

A question to be raised, of course, is the explanation for the therapeutic effect of GCV/IGIV in this clinical setting. Neither GCV or IGIV, when used alone, appears to be consistently efficacious for treatment of CMV-IP after BMT. Based on the hypothesis described in Section II, it is proposed that the pathogenesis of CMV-IP involves T lymphocytes, which appear to be a common effectors for two events, GVHD and IP (see Figure 2). It is well established that the immune system recognizes major histocompatibility complex (MHC) discrepancies, and, through clonal amplification, mediates clinical GVHD (78). For reasons that are not known, prophylactic use of IGIV significantly decreases GVHD (79). Thus, IGIV appears to act as an immune-response modifier and to alter immune recognition of HLA non-identity. It is therefore possible to conjecture that, in the treatment of CMV-IP, IGIV acts by diminishing a host response to CMV infection. The nature of this host response is not known but is presumed to be an immunological event in some way similar to GVHD, namely, the recognition of differences in cell surfaces. During CMV infection in the lung, viral antigen is expressed and recognized by T cells that directly and indirectly contribute to the pulmonary disease. In the treatment regimen, GCV contributes direct inhibition of virus replication and blockade of both late antigen production and subsequent virus spread. Cessation of CMV replication eventually permits termination of the process that the virus has activated in producing interstitial pneumonia.

V. PREVENTION OF CMV-ASSOCIATED DISEASE AFTER BMT

A. Approaches to CMV Disease Prevention

The general methods that could possibly prevent severe CMV infection after BMT include removal of exogenous exposure to CMV, use of prophylactic antiviral agents, and improvement in functional immune recovery post-BMT. Since most severe disease arises from endogenous virus reactivation (80), it is possible to prevent CMV exposure only in the CMV-seronegative recipient of a seronegative donor. The exogenous source of CMV infection is blood-product use, and restriction to use of CMV-seronegative blood-product donors is protective (81). The presence of a CMV-seropositive donor results in approximately the same rate of CMV infection post-BMT regardless of the serologic status of the recipient (80). Hence, the use of seronegative blood products is effective only in the seronegative recipient of marrow from a seronegative donor. In addition to use of screened blood products, blood-product filtration is currently being evaluated as a method for protection of this type of marrow recipient.

The prevention of reactivation of CMV in the seropositive recipient has been the goal of prophylactic antiviral agents. It has been observed that ACV used at a dose of 500 mg/m² IV given three times daily will significantly diminish CMV excretion and CMV-associated disease in selected marrow recipients (82). In this study, a control group of recipients not otherwise eligible to receive ACV for HSV prophylaxis served as controls. Because of this, there is a question of whether the presence of prior infection with HSV could be protective from CMV disease, but clearly the use of ACV had an antiviral effect that would not be explained by prior HSV immunity. These results have been confirmed in renal transplant recipients who received oral ACV at a dose of 800 mg given four times daily and modified for level of renal function (83). ACV clearly has an antiviral effect against CMV and should be considered as a prophylactic agent for prevention of CMV-IP. However, in clinical practice, CMV-IP continues to occur in the face of ACV prophylaxis, and this is a less than optimal agent for prevention of CMV disease.

Similarly, IGIV, although associated with a reduced incidence of CMV-IP when used prophylactically, cannot be expected to reduce the incidence of CMV-IP to low levels. In this regard, studies with more potent antiviral agents such as foscarnet and ganciclovir have been reported (84,85). Foscarnet appeared to prolong the time to first positive CMV culture (39 ± 4 days vs. 58 ± 5 days; $p < 0.01$), but produced significant toxicity when used with cyclosporin A (84). Ganciclovir also has the problem of toxicity, and since marrow toxicity is a major consideration, its use as a prophylactic agent in the BMT recipient will probably require its use after marrow engraftment has occurred (see below).

Another potential mode for prevention of severe CMV disease after BMT is enhancement of immune recovery. There is no basis in experience for this method, but in theory, assuming that defective immune function is a central feature of pathogenesis (see Figure 2), then enhancement of CMV-specific immune function could prevent disease. Two approaches to this type of preventive therapy have been proposed. A method currently in development at the Fred Hutchinson Cancer Research Center is investigating the potential for adoptive T-cell immune therapy using cloned cells with specific cytotoxic function (86). At City of Hope, investigations are in progress to immunize the marrow donor with a CMV subunit peptide vaccine and determine the antiviral effect in the recipient.

B. Effect of Ganciclovir on Asymptomatic CMV Lung Infection

Asymptomatic CMV lung infection is recognized to occur in immunosuppressed persons, and the natural course of this infection is unknown. In AIDS patients, asymptomatic CMV infection determined by BAL is usually not treated, yet its full significance remains to be determined. In BMT recipients, the detection of CMV in BAL from asymptomatic individuals has been reported to be associated with eventual CMV-IP in approximately 61% of

Table 4 Pulmonary CMV Infection and Risk of CMV-IP in Asymptomatic Allogeneic BMT Recipients

Total	BAL CMV + (%)	CMV-IP (%)	Reference[a]
20	13 (65)	5/13 (38)	87
14	9 (65)	6/9 (67)	88
104	40 (38)	12/17[b] (71)	85

[a]Data adapted from these references includes only results of bronchoalveolar lavage (BAL) and subsequent CMV-interstitial pneumonia (CMV-IP) in patients with no respiratory symptoms at the time of the BAL procedure.
[b]These 17 patients were part of a control group randomly assigned to receive no ganciclovir treatment (see text).

patients (Table 4). In a prospective study of asymptomatic allogeneic marrow recipients at City of Hope, 104 subjects received BAL analysis on day +35 post-BMT, and 40 (38%) of these specimens were positive for CMV (85). These individuals were randomly assigned to receive GCV or no treatment using a dosing regimen of 5 mg/kg per day given twice daily for 14 days and then five times weekly until day +120 post-BMT. In the control group, 10 of 15 developed CMV-IP compared to four of 18 treated persons who either developed CMV-IP or died before completion of treatment ($p = 0.015$). In the treated group, two subjects died or nonviral causes and two subjects developed CMV-IP while on treatment. Of these two, one developed CMV-IP after two doses of GCV, and one was removed from GCV because of azotemia. No subject developed CMV-IP after completing the GCV regimen for asymptomatic pulmonary CMV infection. Clearly, GCV can be used as an effective prophylactic agent after BMT, and use of BAL to define a high-risk group for such treatment is a management approach currently recommended by the authors. Other strategies for use of GCV are currently being investigated and include antiviral treatment at the time of first CVM infection from any site or at early times in all CMV-seropositive persons.

ACKNOWLEDGMENTS

This work was supported by United States Public Health Service grants CA 30206 and CA33572. The authors are grateful for the secretarial assistance of Joan Cass.

REFERENCES

1. Neiman PE, Reeves W, Ray G, Flournoy N, Lerner KG, Sale GE, Thomas ED. A prospective analysis of interstitial pneumonia and opportunistic viral infection among recipients of allogeneic bone marrow grafts. J Infect Dis 1977; 136:754-767.

2. Meyers JD, Fluornoy N, Thomas ED. Nonbacterial pneumonia after allogeneic marrow transplantation. A review of ten years' experience. Rev Infect Dis 1982; 4:1119-1132.
3. Craighead JE. Pulmonary cytomegalovirus infection in the adult. Am J Pathol 1971; 63:487-504.
4. Craighead JE, Hanshaw JB, Carpenter CB. Cytomegalovirus infection after renal allotransplantation. J Am Med Assoc 1967; 201:725-728.
5. Betts RF, Freeman RB, Douglas RG Jr, et al. Clinical manifestations of renal allograft derived primary cytomegalovirus infection. Am J Dis Child 1977; 131: 759-763.
6. Rubin RH, Cosimi AB, Tolkoff-Rubin NE, Russell PS, Hirsch MS. Infectious disease syndromes attributable to cytomegalovirus and their significance among renal transplant recipients. Transplantation 1977; 24:458-464.
7. Pollard RB. Cytomegalovirus infections in renal, heart, heart-lung, and liver transplantation. J Pediatr Infect Dis 1988; 7:S97-S102.
8. Meyers JD, Thomas ED. Infection complicating bone marrow transplantation. In Rubin RH, Young LS (Eds), Clinical Approach to Infection in the Compromised Host, Second Ed. Plenum, New York, pp 525-556.
9. Zaia JA. Understanding human cytomegalovirus infection. In Champlin RE, Gale RP (Eds), New Strategies in Bone Marrow Transplantation: UCLA Symposia on Molecular and Cellular Biology New Series, Vol 137. Wiley-Liss, New York, 1990, pp 319-334.
10. Zaia JA, Lang DJ. Cytomegalovirus infection of the fetus and neonate. Neurolog Clin NA 1984; 2:387-410.
11. Jacobson MA, Mills J. Serious cytomegalovirus disease in the acquired immunodeficiency syndrome (AIDS). Ann Intern Med 1988; 108:585-594.
12. Zaia JA. The biology of human cytomegalovirus infection after bone marrow transplantation. Int J Cell Cloning 1986; 4:135-154.
13. Grundy JE, Shanley JD, Griffiths PD. Is cytomegalovirus interstitial pneumonitis in transplant recipients an immunopathological condition? Lancet 1987; 2:996-999.
14. Quinnan GV Jr, Kirmani N, Rook AH, et al. Cytoxic T cells in cytomegalovirus infection. HLA-restricted T lymphocyte and non-lymphotyce cytotoxic responses correlate with recovery from cytomegalovirus infection in bone marrow transplant recipients. N Engl Med 1982; 307:7-13.
15. Collaborative DHPG Treatment Study Group. Treatment of serious cytomegalovirus infections with 9-(1,3-dihydroxy-2-propoxymethyl)guanine in patients with AIDS and other immunodeficiencies. N Engl J Med 1986; 314:801-805.
16. Buhles WC Jr, Mastre BJ, Tinker AJ, Strand V, Koretz SH, and the Syntex Collaborative Ganciclovir Treatment Study Group. Ganciclovir treatment of life- or sight-threatening cytomegalovirus infection: experience in 314 immunocompromised patients. Rev Infect Dis 1988; 10(suppl 3):S495-S505.
17. Reed EC, Bowden RA, Dandiker PS, Lilleby EK, Meyers JD. Treatment of cytomegalovirus pneumonia with ganciclovir and intravenous cytomegalovirus immunoglobulin in patients with bone marrow transplants. Ann Intern Med 1988; 109:783-788.

18. Reed EC, Wolford JL, Kopecky KJ, Likleby KE, Dandliker PS, Todaro JL, McDonald GB, Meyers JD. Ganciclovir for the treatment of cytomegalovirus gastroenteritis in bone marrow transplant patients. Ann Intern Med 1990; 112:505-510.

19. Zaia JA. Viral infections associated with bone marrow transplantation, Forman SJ (Ed). Hematol Oncol Clin North Am 1990; 4(3):603-623.

20. Spruance SL, Schnipper LE, Overall JC Jr, Kern ER, Wester B, Modlin J, Wenerstrom G, Burton C, Arndt KA, Chiu GL, Crumpacker CS. Treatment of herpes simplex labialis with topical acyclovir in polyethylene glycol. J Infect Dis 1982; 146:85-90.

21. Griffiths PD, Grundy JB. Molecular biology and immunology of cytomegalovirus. Biochemistry 1987; 241:313-325.

22. Ho M. Immunology of cytomegalovirus: Immunosuppressive effects during infections. Birth Defects. Original Article Series 1984; 20:131-147.

23. Carney WP, Hirsch MS. Mechanisms of immunosuppression in CMV mononucleosis. II. Virus-monocyte interactions. J Infect Dis 1981; 144:47-54.

24. Dudding LR, Garnett HM. Interaction of strain AD169 and a clinical isolate of cytomegalovirus with peripheral monocytes: the effect of lipopolysaccharide stimulation. J Infect Dis 1987; 155:891-896.

25. Schrier RD, Oldstone MB. Recent clinical isolates of cytomegalovirus suppress human cytomegalovirus-specific human leukocyte antigen-restricted cytotoxic T-lymphocyte activity. J Virol 1986; 59:127-131.

26. Rodgers BC, Scott DM, Mundin J, Sissons JGP. Monocyte-derived inhibitor of interleukin 1 induced by human cytomegalovirus. J Virol 1985; 55:527-532.

27. Kapasi K, Rice GPA. Cytomegalovirus infection of peripheral blood mononuclear cells: Effects on interleukin-1 and -2 production and responsiveness. J Virol 1988; 62:3603-3607.

28. Dudding L, Haskill S, Clark BD, Auron PE, Sporn S, Huang E-S. Cytomegalovirus infection stimulates expression of monocyte-associated mediator genes. J Immunol 1989; 143:3343-3352.

29. Hirsch MS, Schooley RT, Cosimi AB, Russell PS, Delmonico FL, Tolkoff-Rubin NE, Herrin JT, Cantell K, Farrell ML, Rota TR, Rubin RH. Effects of interferon-alpha on cytomegalovirus reactivation syndromes in renal-transplant recipients. N Engl J Med 1983; 308:1489-1493.

30. Piguet PF, Collart MA, Grau GE, Kapanci Y, Vassalli P. Tumor necrosis factor/cachectin plays a key role in bleomycin-induced pneumopathy and fibrosis. J Exp Med 1989; 170:655-663.

31. Khalil N, Bereznay O, Sporn M, Greenberg AH. Macrophage production of transforming growth factor β and fibroblast collagen synthesis in chronic pulmonary inflammation. J Exp Med 1989; 170:727-737.

32. St. Jeor SC, Albrecht TB, Funk FD, Rapp F. Stimulation of cellular DNA synthesis by human cytomegalovirus. J Virol 1974; 13:353-362.

33. Beck S, Barrell GB. 45kDa CMV protein with ≈ 50 homology to Class I MHC. Nature 1988; 331:269-272.

34. Fujinami RS, Nelson JA, Walker L, Oldstone MA. Sequence homology and immunologic cross-reactivity of human cytomegalovirus with HLA-DR β chain: a means for graft rejection and immunosuppression. J Virol 1988; 62:100-105.

35. Pande H, Terramani T, Churchill MA, Hawkins GG, Zaia J. Regulation of fibronectin gene expression by human cytomegalovirus. J Virol 1990; 64:1366-1369.

36. Crabtree GR. Contingent genetic regulatory events in T lymphocyte activation. Science 1989; 243:355-361.

37. Albrecht T, Boldogh I, Fons M, Lee CH, AbuBakar S, Russell JM, Au WW. Cell-activation responses to cytomegalovirus infection relationship to the phasing of CMV replication and to the induction of cellular damage. Subcellular Biochem 1989; 15:157-202.

38. Albrecht T, Boldogh I, Fons M, AbuBakar S, Deng CZ. Cell activation signals and the pathogenesis of human cytomegalovirus. Intervirology 1990; 31:68-75.

39. Chatila T, Wong R, Young M, Miller R, Terhorst C, Geha RS. An immunodeficiency characterized by defective signal transduction in T lymphocytes. N Engl J Med 1989; 320:696-702.

40. Cherrington JM, Mocarski ES. Human cytomegalovirus ie1 transactivates the α promoter-enhancer via an 18-base-pair repeat element. J Virol 1989; 63:1435-1440.

41. Hunninghake GW, Monick MM, Liu B, Stinski MF. The promoter regulatory region of the major immediate-early gene of human cytomegalovirus responds to T-lymphocyte stimulation and contains functional cyclic AMP-response elements. J Virol 1989; 63:3026-3033.

42. Boldogh I, AbuBakar S, Albrecht T. Activation of proto-oncogenes: an immediate early event in human cytomegalovirus infection. Science 1990; 247:561-564.

43. Duncombe AS, Meager A, Prentice HG, Grundy JE, Heslop HE, Hoffbrand AV, Brenner MK. Gamma interferon and tumor necrosis factor production after bone marrow transplantation is augmented by exposure to marrow fibroblasts infected with cytomegalovirus. Blood 1990; 76:1046-1053.

44. Imagawa DK, Millis JM, Olthoff KM, Derus LJ, Chia D, Sugich LR, Ozawa M, Dempsey RA, Iwaki Y, Levy PJ, Terasaki PI, Busuttil RW. The role of tumor necrosis factor in allograft rejection. I. Evidence that elevated levels of tumor necrosis factor-α predict rejection following orthotopic liver transplantation. Transplantation 1990; 50:219-225.

45. Imagawa DK, Millis JM, Olthoff KM, Seu P, Dempsey RA, Hart J, Terasaki PI, Wasef EM, Busuttil RW. The role of tumor necrosis factor in allograft rejection. II. Evidence that antibody therapy against tumor necrosis factor-α and lymphotoxin enhances cardiac allograft survival in rats. Transplantation 1990; 50:189-193.

46. Symington FW, Pepe MS, Chen AB, Deliganis A. Serum tumor necrosis factor α associated with acute graft-versus-host disease in humans. Transplantation 1990; 50:518-521.

47. Rakusan TA, Juneja HS, Fleischmann WR Jr. Inhibition of hemopoietic colony formation by human cytomegalovirus in vitro. J Infect Dis 1989; 159:127-130.

48. Meyers JE, Fluornoy N, Thomas ED. Risk factors for cytomegalovirus infection after human marrow transplantation. J Infect Dis 1986; 153:478-488.

49. Wingard JR, Chen DY, Burns WH, Fuller DJ, Braine HG, Yeager AM, Kaiser H, Burke PJ, Graham ML, Santos GW, Saral R. Cytomegalovirus infection after autologous bone marrow transplantation with comparison to infection after allogeneic bone marrow transplantation. Blood 1988; 71:1432-1437.
50. Reusser P, Fisher LD, Buckner CD, Thomas ED, Meyers JD. Cytomegalovirus infection after autologous bone marrow transplantation: occurrence of cytomegalovirus disease and effect on engraftment. Blood 1990; 75:1888-1894.
51. Appelbaum FR, Meyers JD, Fefer A, Flournoy N, Cheever MA, Greenberg PD, Hackman R, Thomas ED. Nonbacterial nonfungal pneumonia following marrow transplantation in 100 identical twins. Transplantation 1982; 33:265-268.
52. McDonald GB, Sharma P, Hackman RC, et al. Esophageal infections in immunosuppressed patients after marrow transplantation. Gastroenterology 1985; 88:1111-1117.
53. Verdonck LF, van Heugten H, de Gast GC. Delay in platelet recovery after bone marrow transplantation: impact of cytomegalovirus infection. Blood 1985; 66:921.
54. Emanuel D. Ganciclovir treatment of CMV-associated graft failure. Blood 1989; 74(suppl 1).
55. Meyers JD, McGuffin RW, Neiman PE, Singer JW, Thomas ED. Toxicity and efficacy of human leukocyte interferon for treatment of cytomegalovirus pneumonia after marrow transplantation. J Infect Dis 1980; 141:555-562.
56. Meyers JD, McGuffin RW, Bryson YJ, Cantell K, Thomas ED. Treatment of cytomegalovirus pneumonia after marrow transplant with combined vidarabine and human leukocyte interferon. J Infect Dis 1982; 146:80-84.
57. Wade JC, McGuffin RW, Springmeyer SC, Newton B, Singer JW, Meyers JD. Treatment of cytomegaloviral pneumonia with high-dose acyclovir and human leukocyte interferon. J Infect Dis 1983; 148:557-562.
58. Wade JC, Hintz M, McGuffin RW, Springmeyer SC, Connor JD, Meyers JD. Treatment of cytomegalovirus pneumonia with high dose acyclovir. Am J Med 1982; 73:249-256.
59. Levin MJ, Leary PL. Inhibition of human herpesvirus by combinations of acyclovir and human leukocyte interferon. Infect Immunol 1981; 32:995-999.
60. Spector SA, Tyndall M, Kelley E. Effects of acyclovir combined with other antiviral agents on human cytomegalovirus. Am J Med 1982; 73:36-39.
61. Wade JC, McGuffin RW, Springmeyer SC, Newton B, Singer JW, Meyers JD. Treatment of cytomegaloviral penumonia with high-dose acyclovir and human leukocyte interferon. J Infect Dis 1983; 148:557-562.
62. Shepp DH, Newton BA, Meyers JD. Intravenous lymphoblastoid interferon and acyclovir for treatment of cytomegaloviral pneumonia. J Infect Dis 1984; 150:776-777.
63. Ringden O, Wilczek H, Lonnqvist, Gahrton G, Wahren AB, Lernestedt J-O. Foscarnet for cytomegalovirus infections. Lancet 1985; 1:1503-1504.
64. Shepp DH, Dandiker PS, de Miranda P, et al. Activity of 9-[2-hydroxy-1-(hydroxymethyl)ethoxymethyl]guanine in the treatment of cytomegalovirus pneumonia. Ann Intern Med 1985; 103:368-373.

65. Erice A, Jordan MC, Chace BA, Fletcher C, Chinnock BJ, Balfour HH Jr. Ganciclovir treatment of cytomegalovirus disease in transplant recipients and other immunocompromised hosts. J Am Med Assoc 1987; 257:3082-3087.

66. Winston DJ, Ho WG, Bartoni K, Holland GN, Mitsuyasy RT, Gale RP, Busuttil RW, Champlin RE. Ganciclovir therapy for cytomegalovirus infections in recipients of bone marrow transplants and other immunosuppressed patients. Rev Infect Dis 1988; 10(supplement 3):S547-S553.

67. Crumpacker C, Marlowe S, Zhang JL, Abrams S, Watkins P, and the Ganciclovir Bone Marrow Transplant Treatment Group. Treatment of cytomegalovirus pneumonia. Rev Infect Dis 1988; 10(supplement 3):S538-S546.

68. Reed EC, Dandliker PS, Meyers JD. Treatment of cytomegalovirus pneumonia with 9-[2-hydroxy-1-(hydroxymethyl)ethoxymethyl]guanine in the treatment of cytomegalovirus pneumonia. Ann Intern Med 1986; 105:214-216.

69. Blacklock HA, Griffiths P, Stirk P, Prentice HG. Specific hyperimmune globulin for cytomegalovirus pneumonitis. Lancet 1985; 2:152-153.

70. Reed EC, Bowden RA, Dandiker PS, Gleaves CA, Meyers JD. Efficacy of cytomegalovirus immunoglobulin in marrow transplant recipients with cytomegalovirus pneumonia. J Infect Dis 1987; 156:641-645.

71. Shanley JD, Pesanti EL. The relation of viral replication to interstitial pneumonitis in murine cytomegalovirus lung infection. J Infec Dis 1985; 151:454-458.

72. Wilson EJ, Medearis DN Jr, Hansen LA, Rubin RH. 9-(1,3-dihydroxy-2-propoxymethyl)guanine prevents death but not immunity in murine cytomegalovirus-infected normal and immunosuppressed BALB/c mice. Antimicrob Agents Chemother 1987; 31:1017-1020.

73. Reed EC, Bowden RA, Dandliker PS, Meyers JD. Treatment of cytomegalovirus (CMV) pneumonia in bone marrow transplant (BMT) patients (PTS) with ganciclovir (GCV) and CMV immunoglobulin (CMV-IG). Blood 1987; 70(suppl 1):313a.

74. Bratanow N, Ash RC, Turner P, Smith R, Chitambar C, Hansen R, Casper J, Haasler G. The use of 9(1,3-dihydroxy-2-propoxymethyl)guanine (ganciclovir, DHPG) and intravenous immunoglobulin (IVIG) in the treatment of serious cytomegalovirus (CMV) infections in thirty-one allogeneic bone marrow transplant (BMT) patients. Blood 1987; 70(suppl 1):302a.

75. Emanuel D, Cunningham I, Jules-Elysee K, Brochstein JA, Kernan NA, Laver J, Stover D, White DA, Fels A, Polsky B, Castro-Malaspina H, Peppard JR, Bartus P, Hammerling U, O'Reilly RJ. Cytomegalovirus pneumonia after bone marrow transplantation successfully treated with the combination of ganciclovir and high-dose intravenous immune globulin. Ann Intern Med 1988; 109:777-782.

76. Schmidt GM, Kovacs A, Zaia JA, Horak DA, Blume KG, Nademanee AP, O'Donnell MR, Snyder DS, Forman SJ. Ganciclovir/immunoglobulin combination therapy for the treatment of human cytomegalovirus-associated interstitial pneumonia in bone marrow allograft recipients. Transplantation 1988; 46:905-907.

77. Swenson PD, Kaplan MH. Rapid detection of cytomegalovirus in cell culture by indirect immunoperoxidase staining with monoclonal antibody to an early nuclear antigen. J Clin Microbiol 1985; 21:669-673.
78. Vogelsang GB, Wagner JE. Graft-versus-host disease, Forman SJ (Ed). Hematol Oncol Clin North Am 1990; 4:625-639.
79. Sullivan KM, Kopecky KJ, Jocom J, Fisher L, Buckner CD, Meyers JD, Counts GW, Bowden RA, Petersen FB, Witherspoon RP, Budinger MD, Schwartz RS, Appelbaum FR, Clift RA, Hansen JA, Sanders JE, Thomas ED, Storb R. Immunomodulatory and antimicrobial efficacy of intravenous immunoglobulin in bone marrow transplantation. N Engl J Med 1990; 323:705-712.
80. Meyers J. Prevention of cytomegalovirus infection after marrow transplantation. Rev Infect Dis 1989; 11(suppl 7):S1691-S1705.
81. Bowden RA, Sayers M, Flournoy N, Nehon B, Banaji M, Thomas ED, Meyers JD. Cytomegalovirus immune globulin and seronegative blood products to prevent primary cytomegalovirus infection after marrow transplantation. N Engl J Med 1986; 314:1006-1010.
82. Meyers JD, Reed EC, Shepp DH, Thornquist M, Dandliker PS, Vicary CA, Flournoy N, Kirk LE, Kersey JH, Thomas ED, Balfour HH Jr. Acyclovir for prevention of cytomegalovirus infection and disease after allogeneic marrow transplantation. N Engl J Med 1988; 318:70-75.
83. Balfour HH Jr, Chace BA, Stapleton JT, Simmons RL, Fryd DS. A randomized, placebo-controlled trial of oral acyclovir for the prevention of cytomegalovirus disease in recipients of renal allografts. N Engl J Med 1989; 320:1381-1387.
84. Ringden O, Lonnqvist B, Aschan J, Sundberg B. Foscarnet prophylaxis in marrow transplant recipients. Bone Marrow Transplantation 1989; 4:713.
85. Schmidt GM, Horak DA, Niland JC, Duncan SR, Forman SF, Zaia JA. A randomized, controlled study trial of prophylactic ganciclovir for cytomegalovirus pulmonary infection in allogeneic bone marrow transplant recipients. N Engl J Med 1991; 324:1005-1011.
86. Greenberg P. Adoptive immunotherapy and HCMV infection: future role in protection from disease progression. In Zaia JA, Hooper J (Eds.), Pathogenesis of Human Cytomegalovirus-Associated Diseases, Transplant Proceedings 1991, in press.
87. Leskinen R, Tukainen P, Taskinen P, et al. Bronchoalveolar lavage in the diagnosis of pulmonary complications in bone marrow transplant recipients—preliminary experience. Exp Hematol 1984; 12(suppl 15):24-25.
88. Ruutu P, Ruutu T, Volin L, Tukiainen P, Ukkonen P, Hovi T. Cytomegalovirus is frequently isolated in bronchoalveolar lavage fluid of bone marrow transplant recipients without pneumonia. Ann Intern Med 1990; 112:913-916.

12

Cytomegalovirus Resistance to Ganciclovir

M. Colin Jordan
University of Minnesota Medical School
Minneapolis, Minnesota

Karen K. Biron
The Wellcome Research Laboratories
Burroughs Wellcome Company
Research Triangle Park, North Carolina

I. INTRODUCTION

During the past decade, the acquired immunodeficiency syndrome (AIDS) and the increasing use of organ transplantation have greatly affected the frequency and nature of cytomegalovirus (CMV) infection (1-4). Fortunately, ganciclovir has been available during much of this time as the first antiviral agent that significantly inhibits replication of CMV (5). It might have been anticipated, however, that the chronic and relentless nature of CMV disease in severely immunosuppressed patients would be associated with the eventual development of viral resistance to ganciclovir. Thus, fatal CMV disease due to resistant strains of the virus has now been reported in three patients, two of whom had AIDS (6). However, resistance does not appear to be widespread at the present time despite the frequent use of ganciclovir and the necessity for prolonged or repeated courses of therapy. In this chapter, the current status of ganciclovir resistance among CMV strains will be reviewed and the implications of drug resistance will be discussed.

II. A GANCICLOVIR-RESISTANT LABORATORY CMV MUTANT

The first report describing a strain of CMV resistant to ganciclovir was that of Biron and colleagues in 1986 (7). These investigators plaque-purified a clone of the AD169 laboratory strain of CMV and serially passaged the virus in increasing concentrations of the drug. After several passages, they selected a clone of AD169 (759^r D100-1) that could productively infect human diploid fibroblasts in the presence of concentrations of ganciclovir as high as 100 μM. The amount of ganciclovir required to reduce plaque formation of the mutant virus by 50% (ED$_{50}$) was approximately 10-fold higher than that required to inhibit the parent AD169 strain. Similar differences were found in experiments in which the amounts of virus released by infected cells were quantitated. The ganciclovir-resistant laboratory mutant of AD169 retained its susceptibility to compounds that inhibit the viral DNA polymerase [i.e., phosphonoacetic acid (PAA), phosphonoformic acid (PFA), and aphidocolin], suggesting that mutation of the CMV polymerase gene was not responsible for the resistance that developed.

More recent drug susceptibility studies have indicated the presence of a DNA polymerase alteration in this laboratory mutant based on in vitro cross-resistance to the monophosphate nucleotide analog HPMPC. This drug-resistance phenotype has subsequently been genetically separated from the ganciclovir phosphorylation-deficient phenotype. The resulting virus is only marginally resistant to ganciclovir and is fully competent to induce ganciclovir anabolism in virus-infected cells (V. Sullivan et al., presented at the International Herpes Virus Workshop, Georgetown University, Washington, D.C., August 1990). The intracellular phosphorylation of ganciclovir by the parent resistant mutant 759^{r}D100-1 was found to be reduced by 90% compared to the AD169 virus, whereas normal cellular nucleoside and deoxynucleoside levels were not reduced. Since ganciclovir usually persists in CMV-infected cells at high levels in its triphosphorylated form (7-12), the most likely mechanism for ganciclovir resistance was reduction in the activity of a CMV-encoded enzyme involved in phosphorylation of the drug (7). Similar results were recently reported by Lurain et al. (13).

III. FATAL DISEASE DUE TO GANCICLOVIR-RESISTANT CMV

The experiments of Biron et al. (7) and Lurain et al. (13) indicated that strains of CMV resistant to ganciclovir could be selected in the laboratory. These findings also raised the issue of whether resistant CMV strains might also be recovered from patients undergoing treatment with the drug. As noted in Chapter 1, the vast majority of clinical isolates of CMV are inhibited by

ED_{50} concentrations of the drug ranging from 0.5 to 5.9 μM (14-19). The susceptibility of CMV strains recovered before and after ganciclovir therapy has usually remained unchanged (14,15,19). However, a few CMV strains with relatively high ED_{50} values for ganciclovir have been noted. Shepp et al. (14) isolated a strain of CMV with an ED_{50} for ganciclovir of 11.3 μM from the lung of a marrow transplant recipient. After treatment with the drug, however, the virus was not available for further study. In another report, Cole and Balfour (19) isolated a CMV strain with an ED_{50} for ganciclovir of 7.11 μM from a renal transplant patient who had been treated with acyclovir for 14 days.

Clinically important resistance of CMV to ganciclovir was first reported by Erice and colleagues (6) in 1989. In this study, ganciclovir-resistant strains were recovered on numerous occasions from three patients, all of whom died of progressive CMV disease. All of the patients had received multiple courses of induction and maintenance therapy. The susceptibility to ganciclovir of the early and late CMV isolates recovered from the three patients is shown in Table 1. The CMV strain recovered from patient 1 was already resistant to ganciclovir prior to therapy with the drug. During therapy, the ED_{50} of the infecting CMV strain doubled while the ED_{90} and ED_{99} values increased even more. In patients 2 and 3, the ED_{50} values of the CMV strains recovered from the blood increased by factors of 8.4 and 11.6, respectively, over the pretreatment values. The magnitude of this increase in ganciclovir resistance is remarkably similar to that detected in the laboratory mutant described by Biron et al. (7) and discussed above.

Table 1 Susceptibility to Ganciclovir of Early and Late CMV Isolates of Three Patients

CMV isolates	Source	Day of treatment	ED_{50}[a]	ED_{90}[a]	ED_{99}[a]
Patient 1					
Early	Urine	Pretreatment	14.4	127	752
Late	Blood	79	30.5	457	4162
Patient 2					
Early	Blood	3	2.1	14.1	67
Late	Blood	131	17.7	217	1672
Patient 3					
Early	Blood	2	1.4	23.8	346
Late	Blood	60	16.2	445	6030
AD169 control	—	—	3.8	13.2	35.9

[a]Values expressed as micromoles (μM).

Each of the patients from whom ganciclovir-resistant strains of CMV were recovered experienced a relentlessly progressive downhill course. Although it was suspected that the failure to respond to ganciclovir might have reflected the deterioration of the patients' immune systems, the CMV isolates were tested for their susceptibility to the drug. Because the course of each of these patients is instructive in terms of when to suspect drug resistance, they will be summarized briefly here.

Patient 1 was a 58-year-old woman who developed CMV retinitis as a complication of chronic lymphocytic leukemia. She received a 15-day course of ganciclovir at the usual induction dose. Although the retinitis appeared to stabilize, a blood leukocyte culture on the 12th day of treatment with ganciclovir was positive for CMV. A second course of treatment was required 1 month later, and CMV was recovered from two of three blood cultures during therapy. During a third course of therapy, a retinal detachment occurred and was repaired surgically. Subsequently, the patient experienced persistent fever and her retinitis failed to respond to ganciclovir given at a dose of 5 mg per kilogram every 8 hours for 34 days. During this time, CMV was recovered from 10 of 12 blood cultures. Despite the addition of intravenous immunoglobulin to the ganciclovir therapy, the patient died.

Patient 2 was a 33-year-old homosexual man with AIDS who was admitted with fever and liver dysfunction. Cultures of his blood, urine, oropharynx, and bronchoalveolar lavage fluid and biopsy specimens of liver tissue were positive for CMV. Although the patient defervesced, CMV was recovered from numerous sites, including four of five blood cultures, during therapy. Six weeks later the patient was readmitted with CMV retinitis and fever. A 37-day course of ganciclovir was administered at various doses, but seven of nine blood cultures remained positive for CMV. The patient received ganciclovir for an additional 74 days as an outpatient. He remained febrile most of the time and developed CMV pneumonitis diagnosed by open-lung biopsy. He died of progressive respiratory failure and CMV was recovered from additional blood cultures despite ganciclovir therapy.

Patient 3 was a 28-year-old homosexual man with AIDS and intestinal lymphoma. He received a 10-day course of ganciclovir for CMV colitis. Two months later, he developed CMV viremia and pneumonitis. He responded to a 2-week course of ganciclovir although one of three blood cultures obtained during therapy was positive. Subsequently, CMV retinitis developed despite 82 days of maintenance therapy. Twenty of 28 blood cultures were positive for CMV during this time. The patient then developed persistent fever, and all six blood cultures obtained over the ensuing 53 days of ganciclovir treatment were positive. The patient died suddenly during a febrile episode.

At the University of Minnesota, a fourth patient with progressive disease due to a ganciclovir-resistant strain of CMV was recently encountered. A

66-year-old man with chronic lymphocytic leukemia developed persistent CMV viremia and recurrence of a large ulcerative gastric lesion despite prolonged therapy with high doses of the drug. The CMV isolates recovered from the patient's blood and gastric biopsy had become highly resistant to ganciclovir.

From study of these cases, it is apparent that CMV strains with ED_{50} values for ganciclovir over 14 μM are difficult to eradicate and can be considered resistant to the drug in vivo. In addition, CMV strains resistant to the drug remain fully virulent and are capable of causing fatal disease.

IV. FREQUENCY OF CMV RESISTANCE TO GANCICLOVIR

Little information is currently available concerning the frequency of ganciclovir resistance in strains of CMV recovered from patients treated with the drug. Drew and colleagues (20) monitored prospectively viral isolates recovered from the urine of 72 AIDS patients treated with ganciclovir for CMV retinitis. Over a 7-month period, CMV could not be recovered from the urine in 78-80% of the patients. No ganciclovir-resistant strains were recovered from 33 patients before therapy or from seven culture-positive patients treated for less than 3 months. However, of 13 culture-positive patients treated for more than 3 months, ganciclovir-resistant (ED_{50} greater than 12 μM) strains of CMV were recovered from five. In an additional three of the 13 patients, the CMV isolates recovered had ED_{50} values between 6 and 12 μM. Overall, CMV strains resistant to ganciclovir were isolated from five of the 72 patients treated (6.9%) or from five of 13 (38.4%) patients who shed the virus while receiving the drug. Progression of CMV retinitis could not be correlated with the development of resistance among urinary CMV isolates. In addition, the patients who were shedding resistant strains of CMV did not develop the progressive CMV disease seen with the resistant strains reported by Erice and colleagues (6). Whether this difference reflects better control of the underlying HIV infection in patients receiving zidovudine or other factors is not clear.

V. MECHANISMS INVOLVED IN CLINICAL RESISTANCE TO GANCICLOVIR

A total of 10 ganciclovir-resistant CMV isolates recovered from the patients reported by Erice et al. (6) and by Drew and colleagues (20) have been studied in terms of mechanisms of resistance by Biron et al. (21). When the ganciclovir-resistant clinical isolates were examined for their ability to induce phosphorylation of the drug during infection of cells, a consistent correlation was noted between the in vitro susceptibility of an isolate to ganciclovir and its drug anabolism competency (Table 2). In order to assess the ganciclovir-phosphorylating potential, virus-infected cells were incubated with [^{14}C]-labeled ganciclovir for various times, and the phosphorylated forms present in cell extracts were analyzed by a cation-exchange method (7). To determine whether alteration of the viral DNA polymerase was contributing to the ganciclovir resistance of these isolates, the DNA polymerases from one pair of isolates, those recovered from patient 2 of the study by Erice et al. (6), were examined for comparative inhibition by ganciclovir-triphosphate (Table 3). Plaque-purified virus was derived from the pretherapy, ganciclovir-sensitive and the posttherapy, ganciclovir-resistant isolates for these experiments. The results indicate that the viral DNA polymerases of both the sensitive and resistant virus were equally inhibited by the triphosphates of ganciclovir. Inhibition values for the triphosphate of the related nucleoside analog acyclovir as well for the DNA polymerase inhibitor PAA were comparable and similar to those measured for inhibition of the DNA polymerase of strain AD169.

Taken together, these studies illustrate the importance of the intracellular phosphorylation of ganciclovir in the antiviral activity of this drug. The phenotype of these ganciclovir-resistant isolates is similar to the TK-deficient or

Table 2 Ganciclovir Susceptibility and Intracellular Anabolism

Virus strain[a]	GCV ED$_{50}$ (μM)[b]	Phosphorylated GCV (pmol/10^6 cells)[c]
C8918	10.8	20.6
C8917	11.9	21.6
C8916	12.7	15.7
C8915	27.7	9.4
C8912	2.6	90.6
C8913	8.5	33.8
C8914	31.4	19.5
AD169	3.3	59.9
759^{r}D100-1	31.5	8.4
MRC-5 cells	—	6.5

[a]Virus isolates were obtained from L. Drew, Mount Zion Hospital (19). Laboratory control strains include AD169 and the ganciclovir-resistant mutant 759rD100-1 (7).
[b]Ganciclovir susceptibilities were measured using a DNA hybridization assay (Diagnostic Hybrids, Inc., Athens, OH) in MRC-5 lung fibroblasts (33) (American Type Culture Collection, Rockville, MD).
[c]Virus-infected or uninfected MRC-5 cells were incubated with 25 μM [^{14}C]-ganciclovir for 16 hours, day 4 postinfection. Intracellular anabolism of ganciclovir was measured by cation-exchange methods of cell extracts (7).

Table 3 CMV Polymerase and Hela Polymerase Studies

Enzyme	GCV-TP K_i (μM)[a]	dGTP K_m (μM)	Virus GCV inhibition ED_{50} (μM)[b]
Hela pol	16	0.51	
AD169	0.55	1.1	3.5
Pt 2 early (Cl 17-1-1)[c]	0.31	0.79	2.0
Pt 2 late (Cl 9-4-1)[c]	0.28	0.83	25

[a]K_i values were obtained from the $-x$ intercept of Dixon plots where $-x = K_i(1 + S/K_m)$.
[b]Ganciclovir susceptibilities were measured by a plaque-reduction assay in MRC-5 lung fibroblasts.
[c]Patient 2 as described in Ref. 6.

TK-altered variants of herpes simplex or varicella zoster viruses that arise in AIDS patients under prolonged, selective drug pressure with acyclovir. The in vitro susceptibility patterns of the ganciclovir-resistant isolates to various anti-CMV agents indicate that the viruses remain sensitive to agents that serve as substrates for phosphorylation by cellular enzymes [2'-fluoro-5-iodoarabinosylcytosine (FIAC), 2'-fluoro-5-iodoarabinosyluridine (FIAU), adenine arabinoside (Ara-A)], or to those that do not require initial phosphorylation [(s)-9-(3-hydroxy-2-phosphonyl-methoxypropyl]adenine (HPMPA)], HPMPC, and PFA.

In addition to those biochemical findings, other factors related to mixed populations of CMV strains appear to be involved in the development of drug resistance. In the study by Erice et al. (6), the initially resistant CMV strain recovered from patient 1 persisted throughout multiple courses of ganciclovir therapy. The restriction endonuclease pattern of the CMV DNA was identical for the early and late isolates. In patient 2, resistant virus arising through random mutation was presumably selected after multiple courses of ganciclovir, although no alterations in viral DNA were detected with restriction endonuclease analysis. Careful analyses of the antiviral drug susceptibility curves of these two isolates has suggested the presence of a fraction of virus resistant to araA in the posttherapy isolate (Biron, unpublished data). This araA-resistant phenotype was not retained in the final plaque-purified ganciclovir-resistant virus used for DNA polymerase studies (Table 3).

Chou (personal communication) has now been able to detect genetic differences in the DNA polymerase gene amplified by the polymerase chain reaction from the two strains of CMV recovered from this patient. In this regard, specific alterations in either the herpes simplex or varicella zoster virus DNA polymerase have produced cross-resistance in the resulting virus mutants to both acyclovir and araA (22,23). Additionally, resistance of herpes simplex and varicella zoster viruses to acyclovir or ganciclovir has been shown to result from single-base changes in either the virus-encoded thymidine kinase or DNA polymerase genes (24-26). In patient 3, a genetically distinct new strain of CMV emerged during ganciclovir therapy. The extremely high ED_{90} and ED_{99} values for ganciclovir against the initial CMV strain tested (Table 1) may have been a clue that drug resistance might develop in this patient during therapy. In the case of herpes simplex virus, high pretreatment ED_{90} and ED_{99} values indicate a mixed population of viruses varying in susceptibility to acyclovir (27,28). Prolonged treatment of severely immunocompromised patients with acyclovir may then allow the resistant clone of HSV to emerge. Since patients with AIDS and solid-organ transplant patients are often infected with multiple strains of CMV (29,30), ganciclovir therapy in patient 3 may have selected a resistant clone of virus from the mixed population present prior to therapy.

VI. IMPLICATIONS OF RESISTANCE FOR USE OF GANCICLOVIR

As discussed in Chapters 5-8, ganciclovir treatment of CMV retinitis in patients with AIDS requires a course of induction therapy followed by a protracted period of maintenance therapy. This approach has been shown to delay significantly the progression of retinitis or the appearance of new retinal lesions. Whether maintenance therapy after ganciclovir induction is required for treatment CMV gastrointestinal disease in patients with AIDS is not clear, although it seems likely. On the other hand, recipients of solid-organ transplants appear to have a much lower rate of relapse after treatment of CMV disease with ganciclovir, and maintenance therapy is usually unnecessary (Chapter 9). Perhaps related to these differences, the development of resistance to ganciclovir by CMV has been reported primarily in patients with AIDS. Resistance of CMV to ganciclovir has not been described in solid-organ transplant recipients or in bone marrow transplant patients. These observations suggest that ganciclovir resistance is most likely to develop in patients who require prolonged maintenance therapy or repeated courses of induction therapy. In addition, persistent shedding of CMV during treatment appears to be associated with the development of drug resistance and may actually be an indicator of resistance, in a minority of instances, by the selection mechanisms noted previously (21).

These events would suggest that some degree of prudence in the use of ganciclovir is in order. Injudicious use of the drug should be avoided, and therapy should be reserved for treatment of patients who have or who are very likely to have CMV disease. Thus, patients who are simply shedding the virus in secretions (e.g., urine, saliva, bronchoalveolar lavage fluid, or semen) should not be treated unless other evidence of CMV disease is present. In immunosuppressed patients, treatment with ganciclovir is appropriate whenever CMV infection is documented by detection of typical intranuclear inclusions in biopsied tissue or in bronchoalveolar lavage fluid. Treatment may also be appropriate if CMV antigens are found by immunological staining of an inflammatory lesion (e.g., esophagitis, gastritis, colitis, hepatitis, or pneumonitis). Recovery of virus from peripheral blood leukocytes (viremia) is often but not always associated with the presence of or the subsequent development of CMV disease. For example, protracted asymptomatic CMV viremia has been described without evidence of organ involvement in marrow recipients (31). At the University of Minnesota, a number of asymptomatic solid-organ transplant recipients have been found to be viremic and have not developed CMV disease over period of several months of observation. However, ganciclovir therapy is probably indicated if such viremic patients should become febrile or develop leukopenia, thrombocytopenia, or liver dysfunction (i.e., a "CMV syndrome") (32). For a thorough review of diagnostic procedures available for identifying CMV disease, see Chapter 14.

During treatment with ganciclovir, cultures for CMV are rendered negative in most patients. Viremia is almost invariably eradicated by successful therapy. Persistent viral shedding in bodily secretions, however, is not usually due to the development of ganciclovir-resistant strains of CMV. On the other hand, positive viral cultures from peripheral blood leukocytes ("breakthrough viremia"), especially if associated with fever or other symptoms and signs, may well reflect the development of CMV resistance. Based on experience reported to date, persistence of viremia while the patient is receiving ganciclovir is an indication for viral susceptibility testing. (See Chapter 14 for a review of viral-susceptibility testing procedures.) Thus, patients receiving ganciclovir should be monitored with periodic blood cultures in order to detect drug resistance in its early stages.

Several studies are under way that will provide important information on the optimal use of ganciclovir. For example, the most appropriate treatment regimen for CMV retinitis in patients with AIDS has not yet been fully defined. Should all AIDS patients with retinitis be treated immediately, or should those with peripheral lesions that are not an immediate threat to vision be observed and treated only if the lesion progresses? Taking into account drug toxicity, cost, inconvenience, infectious complications of indwelling intravenous access devices, and the possible development of ganciclovir resistance, which approach is in the best interests of the patient on a long-term basis? On many occasions, however, the hand of the clinician is forced toward long-term ganciclovir therapy in certain patients. These instances include relapse of chorioretinitis, the appearance of a new retinal lesion, persistent viremia with high spiking fever, or the development or relapse of visceral organ involvement. Although these are the precise circumstances in which CMV resistance to ganciclovir appears most likely to develop, the physician has no choice except to treat the patient.

Fortunately, strains of CMV that have developed resistance to ganciclovir to date have retained their susceptibility to such antiviral agents as PFA (foscarnet), HPMPC, and HPMPA (21). In the future, the clinician may have a choice of effective drugs for treatment of CMV disease, with selection tailored to the individual patient on the basis of known efficacy and toxicity data. It is also possible that antiviral agents active against CMV may be used in combination or in alternating regimens to prevent the selection of drug-resistant CMV strains.

VII. CONCLUSIONS

In summary, ganciclovir-resistant strains of CMV have been produced in the laboratory and have been recovered from patients with fatal CMV disease. In both instances, resistance to ganciclovir is associated with failure of the virus to convert the drug to its triphosphorylated form within infected cells. At the present time, resistance to ganciclovir is extremely rare among CMV strains recovered from patients who have not been treated with the drug. However, resistance may develop in CMV strains recovered from patients who have received multiple courses or prolonged periods of therapy. Further studies are necessary to determine the importance of CMV ganciclovir resistance and to define optimal treatment strategies with the drug.

ACKNOWLEDGMENTS

The authors thank Jo-Ellyn Pilarski for preparation of the manuscript. This chapter was supported by Public Health Service NIH grants HL35374, AM 13083, and CA21737 and by the George Nelson Fund.

REFERENCES

1. Jacobson MA, Mills J. Serious cytomegalovirus disease in the acquired immunodeficiency syndrome (AIDS). Ann Intern Med 1988; 108:585-594.
2. Drew WL. Cytomegalovirus infection in patients with AIDS. J Infect Dis 1988; 158:449-456.
3. Ho M. Cytomegalovirus. In Mandell GL, Douglas RG, Bennett JE (Eds), Principles and Practice of Infectious Diseases, 3rd ed., Churchill Livingstone, New York, 1990, pp 1159-1172.
4. Jordan MC. Cytomegalovirus infections. In Hoeprich PD, Jordan MC (Eds), Infectious Diseases, 4th ed. Lippincott, Philadelphia, 1989, pp 805-812.
5. Fletcher CV, Balfour, Jr. HH. Evaluation of ganciclovir for cytomegalovirus disease. Drug Intell Clin Pharm 1989; 23:5-11.

6. Erice A, Chou S, Biron KK, Stanat BS, Balfour HH Jr, Jordan MC. Progressive disease due to ganciclovir-resistant cytomegalovirus in immunocompromised patients. N Eng J Med 1989; 320:289-293.

7. Biron KK, Fyfe JA, Stanat SC, Leslie LK, Sorrell JB, Lambe CU, Coen DM. A human cytomegalovirus mutant resistant to the nucleoside analog 99-{[2-hydroxy-1-(hydroxymethyl) ethoxy]methyl}guanine (BWB759U) induces reduced levels of BWB759U triphosphate. Proc Natl Acad Sci 1986; 83:8769-8773.

8. Mar EC, Chiou JF, Cheng YC, Huang ES. Inhibition of cellular DNA polymerase and human cytomegalovirus-induced DNA polymerase by the triphosphates of 9-(2-hydroxyethoxymethyl)guanine and 9-(1,3-dihydroxy-2-propoxymethyl)guanine. J Virol 1985; 53:776-780.

9. Biron KK, Stanat SC, Sorrell JB, Fyfe JA, Keller PM, Lambe CU, Nelson DJ. Metabolic activation of the necleoside analog 9-{[2-hydroxy-1-(hydroxymethyl)-ethoxy]methyl}guanine in human diploid fibroblasts infected with human cytomegalovirus. Proc Natl Acad Sci USA 1985; 82:2473-2477.

10. Lewis RA, Watkins L, St. Jeor S. Enhancement of deoxyguanosine kinase activity in human lung fibroblast cells infected with human cytomegalovirus. Molec Cellular Biochem 1985; 65:67-71.

11. Meyer H, Brugemann CA, Dormans PHK, van Boven CPA. Human cytomegalovirus induces a cellular deoxyguanosine kinase, also interacting with acyclovir. FEMS Microbiol Lett 1984; 25:283-287.

12. Smee DF. Interaction of 9-(1,3-dihydroxy-2-propoxymethyl) guanine with cytosol and mitochondrial deoxyguanosine kinases: possible role in anti-cytomegalovirus activity. Molec Cell Biochem 1985; 69:75-81.

13. Lurain NS, Tatarowicz WA, Read GS, Thompson KD. Characterization of mutants of human cytomegalovirus resistant to ganciclovir. Second International Cytomegalovirus Workshop, San Diego, California, March 27-30, 1989, abstract 66.

14. Shepp DH, Dandliker PS, de Miranda P, et al. Activity of 9-[2-hydroxy-1-(hydroxymethyl)ethoxymethyl]guanine in the treatment of cytomegalovirus pneumonia. Ann Intern Med 1985; 103:368-373.

15. Felsenstein D, D'amica DJ, Hirsch MS, et al. Treatment of cytomegalovirus retinitis with 9-[2-hydroxy-1-(hydroxymethyl) ethoxymethyl]guanine. Ann Intern Med 1985; 103:377-380.

16. Mar EC, Cheng YC, Huang ES. Effect of 9-(1,3-dihydroxy-2-propoxymethyl)guanine on human cytomegalovirus replication *in vitro*. Antimicrob Agents Chemother 1983; 24:518-521.

17. Tyms AS, Davis JM, Jeffries DJ, Meyers JD. BWB759U, an analogue of acyclovir, inhibits human cytomegalovirus *in vitro*. Lancet 1984; 2:924-925.

18. Plotkin SA, Drew WL, Felsenstein D, Hirsch MS. Sensitivity of clinical isolates of human cytomegalovirus to 9-(1,3-dihydroxy-2-propoxymethyl)guanine. J Infect Dis 1985; 152:833-834.

19. Cole NL, Balfour HH Jr. *In vitro* susceptibility of cytomegalovirus isolates from immunocompromised patients to acyclovir and ganciclovir. Diagn Microbiol Infect Dis 1987; 6:255-261.

20. Drew WL, Miner RC, Mehalko S, Gullett J. CMV resistance in patients receiving ganciclovir. 29th Interscience Conference on Antimicrobial Agents and Chemotherapy, Houston, Texas, September 17-20, 1989, abstract 61.

21. Biron KK, Stanat SC, Reardon J, Erice A, Balfour HH Jr, Jordan MC. Ganciclovir-resistant clinical isolates of CMV: antiviral susceptibility profiles and mode of resistance studies. Second International Cytomegalovirus Workshop, San Diego, California, March 27-30, 1989, abstract 65.

22. Gibbs JS, Chiou HC, Bastow KF, Cheng Y-C, Coen DM. Identification of amino acids in herpes simplex virus DNA polymerase involved in substrate and drug recognition. Proc Natl Acad Sci USA 1988; 85:6672-6676.

23. Knopf CW, Weisshart K. The herpes simplex virus DNA polymerase: analysis of the functional domains. Biochim Biophys Acta 1988; 951:298-314.

24. Larder BA, Darby G, Virus drug-resistance: mechanisms and consequences. Antiviral Res 1984; 4:1-42.

25. Larder BA, Kemp SD, Darby G. Related functional domains in virus DNA polymerases. EMBO J 1987; 6:169-175.

26. Kit S, Sheppard M, Ichimura H, et al. Nucleotide sequence changes in thymidine kinase gene of herpes simplex virus type 2 clones from an isolate of a patient treated with acyclovir. Antimirob Agents Chemother 1987; 31:1483-1490.

27. Parris DS, Harrington JE. Herpes simplex virus variants resistant to high concentrations of acyclovir exist in clinical isolates. Antimicrob Agents Chemother 1983; 22:71-77.

28. Hill E, Lobe DC, Burns WH, Ellis MN. *In vitro* studies of pretherapy HSV-1 isolates recovered from bone marrow transplant patients. In Abstracts of the 27th Interscience Conference on Antimicrobial Agents and Chemotherapy, New York, October 4-7, 1987. American Society for Microbiology, Washington, DC, 1987, p 299.

29. Drew WL, Sweet ES, Miner RC, Mocarski ES. Multiple infections by cytomegalovirus in patients with acquired immunodeficiency syndrome: documentation by Southern blot hybridization. J Infect Dis 1984; 150:952-953.

30. Spector SA, Hirata KK, Neuman TR. Identification of multiple cytomegalovirus strains in homosexual men with acquired immunodeficiency syndrome. J Infect Dis 1984; 150:953-956.

31. Zaia JA, Forman SJ, Gallagher MT. Prolonged human cytomegaloviremia following bone marrow transplantation. Transplantation 1984; 37:315-317.

32. Peterson PK, Balfour HH Jr, Marker SC, Fryd DS, Howard RJ, Simmons RL. Cytomegalovirus disease in renal allograft recipients: a prospective study of clinical features, risk factors, and impact on renal transplantation. Medicine 1980; 59:283-300.

13

Combined Ganciclovir and Granulocyte-Macrophage Colony-Stimulating Factor in the Treatment of Cytomegalovirus Retinitis in AIDS Patients

Rationale for and Preliminary Results from a Phase II Randomized Trial (ACTG 073)

W. David Hardy

AIDS Clinical Research Center
UCLA School of Medicine
Los Angeles, California

ACTG 073 Treatment Group: **Stephen A. Spector, Wayne Dankner, Bruce Polsky, Clyde Crumpacker, Gary Holland, William Freeman, Murk-Hein Heinemann, George Sharuk, Vasilios Avramis, James Connor, and Judith Feinberg**

I. INTRODUCTION

Cytomegalovirus (CMV) infection is common in persons infected with the human immunodeficiency virus (HIV) (1). Clinical manifestations of this usually latent infection become increasingly recognized as HIV-mediated immunodeficiency reaches its advanced stages (2). CMV retinopathy is the most frequent clinical manifestation of CMV infection diagnosed in patients with AIDS (3). This relentlessly progressive disease occurs in 20 to 25% of these patients, making it the most common ophthalmic opportunistic infection and cause of blindness in AIDS patients (4). Prior to 1984, the natural history of CMV retinitis was essentially unaltered by several therapeutic attempts with agents such as acyclovir (5), adenosine arabinoside (6), and alpha-interferon (7).

II. BACKGROUND

Ganciclovir (GCV, formerly DHPG, BW B759U) is effective in the treatment of CMV retinitis in AIDS patients. This conclusion is based on reports from several open-label clinical trials carried out by numerous investigators (8-13) as well as a retrospective comparison of ganciclovir-treated versus untreated historical control patients (14). Ophthalmological response rates of CMV retinopathy to ganciclovir in these open-label trials have been reported to vary from 82% to as high as 100% of patients treated. In one of these studies (8), a complete ophthalmological response, defined as stabilization of all existing retinal lesions, decrease in retinal opacification, resolution of hemorrhage and vasculitis, and development of no new retinal lesions, was observed in 28 of 32 (88%) AIDS patients treated with 14- to 20-day course of ganciclovir. Three of 32 (9%) patients were considered to have an incomplete response due to continued lesion opacification with no enlargement in size or continued enlargement of lesion size with decrease in opacification, hemorrhage, and vasculitis. One of these 32 patients (3%), who had extensive bilateral retinal disease, had no detectable ophthalmological response. In patients treated with ganciclovir, visual acuity was noted to improve by more than two lines on the Snellen chart in five of 34 (15%), to remain stable in 25 of 34 (73%), and to decrease by more than two lines on the Snellen chart in four of 34 (12%). Thus, ganciclovir therapy is associated not only with ophthalmologically detectable stabilization of CMV retinal lesions, but also with patient-reported improvement or stabilization of visual acuity. The above studies provided the basis for the licensure of ganciclovir by the U.S. Food and Drug Administration for the treatment of CMV retinitis in patients with AIDS in July 1989.

Ganciclovir's efficacy in suppressing CMV shedding in body fluids of infected patients is also well established. Laskin and colleagues (9) reported that pretreatment CMV viremia and viruria were completely suppressed in 30 of 34 (88%) viremic patients and 56 of 72 (78%) viruric patients at median 3 and 5 days, respectively, after the initiation of ganciclovir therapy.

While ganciclovir has demonstrated efficacy in the stabilization of CMV retinopathy and preservation of vision as well as in suppression of CMV viremia and viruria, its therapeutic success has been limited both by the natural occurrence of neutropenia in AIDS patients with CMV infection and by ganciclovir-associated neutropenia. Patients with AIDS are frequently noted to be neutropenic; this probably results from several HIV-related myelosuppressive factors (15). CMV infection itself can also contribute to neutropenia in these patients (16).

The accumulated experience derived from over 8000 immunocompromised patients (85% with AIDS) treated with ganciclovir for sight- or life-threatening CMV infections has evidenced several minor adverse effects, the great majority of which have occurred infrequently. Leukopenia, the most commonly reported adverse event, occurred in 24% of ganciclovir-treated patients. This was followed by thrombocytopenia, in 6% of patients. Nadir absolute neutrophil counts (ANCs) between 500 and 1000 cells/ml were noted in 22% of patients treated with ganciclovir and ANCs less than 500 cells/ml were reported in 16% of treated patients. Nadir platelet counts between 20,000 and 50,000/ml have occurred in 10% of ganciclovir-treated patients, and platelet counts less than 20,000/ml were reported in 9% of patients (17). In the UCLA study, neutropenia (ANC < 1000 cells/ml) occurred in 12 of 40 (30%) patients during ganciclovir induction therapy and in 10 of 26 (38%) patients during maintenance therapy (8).

Development of neutropenia is the most frequent reason given for discontinuing or interrupting ganciclovir treatment. In a sample of 522 AIDS patients with CMV infections, ganciclovir treatment was discontinued or interrupted due to an adverse event in 169 (32%) patients, for a cumulative total of 246 episodes. Of these 246 treatment discontinuations or interruptions, 159 (65%) episodes were due to neutropenia. Thirty episodes (12%) of ganciclovir treatment interruptions were due to nervous system adverse events (primarily complaints of transient dizziness or confusion) and in 22 episodes (9%) due to thrombocytopenia (17).

Discontinuation of ganciclovir treatment is associated not only with re-emergence of previously suppressed CMV viremia but also reactivation of CMV retinal lesions. Masur et al. (18) reported the recurrence of CMV viremia in seven of eight patients treated with ganciclovir within 2 to 16 days after discontinuing treatment. In the UCLA ganciclovir treatment experience, reactivation of previously quiescent CMV retinopathy occurred in 10 of 10 patients at a median of 3 weeks following cessation of initial induction treatment without immediate maintenance therapy. When ganciclovir maintenance therapy was interrupted (most commonly due to neutropenia), reactivation of previously stable retinal disease occurred in nine of nine patients within 1 to 4 weeks (8). Thus, ganciclovir's efficacy against CMV infection is clearly virustatic, not virucidal. Treatment interruptions are associated with progression of retinopathy and irreversible loss of vision.

Treatment strategies designed to decrease the weekly maintenance dosage of ganciclovir (most commonly to improve neutrophil tolerance) have been associated with decreased efficacy compared to full-dose maintenance therapy. Among 121 AIDS patients treated with ganciclovir for CMV retinitis, the mean time to ophthalmologically detectable progression of retinopathy (based on Kaplan-Meier plots) was 37 days in 41 patients receiving no maintenance therapy, 31 days in 10 patients receiving 10 to 20 mg/kg per week of ganciclovir maintenance therapy, and 145 days in 70 patients receiving 25 to 35 mg/kg per week of ganciclovir maintenance therapy. Statistical significance ($p = 0.0001$ by log-rank test) was achieved comparing both the untreated and the low-dose patients to the high-dose patients in this retrospective analysis (17). Thus, an evident dose-response relationship for ganciclovir maintenance therapy exists. Decreasing the dosage clearly compromises the sight-preserving effects of ganciclovir treatment.

The primary reason for discontinuous or reduced-dose regimens of ganciclovir is neutropenia. A therapeutic approach that could ameliorate or prevent neutropenia would offer a means of improving ganciclovir treatment. Over the past 7 years, hematopoietic growth factors have been characterized, cloned, and clinically developed to make them available as therapeutic adjuvants for myelosuppressive therapies (19). Granulocyte-macrophage colony stimulating factor (GM-CSF), one of the first CSFs to be cloned and synthetically produced, has several properties that recommend it as a myelosupportive agent. In in vitro studies (20-22), recombinant human GM-CSF (rHuGM-CSF) has been noted to:

1. Stimulate the proliferation and differentiation of granulocytes and macrophages
2. Increase the survival of neutrophils and eosinophils
3. Enhance phagocytic and cytocidal activity against bacteria, yeasts, and tumor cells
4. Prime neutrophils for enhanced oxidative metabolism
5. Enhance neutrophil chemotaxis

The in vitro effect of rHuGM-CSF on HIV expression in monocytoid cell lines and primary monocyte cultures remains controversial, with reports of HIV suppression (23) as well as proliferation (24). Enhanced anti-HIV effects of combined GM-CSF and zidovudine (ZDV) have been reported by two groups of investigators (25,26). This enhancement may be due to an increased uptake of thymidine nucleosides and increased intracellular levels of nucleoside triphosphates in cells exposed to GM-CSF (26). In vivo effects of GM-CSF both with and without zidovudine are under investigation in this study and others.

The phase I, dose-escalating clinical trial of rHuGM-CSF in leukopenic AIDS patients reported by Groopman et al. (27) demonstrated that intravenous administration of this recombinant growth factor clearly proliferates granulocytic-myeloid cell lines in vivo. In this study the numbers of both mature and band neutrophils were increased in a dose-dependent manner. Eosinophils and, to a lesser extent, monocytes, were also noted to increase in number (27). In vitro neutrophil function was also noted to be enhanced in these patients (28). The results of this trial provided the basis for further therapeutic exploitation of the myeloid-stimulating properties of rHuGM-CSF in AIDS patients with both naturally occurring and treatment-associated neutropenia.

Grossberg et al. reported the preliminary results of a compassionate-use protocol that made GM-CSF available as a "rescue" adjuvant therapy to AIDS patients with CMV retinitis who became neutropenic (ANC <500/ml) with ganciclovir treatment. In this report, all 16 evaluable patients who received concomitant GM-CSF therapy were able to resume and tolerate ganciclovir therapy at doses of 5 to 10 mg/kg per day for as long as 8 months. Combined ganciclovir/GM-CSF therapy was reported to be generally well tolerated, and progression of CMV retinitis was prevented in "virtually all patients" treated (29).

Encouraged by these early reports, a phase II randomized study sponsored by the AIDS Treatment Program of the National Institute of Allergy and Infectious Diseases comparing the safety, tolerance, and efficacy of combined ganciclovir and GM-CSF to those of ganciclovir alone for treatment of newly diagnosed, sight-threatening CMV retinitis in AIDS patients was initiated in April 1989 (ACTG Protocol 073). Four AIDS Clinical Trials Units—the University of California at Los Angeles, the University of California at San Diego, Memorial Sloan-Kettering Cancer Center, and Harvard University-Beth Israel Hospital—are conducting this study. The following data are from a preliminary analysis of this ongoing study as of June 1990.

The experimental design and study medication regimens used in protocol 073 are shown in Figure 1. All patients receive induction ganciclovir therapy dosed at 5 mg/kg every 12 hours IV for 14 days followed by maintenance therapy dosed at 5 mg/kg once a day, 7 days a week. One-half of the patients are randomized to receive concomitant GM-CSF, given by subcutaneous

ACTG 073

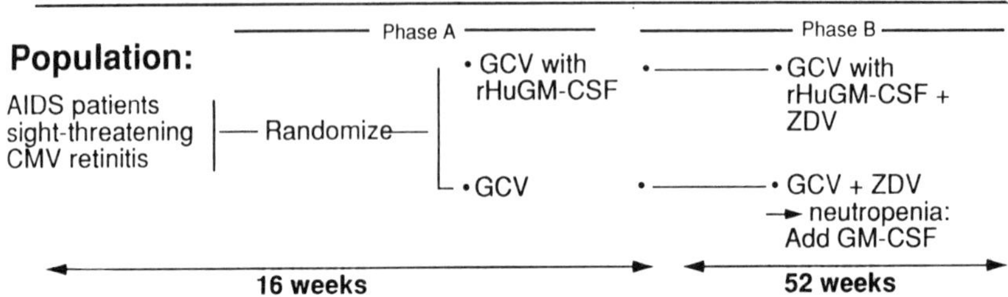

Dose: Phase A:

GCV 5 mg/kg bid IV × 14 days, then GCV 5 mg/kg/day IV × 14 weeks
rHuGM-CSF titrated to maintain ANC at 2,500–5,000 cells/µL by
incremental escalation of doses of 1.0, 2.0, 4.0, 8.0 µg/kg/day SC

Phase B:

ZDV 600 mg/day introduced after Phase A, GM-CSF titrated as in
Phase A, rHuGM-CSF introduced to GCV/ZDV if neutropenia occurs

Figure 1 Experimental design and study medication regimens used in ACTG Protocol 073.

injection, beginning at a dose of 1 μg/kg per day, escalated progressively based on individual patient response, to 2, 4, and then 8 μg/kg per day in order to reach and maintain a target ANC of 2500-5000/ml. The first part of the study, phase A, is 16 weeks in duration (2 weeks of induction therapy followed by 14 weeks of maintenance therapy). In phase B of the study, ZDV dosed at 600 mg/day is added to all study patients' regimens. Patients receiving ganciclovir with ZDV who become neutropenic (ANC <750/ml on two consecutive occasions) also receive "rescue" GM-CSF.

III. PRIMARY OBJECTIVES

The primary objectives of this study are to:

1. Determine the safety and tolerance of combined GCV/CM-CSF (and GCV/GM-CSF/ZDV)
2. Observe the occurrence, severity, and time to neutropenia in patients treated with GCV/GM-CSF vs. patients treated with GCV alone and, in phase B, GCV/GM-CSF/ZDV vs. GCV/ZDV
3. Monitor the number and duration of episodes of GCV therapy interruption due to neutropenia in the two treatment cohorts
4. Define the pharmacokinetics of combined GCV/GM-CSF

IV. SECONDARY OBJECTIVES

The secondary objectives are to:

1. Compare the efficacy of GCV/GM-CSF vs. GCV alone on suppression of CMV retinopathy (i.e., time to first progression of retinitis)
2. Compare the effect of GCV/GM-CSF vs. GCV on:
    A. Suppression of CMV infection by standard buffy coat and urine cultures and in situ hybridization studies
    B. HIV infection by serum p24 antigen detection, HIV plasma culture, and quantitative cell dilution and in situ hybridization

Neutrophil counts are quantitated 3 times a week during the induction therapy and twice weekly during the maintenance therapy. In addition, standard chemistry, CMV cultures, and HIV detection parameters listed above are monitored on a regular basis. As per protocol, ganciclovir infusions are withheld if the ANC falls below 500/ml on two consecutive occasions at least 24 hours apart. Infusions are reinitiated when the ANC rises above 750/ml again on two consecutive occasions 24 hours apart. Consecutive but separated ANCs are used to manage ganciclovir therapy in order to base dosing changes on trends in neutrophil response as opposed to isolated, perhaps errant, fluctuations in neutrophil counts. Ganciclovir therapy is also withheld for platelet counts less than 25,000/ml. GM-CSF dosage is escalated to the next higher level if the ANC remains below 2500/ml on two consecutive occasions within a 5-day period. If the ANC increases to greater than 5000/ml on two consecutive occasions within 5 days, the dosage of GM-CSF is decreased by 25%. The 5-day period for monitoring the effect of GM-CSF on neutrophils is necessary in order not to under- or overdose this hematopoietic hormone, but rather to maintain the ANC within a physiological range. If the ANC rises above 10,000/ml, GM-CSF is withheld until it falls below 5000/ml, at which time GM-CSF dosing is reinitiated at a 25% dose reduction. This regimen for dose modification of GM-CSF is highly dependent on individual patient response to this hematopoietic hormone. The typical dosing pattern of GM-CSF in the majority of patients has been satisfactory maintenance of an ANC between 2500 and 5000/ml with 1 μg/kg per day during the initial 7 to 10 days of induction therapy. Toward the end of or following induction, however, most patients have required a dose escalation to 2 or 4 μg/kg per day in order to keep the neutrophil count within the targeted range. Three out of 15 patients randomized to GM-CSF have required dose escalations to 8 μg/kg per day or greater (maximum 12 μg/kg per day) to maintain the target neutrophil count. The mean dosage of GM-CSF has been approximately 5 μg/kg per day in the 15 patients receiving combined GCV/GM-CSF.

Table 1 Patient Demographics (ACTG
Protocol 073)

No. of patients	38
Age (years)	
Mean	39
Range	26-68
Sex	
Male	37 (97%)
Female	1 (3%)
Race/ethnicity	
White	30 (79%)
Black	1 (3%)
Hispanic	7 (18%)
HIV exposure	
Gay/bisexual	33 (87%)
IV drug use	6 (16%)
Transfusion	3 (8%)
Heterosexual	3 (8%)
IV drug use	
Never	32 (84%)
Previous	5 (13%)
Current	1 (3%)
Previous AIDS-opportunistic inf.	
Yes	36 (95%)
No	2 (5%)

Demographic characteristics of the 38 patients enrolled in the trial to date
are shown in Table 1. The majority of patients in this trial are young men,
with one woman enrolled, and are primarily white or hispanic. Gay or bi-
sexual men account for the majority of study participants, with intravenous
drug users, transfusion recipients, and heterosexual contacts also represented.
Six of the 38 patients have a previous or current history of intranveous drug
use. And of special note, 36 of the 38 patients (95%) have had a previous
history of an AIDS-defining opportunistic infection, demonstrating the advanced stage of HIV disease in this patient population. Baseline laboratory
values for study patients are shown in Table 2. Of note, study participants
have had a mean neutrophil count of 2149/ml at study entry, with a range
of 714 to 5358/ml. The mean CD_4+ lymphocyte count for these patients
has been 40 cells/ml with a range of 0 to 251 cells/ml, thus also reflecting
the severe degree of immune deficiency in these patients.

Table 2 Baseline Laboratory Values (ACTG Protocol 073) ($n = 38$)

	Mean	Range
Hemoglobin (g/dl)	11.0	6.7-15.1
Total WBC (/ml)	2746	1000-7000
Neutrophils (/ml)	2149	714-5358
Platelets (/ml)	178,000	60,000-339,000
Creatinine (mg/dl)	0.9	0.6-1.3
CD4+ lymphocytes (/ml)	40	0-251

V. PRELIMINARY RESULTS

A. Pharmacokinetics

In order to investigate potential drug-drug interactions between ganciclovir and GM-CSF, two 12-hour washouts following steady-state ganciclovir infusions have been carried out, one before and one after at least three doses of GM-CSF, in the first eight patients randomized to combined therapy. Preliminary pharmacokinetic findings indicate that there is no significant alteration of the disposition of ganciclovir by GM-CSF.

Table 3 summarizes the key preliminary results from protocol 073. Of the 38 patients randomized in this study, 36 have been evaluable; 21 have been randomized to ganciclovir alone and 15 to combined ganciclovir and GM-CSF. Mean follow-up time on study has been approximately 20 weeks for both groups of patients. Neutropenia, defined as an ANC less than 750/ml, has occurred in 12 of 21 (57%) ganciclovir-treated patients, for a cumulative total of 68 episodes. In the patients receiving GCV/GM-CSF, neutropenia has occurred in six of 15 (40%) patients, for a cumulative total of 20 episodes. Of note, in three of these six patients, compliance with GM-CSF subcutaneous injections was erratic due to various practical administration problems (e.g., one patient was a right-upper-extremity amputee who was dependent on his housemates for injection of his GM-CSF). Ganciclovir infusions have been held due to persistent neutropenia (ANC < 500/ml on two consecutive occasions) in seven of 21 (33%) ganciclovir patients for a mean duration of 10.1 days. In the GCV/GM-CSF patients, ganciclovir infusions have been held due to neutropenia in four of 15 (26%) patients for a mean duration of 5.5 days. As a preliminary marker of efficacy, time to first ophthalmologically detectable progression of CMV retinitis has been monitored. Progressive retinopathy has been noted in nine of 21 (43%) ganciclovir-treated patients and six of 15 (40%) GCV/GM-CSF-treated patients. The mean time to first

Table 3 Preliminary Results (ACTG Protocol 073) ($n = 36$)

	GCV	GCV/GM-CSF
No. of evaluable patients	21	15
Follow-up (days)		
Mean	137	145
Range	28-386	3-374
Neutrophils <750/ml		
No. of patients	12 (57%)	6 (40%)
No. of episodes	68	20
GCV held due to ANC <500/μl		
No. of patients	7 (33%)	4 (26%)
No. of days (mean)	10.1	5.5
Duration in days	3, 5, 7, 9, 9, 17, 21	4, 5, 6, 7
Retinitis progression		
No. of patients	9 (43%)	6 (40%)
No. of days (mean)	102	156
Platelets <50,000/ml		
No. of patients	4 (19%)	2 (13%)
No. of episodes	18	10
GCV held due to platelets <25,000		
No. of patients	2 (10%)	2 (13%)
Duration (days)	6, 8	7, 8
Eosinophils >13% of WBC		
No. of patients	6 (29%)	10 (66%)
No. of episodes	38	132

progression in the ganciclovir patients has been 102 days, and in the GCV/
GM-CSF patients 156 days. Due to the small numbers of patients enrolled
in the study to date, no formal statistical analysis of these data has been
completed.

Additional laboratory data are summarized in Table 3. Approximately
equal numbers of patients in each treatment group have developed either
moderate or severe thrombocytopenia (platelets <50,000/ml). Both of these
patients in the GCV/GM-CSF group also developed severe thrombocytopenia
(platelets <25,000/ml). Eosinophilia (eosinophils >13% of total leukocytes)
has been seen in six of 21 (29%) ganciclovir patients for a total cumulative
number of episodes of 38, compared to 10 of 15 (66%) GCV/GM-CSF patients, for a total cumulative number of episodes of 132. The development
of eosinophilia seems to be much more commonly associated with GCV/GM-
CSF than with ganciclovir alone. No evidence of tissue infiltration or other
clinically relevant adverse effects related to eosinophilia has been noted in
these patients.

Patient-reported symptoms as well as adverse clinical events have also been closely monitored. Of the five most commonly reported symptoms associated with GM-CSF, namely fatigue, fever, headache, myalgias, and bone pain, only myalgias have been more commonly reported by GM-CSF-treated patients. Bacterial infections, potentially resulting from either GCV-associated neutropenia or neutrophil migration inhibition by GM-CSF, have been diagnosed in 13 of 21 (62%) ganciclovir patients, with seven of these (33%) being bacteremias related to central venous catheters. Bacterial infections have occurred in seven of 15 (47%) GM-CSF patients, with five of these (33%) being bacteremias associated with central venous catheters. Thus, no predominance of bacterial infections, particularly ones related to central venous catheters, seems to be occurring in one patient group over the other.

Pretreatment buffy-coat cultures for CMV have been positive in 17 of 38 (45%) study patients, and CMV viruria has been detected in 19 of 38 (50%) patients. Both viremia and viruria have been suppressed in all patients treated with either regimen. Breakthrough CMV viremia has been documented in one patient who was initially randomized to ganciclovir alone and later treated with ganciclovir, zidovudine, and GM-CSF, after 8 months on study. CMV viruria was also noted in one patient initially randomized to ganciclovir plus GM-CSF after 10 months on study. In vitro ganciclovir sensitivity for both of these CMV isolates is pending.

Preliminary results of serial in situ hybridization studies examining CMV nucleic acid expression in polymorphonuclear as well as mononuclear leukocytes utilizing CMV genomic probes have not revealed any increase in the detection of CMV nucleic acids in leukocytes from patients treated with or without GM-CSF (Wayne Dankner, Stephen Spector, personal communication).

In phase B of the study, 10 patients, six originally randomized to ganciclovir alone and four to GCV/GM-CSF, have begun zidovudine (600 mg/day) after completing the initial 16 weeks of study (phase A). Five of the six ganciclovir patients became neutropenic (ANC <750/ml on two consecutive occasions) within 2, 2, 9, 28, and 98 days, respectively, and began "rescue" GM-CSF while continuing GCV/ZDV. One patient has tolerated GCV/ZDV without severe neutropenia for 18 weeks to date. The three medications have been generally well tolerated, with no new adverse effects observed. The mean GM-CSF dosage required to maintain an ANC of 2500 to 5000/ml has been approximately 6 μg/kg per day for these five patients. Zidovudine therapy has been continued with ganciclovir reinduction (10 mg/kg per day) in five of these patients, with a small increase in GM-CSF required to maintain target ANCs. Zidovudine has been dose-reduced in three patients due to persistent anemia. Two patients have developed eosinophilia (eosinophils

>30% of total leukocytes) with introduction of GM-CSF after ZDV. Eosinophil counts have fluctuated between 15 and 60% in these patients.

A concern regarding the use of GM-CSF in AIDS patients is the potential for proliferation of HIV in latently infected monocyte/macrophages. Multiple assays to quantitate HIV infection in study patients are currently under investigation, including serum HIV p24 antigen quantitation, HIV plasma viremia cultures, and quantitative cell dilution, as well as HIV in situ hybridization studies. Preliminary analysis of the serum HIV p24 antigen studies are presented in Figures 2-5. All serial specimens have been run in batched assays using the Abbott EIA kit and Virology Research Laboratory (VRL) standard. Figure 2 depicts the results of serial p24 antigen studies in eight patients randomized to ganciclovir alone with baseline p24 antigen levels less than 30 pg/ml (lower limit of detection for the assay). In six of these patients, no change in the detection of p24 antigenemia has been observed. Of note, in one patient (UCLA RT), p24 antigen level dropped with the introduction of AZT at week 16 of study; following persistent neutropenia and the introduction of GM-CSF, an increase in p24 antigen level to greater than 1000 pg/ml was seen by week 34 of study. In another patient (USCD 003) who has also received combined ganciclovir, zidovudine, and subsequently GM-CSF, no change in p24 antigen level has been detected over 52 weeks of study.

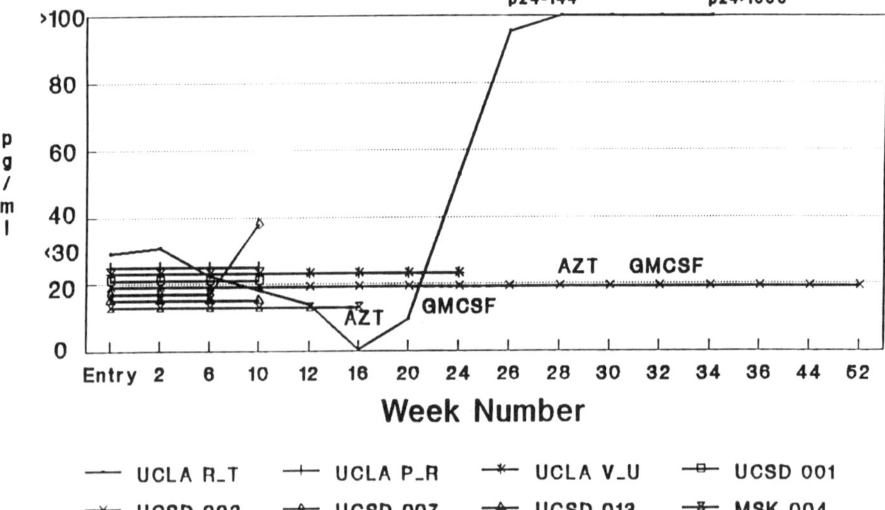

Figure 2 HIV p24 antigen in ganciclovir patients with baseline p24 antigen levels less than 30 pg/ml.

Figure 3 depicts the results of p24 antigen levels in patients randomized to ganciclovir alone whose baseline p24 antigen levels were greater than 30 pg/ml. These serial values over 10 to 36 weeks illustrate variable patterns. One patient (UCLA DR) has had a marked rise in his p24 antigen level to greater than 1000 pg/ml while on ganciclovir therapy alone. HIV p24 antigen levels from another patient (UCSD 005), which were greater than 1000 pg/ml at baseline, dropped with the institution of zidovudine at week 20 of study and continued to drop with the introduction of GM-CSF at week 28 of study. Figure 4 demonstrates the results of p24 antigen levels from patients initially randomized to ganciclovir plus GM-CSF whose entry p24 antigen values were less than 30 pg/ml. In all four of these patients, these levels have remained less than 30 pg/ml over a follow-up period of 8 to 42 weeks. Finally, Figure 5 demonstrates results of p24 antigen levels in patients initially randomized to ganciclovir plus GM-CSF with entry levels greater than 30 pg/ml. Again, a variable response has been witnessed in these patients. In one patient (UCLA RV), a sharp rise in p24 antigen level to greater than 1000 pg/ml was noted at the second week of study. Unfortunately, no further specimens from this patient are available for analysis after week 2. Another patient (UCLA GM), whose entry p24 antigen level was greater than 1000 pg/ml, demonstrated a spontaneous fall to approximately 100 pg/ml at week 16 of

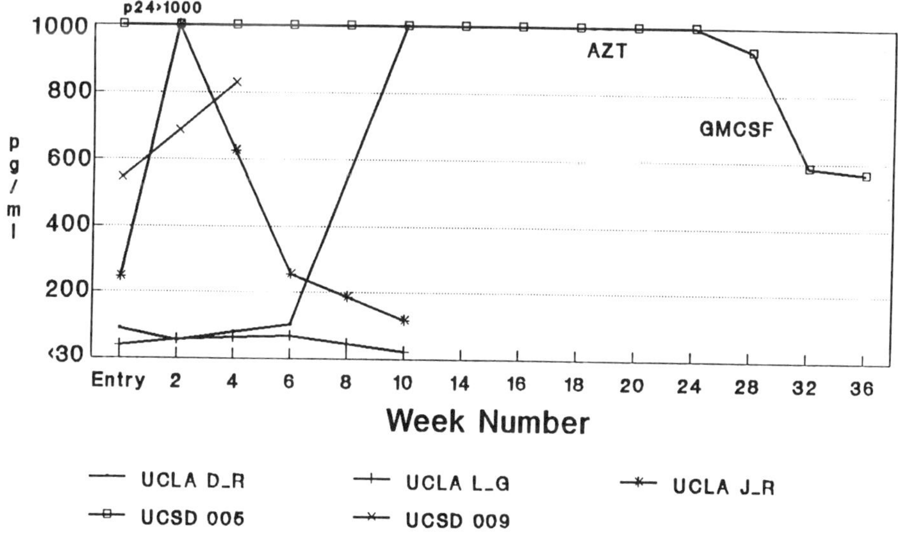

Figure 3   HIV p24 antigen in ganciclovir patients with baseline p24 antigen levels greater than 30 pg/ml.

 Hardy et al.

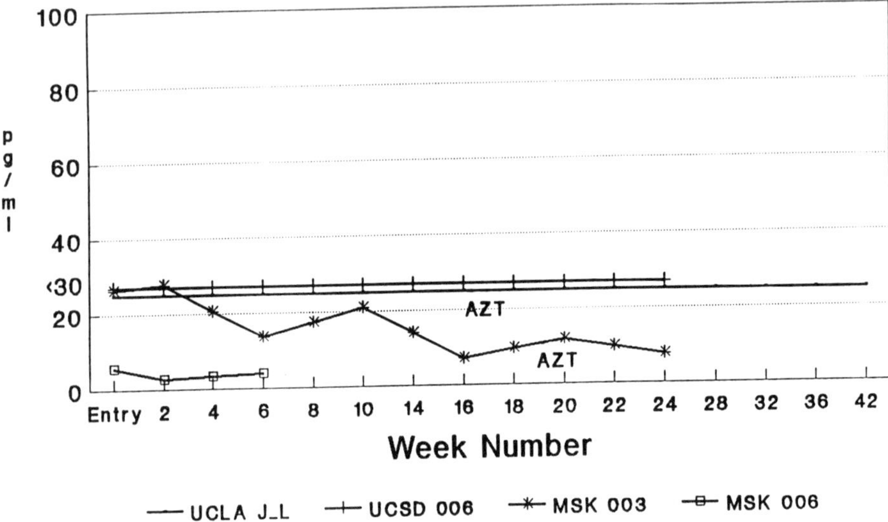

Figure 4   HIV p24 antigen in ganciclovir/GM-CSF patients with baseline p24 antigen levels less than 30 pg/ml.

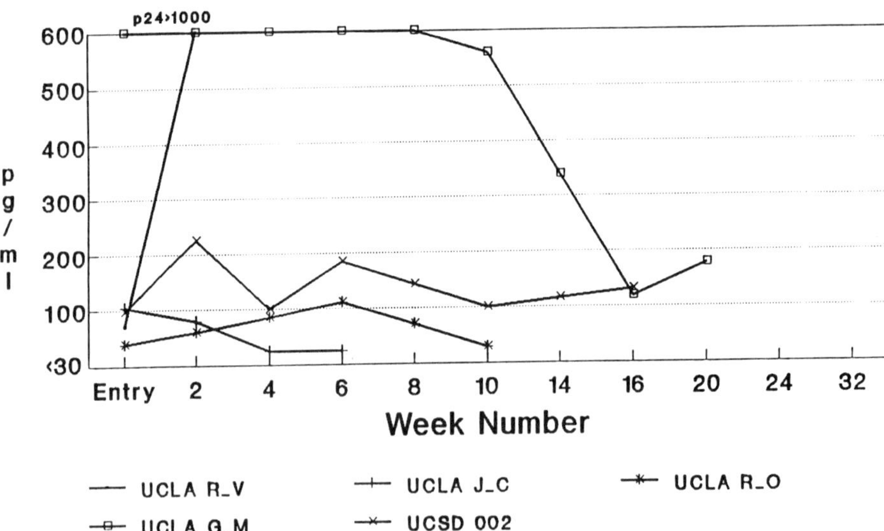

Figure 5   HIV p24 antigen in ganciclovir/GM-CSF patients with p24 antigen levels greater than 30 pg/ml.

study with GCV/GM-CSF alone. Results of other HIV quantitation assays are pending at this time.

B. Preliminary Conclusions

Based on experience with the first 36 evaluable patients enrolled in this study, the following preliminary conclusions can be made:

1. GM-CSF is well tolerated as a concomitant medication with ganciclovir. More frequent adverse events or laboratory abnormalities observed with the patients receiving GM-CSF include myalgias and eosinophilia.
2. Based on detailed pharmacokinetic analyses, there appear to be no evident drug-drug interactions between ganciclovir and GM-CSF.
3. There has been a trend, with GM-CSF administration, toward a decrease in both the proportion of patients experiencing and the total cumulative number of episodes of ganciclovir-associated neutropenia. The mean duration of ganciclovir treatment interruptions has also been decreased from 10.1 days in ganciclovir-treated patients to 5.5 days in GCV/GM-CSF patients.
4. While the proportion of patients with progressive CMV retinopathy has been similar for the two treatment groups, GM-CSF-treated patients have had a longer mean time to first progression than patients treated with ganciclovir alone. Kaplan-Meier plots of time to first progression will need to be constructed in order to evaluate these findings more critically.
5. Based on preliminary HIV p24 antigen studies, no consistent increase in proliferation of HIV infection has been observed in GCV/GM-CSF-treated patients compared to patients treated with ganciclovir alone.

Completion of this study will provide important data further defining the utility of GM-CSF as a therapeutic adjuvant to myelosuppressive therapies in AIDS patients. Of particular interest will be the results of additional studies (HIV plasma viremia cultures and in situ hybridization) evaluating the in vivo effect of GM-CSF on HIV infection. If GM-CSF/GCV therapy is found to have a significant impact on the prevention of treatment-associated neutropenia, then enhanced tolerance of ganciclovir and more effective suppression of CMV infection would be expected. This could then be translated into increased duration of progression-free time for patients with CMV retinitis, prolonged preservation of vision, and enhanced quality of life.

ACKNOWLEDGMENT

This work was supported by the UCLA AIDS Clinical Trials Unit (NIAID Al-27660) and the UCLA AIDS Clinical Research Center (California State Task Force on AIDS, 89C-CC86LA).

REFERENCES

1. Mintz L, Drew WL, Miner RC, Braff EH. Cytomegalovirus infections in homosexual men: an epidemiologic study. Ann Intern Med 1983; 98:326-329.
2. Quinnan GV Jr, Masur H, Rook AH, et al. Herpes virus infections in the acquired immune deficiency syndrome. JAMA 1984; 252:72-77.
3. Jacobson MA, Mills J. Serious cytomegalovirus disease in the acquired immunodeficiency syndrome (AIDS): Clinical findings, diagnosis and treatment. Ann Intern Med 1988; 108:585-594.
4. Holland GN, Pepose JS, Pettit TH, et al. Acquired immune deficiency syndrome: ocular manifestations. Ophthalmology 1983; 90:859-873.
5. Schulman JA, Peyman GA, Fiscella RG, Pulido J, Sugar J. Parenterally administered acyclovir for viral retinitis associated with AIDS (letter). Arch Ophthalmol 1984; 102:1750.
6. Egbert PR, Pollard RB, Gallacher JG, Merigan TC. Cytomegalovirus retinitis in immunosuppressed hosts. Natural history and effects of treatment with adenosine arabinoside. Ann Intern Med 1980; 93:655-664.
7. Chou S, Dylewski JS, Gaynon MW, Egbert PR, Merigan TC. Alpha-interferon administration in cytomegalovirus retinitis. Antimicrob Agents Chemother 1984; 25:25-28.
8. Holland GN, Sidikaro Y, Kreiger AE, Hardy WD, et al. Treatment of cytomegalovirus retinopathy with ganciclovir. Ophthalmology 1987; 94:815-823.
9. Laskin OL, Cederberg DM, Mills J, Eron LJ, et al. Ganciclovir for the treatment of serious infections caused by cytomegalovirus. Am J Med 1987; 83:201-207.
10. Palestine AG, Stevens G Jr, Lane HC, et al. Treatment of cytomegalovirus retinitis with dihydroxy propoxymethyl guanine. Am J Ophthalmol 1986; 101: 95-101.
11. Henderly DE, Freeman WR, Causey DM, Rao NA. Cytomegalovirus retinitis and response to therapy with ganciclovir. Ophthalmology 1987; 94:425-434.
12. Collaborative DHPG Treatment Study Group. Treatment of serious cytomegalovirus infections with 9-(1,3-dihydroxy-2-propoxymethyl)guanine in patients with AIDS and other immunodeficiencies. N Engl J Med 1986; 314:801-805.
13. Jabs DA, Newman C, De Bustros S, Polk BF. Treatment of cytomegalovirus retinitis with ganciclovir. Ophthalmology 1987; 94:824-830.
14. Holland GN, Buhles WC, Mastre B, Kaplan HJ, et al. A controlled, retrospective study of ganciclovir treatment for cytomegalovirus retinopathy. Arch Ophthalmol 1989; 107:1759-1766.
15. Castella A, Croxson TX, Mildvan D, Witt DH, Zalusky R. The bone marrow in AIDS: a histologic, hematologic and microbiologic study. Am J Clin Pathol 1987; 84:425.

16. Rakusan TA, Juneja H, Fleischmann WR Jr. Inhibition of hematopoietic colony formation by human cytomegaloviris in vitro. J Infect Dis 1989; 159:127-30.
17. Investigator's monograph on ganciclovir, Syntex document RS-21592, DM0102, 5th ed. Institute of Clinical Medicine, Syntex Research, Palo Alto, CA, December 1987.
18. Masur H, Lane HC, Palestine A, et al. Effect of 9-(1,3-dihydroxy-2-propoxy-methyl)guanine on serious cytomegalovirus disease in eight immunosuppressed homosexual men. Ann Intern Med 1986; 104:41-44.
19. Golde D. Hematopoietic growth factors. In Golde D (Ed), Hematology/Oncology Clinics of North America—Hematopoietic Growth Factors. WB Saunders, Philadelphia, 1989, pp XI-XII.
20. Gasson JC, Weisbart RH, Kaufman SE, et al. Purified human granulocyte-macrophage colony-stimulating factor: direct action on neutrophils. Science 1984; 226:1339-1342.
21. Metcalf D, Begley CG, Johnson GR, et al. Biologic properties in vitro of a recombinant human granulocyte-macrophage colony-stimulating factor. Blood 1986; 67:37.
22. Weisbart RH, Golde DW, Clark SC, et al. Human granulocyte-macrophage colony-stimulating factor is a neutrophil activator. Nature 1985; 314:361.
23. Hammer SM, Gillis JM, Groopman JE, Rose RM. In vitro modification of human immunodeficiency virus infection by granulocyte-macrophage colony-stimulating factor and gamma interferon. Proc Natl Acad Sci USA 1986; 83:8734-8738.
24. Folks TM, Justement J, Kinter A, et al. Cytokine-induced expression of HIV-1 in a chronically infected promonocytic cell line. Science 1987; 238:800-802.
25. Hammer SM, Gillis JM. Synergistic activity of granulocyte-macrophage colony-stimulating factor and 3'-azido-3' deosythymidine against human immunodeficiency virus in vitro. Antimicrob Agents Chemother 1987; 31:1046-1050.
26. Perno C, Yarchoan R, Cooney DA, et al. Replication of human immunodeficiency virus in monocytes. GM-CSF potentiates viral production yet enhances the antiviral effect mediated by AZT and other dideoxynucleoside congeners of thymidine. J Exp Med 1989; 169:933-951.
27. Groopman JE, Mitsuyasa RT, De Leo MJ, et al. Effect of recombinant human granulocyte-macrophage colony-stimulating factor on myelopoiesis in the acquired immunodeficiency syndrome. N Engl J Med 1987; 317:593-598.
28. Baldwin CG, Gasson JC, Quan SG, et al. GM-CSF enhances neutrophil function in AIDS patients. Proc Natl Acad Sci USA 1988; 85:2763-2766.
29. Grossberg HS, Bonnem EM, Buhles WC. GM-CSF with ganciclovir for the treatment of CMV retinitis in AIDS (letter). N Engl J Med 1989; 320:1560.

14

Diagnosis of Cytomegalovirus Infection and Virologic Monitoring of Ganciclovir Therapy

Stephen A. Spector
University of California, San Diego
and University of California, San Diego Medical Center
San Diego, California

I. INTRODUCTION

Human cytomegalovirus (CMV) is a betaherpesvirus that has a slow replication cycle, may persist for a prolonged time following infection, and after primary infection establishes latency (see Ref. 1 for review). The clinical manifestations associated with CMV affect all ages and range from asymptomatic to severe and life-threatening. CMV diagnosis is often complex and varies with the age of the patient and the clinical disease involved. A systematic approach to making a rapid and specific CMV diagnosis is an essential component for the institution of appropriate antiviral therapy. Often the clinician, having detected CMV in a clinical specimen, must determine if the patient is merely shedding the virus or has invasive visceral CMV disease. In this chapter, the methods currently available for establishing CMV-related disease and an approach to the institution and monitoring of ganciclovir therapy are reviewed.

II. DIAGNOSIS OF CMV INFECTION

A. Tissue Specimen

The diagnosis of CMV-related disease is often most accurately accomplished by identification of the virus in biopsy material obtained from the affected organ or tissue site. Although there have been extensive efforts to develop less invasive procedures for definitively establishing CMV diagnosis, including detection of the virus in blood cells, urine, saliva, or bronchoalveolar lavage (BAL), these procedures in most situations are less predictive of disease than direct tissue examination.

Histopathology

Following tissue biopsy, microscopic examination of sections stained with either hematoxylin and eosin or Wright-Giemsa demonstrate characteristic large cells with intranuclear and occasionally intracytoplasmic inclusions (Figure 1). The nuclear inclusion is often surrounded by a clear halo. Ultrastructural studies of the nuclear inclusions show herpesvirus capsids; the cytoplasmic inclusions are formed by aggregates of dense material surrounding enveloped virions (2). Although the presence of characteristic cytomegalic cells are suggestive of CMV infection, confirmation that CMV is the causa-

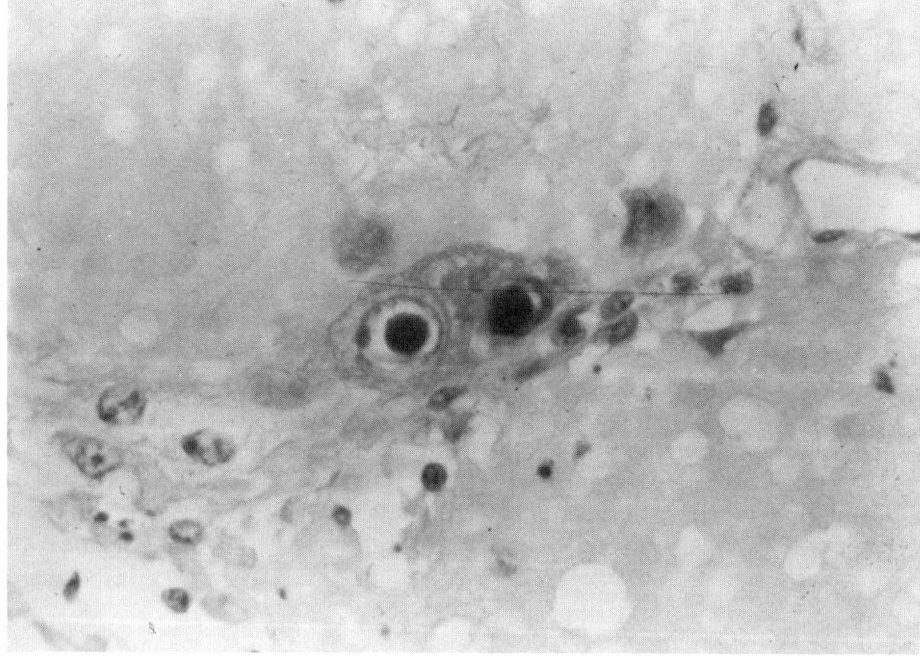

Figure 1 Lung biopsy specimen from a bone marrow transplant recipient whose chest radiograph had a diffuse interstitial pneumonia. Cytomegalic cells are typical of those seen with CMV pneumonia.

tive agent should be carried out by immunocytochemistry, in situ hybridization, or culture. Additionally, because CMV can infect tissue without producing cytologic changes, at least one of these other procedures should be performed on any tissue specimen suspected of being infected with CMV.

Immunocytochemistry

Both monoclonal and polyclonal antibodies are available commercially for the detection of CMV in tissue specimens (3-6). The polyclonal antibodies have the advantage of frequently still retaining their ability to detect CMV antigens present in fixed tissues, whereas the specific epitope for many monoclonal antibodies is destroyed during fixation. However, the specificity of monoclonal antibodies usually makes them the reagents of choice, particularly when frozen sections are being examined. The main advantages of immunocytochemical detection are its rapidity and the availability of well-characterized and standardized reagents. Immunostaining procedures are routinely performed in most pathology and viral diagnostic laboratories, and combined with histopathology are the cornerstone of tissue diagnosis for CMV at most institutions.

In Situ Hybridization

The presence of CMV in tissue specimens can also be determined by in situ hybridization using RNA or DNA probes that recognize CMV-specific nucleic acid sequences (6-9). Although probes labeled isotopically (usually with ^{35}S) can be used for clinical applications, probes labeled with biotin-avidin or other nonisotopic detection systems are more rapid, permitting the detection of CMV in tissue specimens within 24-48 hours (7). Because in situ hybridization can be applied to tissue processed for routine pathological studies by formalin fixation and paraffin embedding, it is the preferred procedure for fixed tissue. In some laboratories, in situ hybridization and immunocytochemistry have been used to detect CMV in tissues where the virus is apparently latent (6,10). In such situations, clinical interpretation of results may be difficult and requires quantitation of a positive response in order to correlate laboratory findings with clinical disease. In most laboratories, the sensitivity of these procedures is usually insufficient to detect latent infection; however, controls including tissue from both healthy CMV seronegatives and seropositives should be evaluated with each clinical specimen.

B. Tissue Culture Diagnosis

Direct viral culture of CMV remains a valuable technique for diagnosis. As the virus replicates, cytopathic effects (CPE) result, with characteristic plaque formation (11). Although direct tissue-culture isolation is accurate, the time required for the development of characteristic CPE may be from 2 to 6 weeks following tissue culture inoculation. In one study, the mean time to culture positivity for urine specimens obtained from bone marrow transplant recipients was 9 days, whereas a mean time of approximately 4 weeks was required for buffy-coat samples (8).

Modification of the viral culture technique has made possible the detection of infectious virus present in cell culture (12-18). In this procedure, the clinical specimen is centrifuged onto fibroblast-coated shell vials (Figure 2) (17,18). After an incubation of approximately 16 to 18 hours, monoclonal antibodies specific to the 72-KDa major immediate-early (IE) CMV protein are used to detect IE antigen expression (Figure 3). This technique detects over 90% of specimens that will ultimately be shown to be CMV-culture-positive. If the centrifugation step is not performed, the sensitivity of the procedure decreases to approximately 70 to 75%. The major problem associated with the shell-vial procedure has been that centrifugation of specimens onto fibroblasts may result in disruption of the fibroblast monolayer, making the specimen unusable. Additionally, the procedure requires the maintenance of cell cultures and a trained technologist to interpret results.

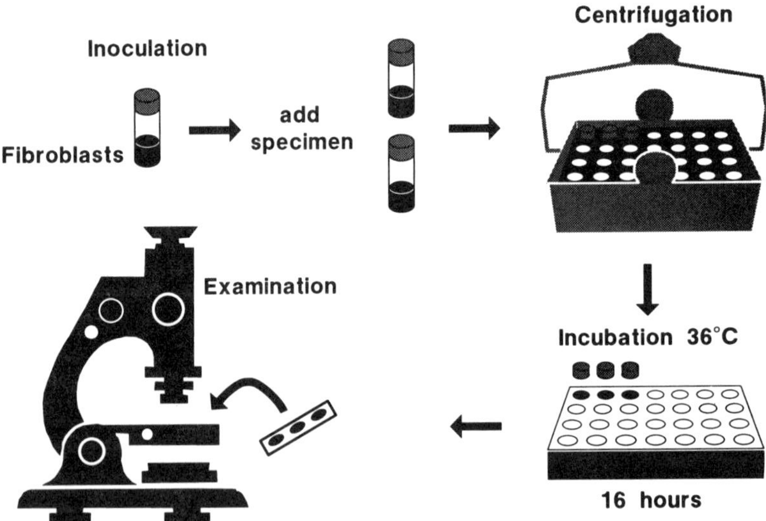

Figure 2 Schematic representation of the shell-vial technique for detection of CMV infection. Virus-containing material is centrifuged onto shell vials with fibroblasts growing on the bottom. Monoclonal antibodies are used to detect immediate-early (IE) CMV antigens after a 16-24-hour incubation. (From Ref. 18; adapted from Ref. 17.)

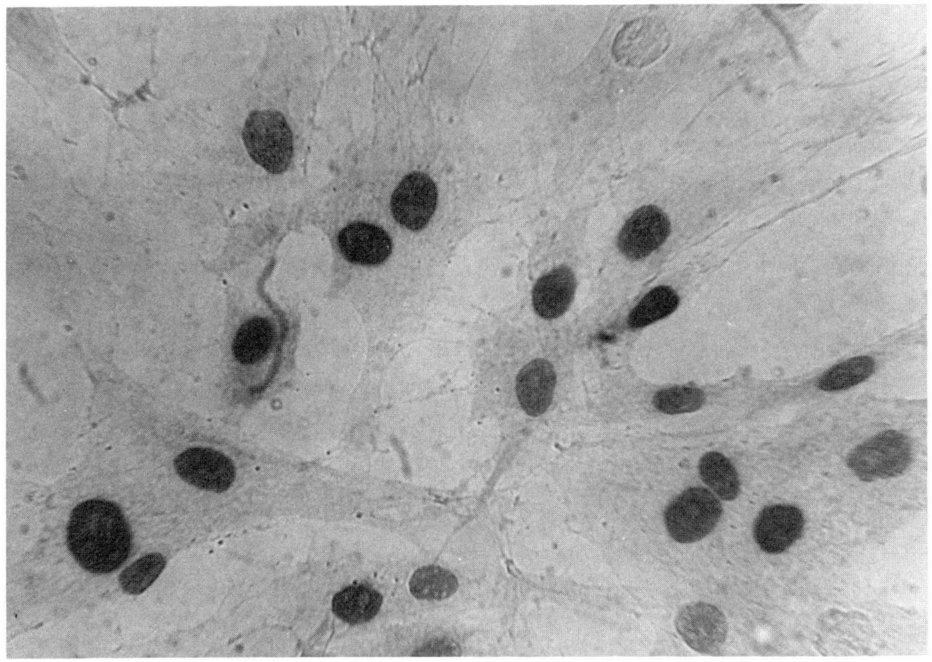

Figure 3 Human fibroblast cultures incubated in the presence of a specific mono-clonal antibody directed against CMV IE proteins using the procedure outlined in Figure 2. (From Ref. 18.)

C. Serological Diagnosis

Assays have been developed for the detection of CMV-specific IgG anti-bodies, including complement fixation (CF) (19,20), anticomplement immu-nofluorescence (ACIF) (21,22), indirect immunofluorescence (IFA) (23), immune adherence hemagglutination assay (24,25), indirect hemagglutina-tion (IHA) (26), neutralization (27,28), latex agglutination (29-31), and en-zyme immunoassays (EIA) (32-36). Most clinical laboratories currently use an EIA procedure because of its sensitivity, reproducibility, and ease of per-formance; although fluorescent, IHA, and latex agglutination assays have compared favorably (37-41). Similarly, a number of tests are available for detection of CMV IgM antibodies, but, again, most laboratories perform an EIA test for detection (42-46). The correlation of antibody findings with clinical disease is often difficult. In this regard, although the detection of a fourfold or greater rise of CMV IgG titers or the presence of CMV IgM is often used to detect a recent CMV infection or reactivation, they do not establish clinical disease. In most situations, therefore, including those involving patients with AIDS and patients who have received organ transplants, serological tests are not useful for establishing CMV as the etiologic cause of a specific clinical disease. However, measurement of CMV IgG can be useful for establishing previous infection and for establishing primary infection.

D. Detection of CMV-Specific Nucleic Acid

Slot/Dot Blot Hybridization

DNA/DNA or DNA/RNA hybridization have been used for the detection of CMV-specific nucleic acid in many laboratories (47-50). The clinical application of this procedure for the diagnosis of CMV disease remains unclear. Recent advances in the use of nonisotopic detection systems and nucleic acid quantitation promise to make this procedure more applicable to clinical diagnosis. In one study of bone marrow transplant recipients, eight of 15 patients identified as being viremic by detection of CMV DNA in their peripheral blood leukocytes developed CMV pneumonia (51). The viremia preceded pneumonia by a mean of over 6 weeks, suggesting that prophylaxis of these patients early in their viremia might have prevented visceral disease. In another study, quantitation of CMV DNA in leukocytes of viremic patients with AIDS or following either bone marrow or solid-organ transplantation was predictive of those individuals who developed organ disease (52). Although these studies are promising, dot/slot blot hybridization for the diagnosis of CMV is routinely performed in only a few viral diagnostic laboratories and is generally unavailable to most clinicians.

DNA Amplification by Polymerase Chain Reaction (PCR)

The ability to amplify small fragments of DNA a millionfold has led to a great deal of excitement and enthusiasm by investigators interested in the application of nucleic acid detection to clinical diagnosis. Much research has demonstrated that the PCR approach can be used for the detection of CMV (53-57); however, the very sensitivity of PCR has complicated its use as a diagnostic tool for CMV-related disease. More than ever, the fundamental question to the clinician, following detection of CMV DNA by PCR, is what the clinical significance is. Thus, except for specific clinical situations in which the presence of CMV correlates with disease, the application of PCR is limited. There is still room for optimism, however, regarding the use of PCR as a helpful technique for establishing CMV disease. Methods of product quantitation will be particularly important for future applications. Additionally, detection of CMV RNA by reverse transcription PCR may be of value in predicting CMV disease. Technical considerations, including the prevention of product carryover leading to falsely positive results, will need to be resolved. All these issues are currently being extensively investigated by numerous groups in academia and industry, and PCR is likely to become a useful tool for CMV diagnosis.

E. Specific Diagnoses

Because the diagnosis of CMV disease varies with the age of the patient and the clinical disease under consideration, this section reviews the approaches to establish different CMV diagnoses. Figure 4 schematically outlines a systematic approach to the diagnosis of serious CMV disease in high-risk patients. In certain situations, although the diagnosis of CMV as the etiologic agent is equivocal, there may be sufficient evidence to warrant antiviral treatment. The ultimate decision regarding the institution of ganciclovir (or another anti-CMV) therapy is usually decided by the likelihood of CMV disease, the potential seriousness of the infection, and the risks associated with therapy.

Congenital Cytomegalic Inclusion Disease

Infants congenitally infected with CMV who have symptomatic disease, including hepatomegaly, splenomegaly, petechiae or purpura, microcephaly, chorioretinitis, cerebral calcifications, hearing impairment, and other serious or life-threatening manifestations, may be candidates for antiviral treatment. At present, however, no antiviral therapy has been demonstrated to improve the outcome of such infants. Studies with ganciclovir are currently under way. The diagnosis of congenital CMV infection in such infants who are less than 3 weeks old can be accomplished by isolating CMV or detecting CMV-specific nucleic acid from the baby (Figure 5) (58). Urine specimens are most commonly used, but virus can also be isolated from throat wash, blood, or other specimens. The detection of CMV-IgM is also diagnostic within 21 days of birth, but may be absent in as many as 30% of congenitally infected infants (59-61). Babies older than 3 weeks who have clinical findings suggestive of congenital CMV with positive cultures or IgM for the virus can be presumed to have congenital CMV in the absence of another identified source; however, in such situations postnatally acquired CMV is possible.

CMV Retinitis

As described in Chapter 6, the diagnosis of CMV retinitis can be established by an experienced ophthalmologist without difficulty, particularly in immunocompromised patients with whom there is a high index of suspicion. Once the diagnosis of retinitis is established, the treatment options for such patients are reviewed (Chapters 5, 6, and 13).

CMV Gastrointestinal Disease

The diagnosis of gastrointestinal disease caused by CMV is described in detail in Chapter 9. Multiple biopsy sites are encouraged to establish the diagnosis

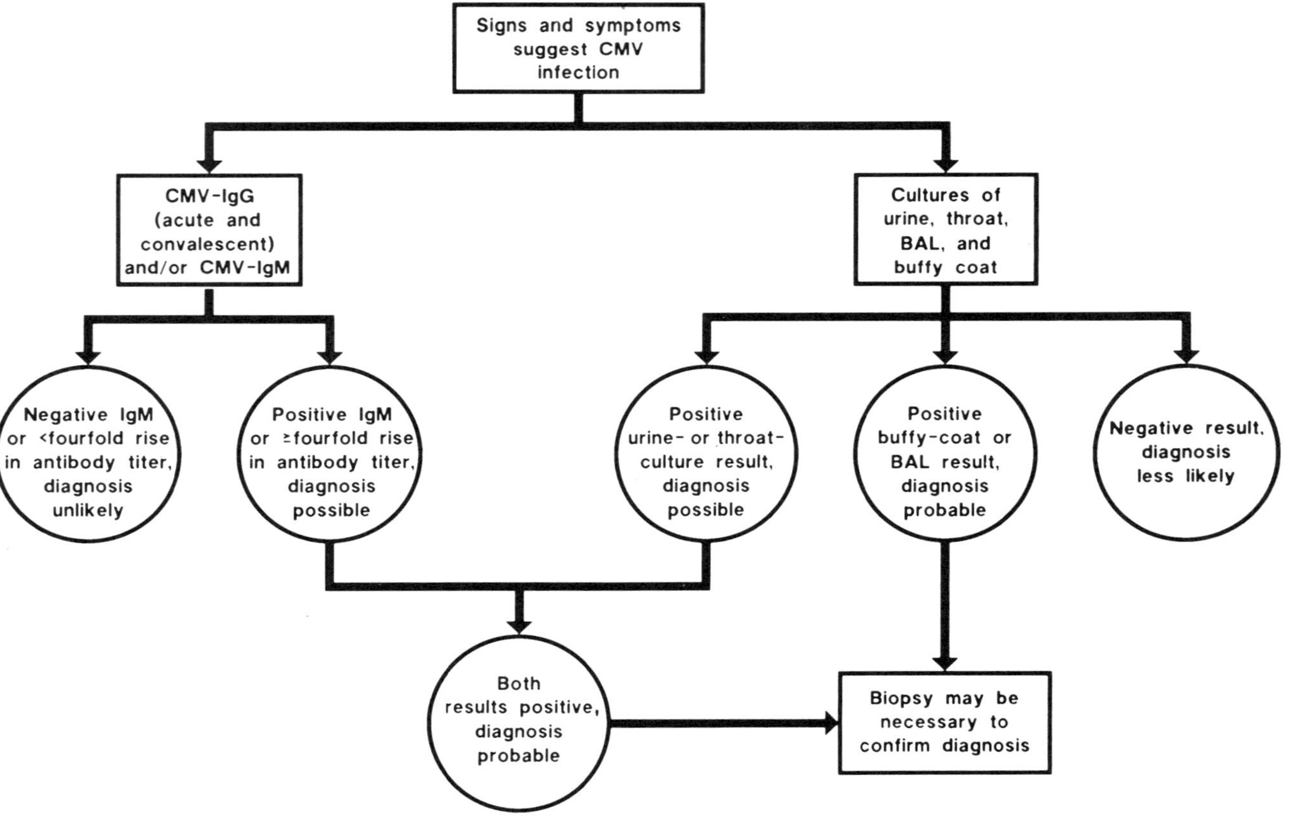

Figure 4 A general approach to the diagnosis of acute CMV infection. (From Ref. 18.)

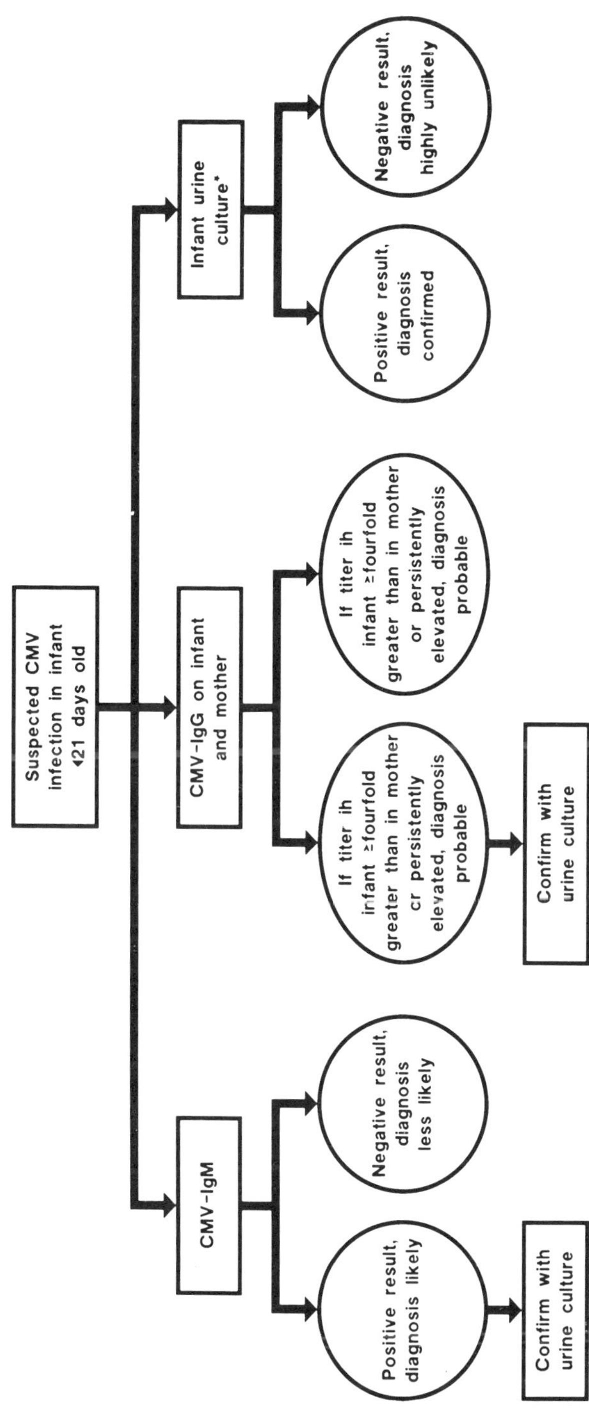

Figure 5 A general approach to the diagnosis of congenital CMV infection.

rigorously. In patients with AIDS, Dieterich et al. and others (62,63) have found that the two factors most closely associated with intestinal infection are diarrhea and extraintestinal CMV. As previously discussed in Chapter 9, ulcerative lesions identified in the GI tract, although most commonly associated with CMV, can also be direct HIV infection of the esophagus or colon. Histopathology, immunohistochemical techniques, and in situ hybridization are all useful in helping to establish the diagnosis of CMV gastrointestinal disease.

CMV Pneumonia

Among the most challenging clinical diseases in which to establish CMV as the etiologic agent is pneumonia. Particular difficulty exists because the likelihood of CMV being an acute pathogen of pneumonia appears to vary significantly for different patient groups. For example, following organ transplantation, CMV pneumonia is a common cause of severe and often fatal disease (64-71). In particular, bone marrow transplant recipients are at high risk for developing CMV pneumonia (64-66). On the other hand, CMV retinitis is relatively uncommon in patients following bone marrow transplantation. In contrast, patients with AIDS, although they frequently have CMV present in BAL specimens or in lung tissue, rarely develop acute CMV pneumonia (72,73). Thus, identification of CMV in lung biopsy tissue in patients following organ transplantation should be considered diagnostic for CMV disease, while the same specimen obtained from a patient with AIDS should be considered diagnostic only when no other pathogens are identified.

Numerous studies have attempted to establish the diagnosis of CMV pneumonia without performing a lung biopsy. The most popular approach has been to obtain BAL fluid during bronchoscopy (74-78). This fluid is then examined by tissue culture, shell-vial culture, direct cytology, IFA, in situ hybridization, slot/dot blot hybridization, or PCR. Each approach has been proposed by some groups as being most predictive of CMV pneumonia. However, an increasing number of studies have indicated that many patients may have CMV-positive BAL specimens without having acute CMV pneumonia. Generally, the most sensitive procedures (e.g., PCR) have the highest sensitivity for detecting CMV pneumonia, but also have the highest percentage of positive results without the presence of disease. Cytology, on the other hand, is the least sensitive, but when clearly positive is most likely to be associated with CMV pneumonia. The combination of cytology with immunofluorescent staining with monoclonal antibody specific for IE antigens is probably the most useful diagnostic approach at present. In this regard, in one study the detection of >0.5% of cells in BAL specimens obtained from bone marrow transplant recipients was highly correlated with the presence of CMV pneumonia. In a recent study by Zaia (79), asymptomatic bone marrow transplant recipients had BAL specimens obtained for CMV 35 days following transplantation. Of those individuals identified as CMV-positive on BAL culture, ~70% developed CMV pneumonia. Even more importantly, those patients randomized to receive ganciclovir therapy had no episodes of CMV pneumonia (see Chapter 10). Thus, bronchoscopy 35 days following bone marrow transplantation can be used as a predictor of those individuals at risk for developing CMV pneumonia and for initiating ganciclovir therapy.

CMV Polyradiculopathy

Peripheral nervous system dysfunction is commonly seen in patients with AIDS. The most common is a sensory neuropathy of uncertain etiology but probably relating to direct infection with HIV (80,81). The second peripheral nervous system abnormality is caused by CMV, has a typical clinical presentation, and appears to respond to ganciclovir therapy (81-83). Most patients presenting with this syndrome complain initially of paresthesias with numbness or tingling in the toes that subsequently spreads proximally. Sensory symptoms are usually symmetrical and progress over weeks but sometimes more rapidly. Patients with CMV polyradiculopathy may have previous retinitis or colitis, but frequently have had no other clinical manifestations relating to CMV. The laboratory findings and clinical manifestations found with CMV polyradiculopathy have been presented by Miller (81) and are summarized in Table 1. Of note is the cerebrospinal fluid pleocytosis, which has

Table 1 Clinical and Laboratory Findings Associated with CMV Polyradiculopathy in Patients with AIDS (Mean values with range or number with positive finding/number evaluated)

CSF-cell count	449 (29-1500)
% PMNs	71 (58-94)
Protein, mg/dl	274 (113-630)
Glucose, mg/dl	29 (15-47)
CMV culture positive	4/7
CMV at autopsy	5/5
Acute denervation (EMG)	7/7
Small evoked M-waves	7/7
Progressive severe weakness	7/7
Early sacral paresthesias	7/7
Early urinary retention	7/7
CMV retinitis	3/7
Sensory level	2/7
Duration of illness (days)	40 (29-56)

Source: Adapted from Ref. 81.

a predominance of polymorphonuclear leukocytes, an elevated protein, and a low glucose. Although most patients with CMV polyradiculopathy have progressive disease and death, we and others have treated patients early in their disease course with ganciclovir and have observed improvement in function. For this reason, the diagnosis of CMV polyradiculopathy should be made on clinical grounds, with the initiation of anti-CMV therapy before culture results are obtained. Most patients in my experience are CMV-culture-positive from the CSF.

III. VIROLOGIC MONITORING OF GANCICLOVIR THERAPY

Prior to the initiation of ganciclovir therapy, all patients should have a leukocyte (buffy-coat) and urine culture for CMV. These cultures document the state of viral shedding at the time of ganciclovir therapy and are helpful in the evaluation of the subsequent antiviral effect of treatment. Virologic studies indicate that over 90% of patients will become CMV-culture-negative from their blood within a week of instituting ganciclovir therapy and that there is a significant decrease in urinary shedding, with most patients becoming CMV-culture-negative while receiving 2 to 3 weeks of induction therapy at 5 mg/kg per dose every 12 hours. I have recently reviewed the first 19 patients treated at the UCSD ACTU on protocol 073, which evaluates the use of GM-CSF with ganciclovir for patients with CMV retinitis (see Chapter 13 for details). In these 19 patients, who were treated for more than 3 months (mean of 6 months), only two patients had positive cultures for CMV (one in urine and one in blood). All others remained CMV-culture-negative while receiving ganciclovir therapy. Despite failing to have virologic relapse, nine patients reactivated their CMV retinitis while receiving maintenance therapy (ganciclovir 5 mg/kg/day). In eight of these patients, reinduction with ganciclovir was attempted and proved successful in each. Both published and unreported data support that most patients who reactivate their CMV retinitis do not have resistant viruses and can be reinduced with higher doses of ganciclovir (see Chapter 12). However, patients who do reactivate their retinitis should have viral cultures for CMV. Patients who have persistently positive cultures without clinical improvement should be suspected of having developed ganciclovir resistance and should have their pre- and posttreatment viruses tested for resistance (see Chapter 1). At present, treatment with foscarnet should be considered in such cases.

Treatment of patients with AIDS or organ transplant recipients with CMV disease other than retinitis in AIDS patients usually does not require prolonged maintenance therapy with ganciclovir. However, relapse of disease is common in AIDS patients with CMV gastrointestinal disease, as well as other end-organ disease. In such cases, once recurrent CMV disease is documented, repeat treatment with ganciclovir is warranted. When patients have not undergone extended treatment with ganciclovir, the development of resistant virus will likely be uncommon. Thus, these clinical situations should not require changing to other therapeutic agents unless the patient fails to respond to reinduction with ganciclovir 5 mg/kg per dose every 12 hours.

IV. SUMMARY

Advances in methodology to accomplish CMV diagnosis and the expanded list of clinical conditions identified as being caused by the virus have dramatically expanded the need for treatment of patients with serious CMV disease. Currently, the only drug available with documented clinical efficacy for many conditions associated with CMV is ganciclovir. However, as has been frequently reviewed in this book as well as in numerous published reports, ganciclovir treatment frequently results in neutropenia and thrombocytopenia. Other potential serious toxicities associated with ganciclovir administration mandate that this drug be used only in settings where CMV disease has been clearly documented. Overwhelming clinical evidence supports the use of ganciclovir for serious and life-threatening CMV infections. Thus, rapid and specific CMV diagnosis is essential and should frequently be followed by the immediate initiation of antiviral therapy. In this chapter, I have reviewed the essential components for establishing CMV as the etiologic agent in many of the most common clinical conditions associated with CMV. It is important to note that peripheral cultures positive for CMV, particularly positive buffy-coat cultures, are suggestive of CMV disease but are not confirmatory. A systematic approach as outlined in Figure 4 will help to identify those patients who require CMV treatment. Once therapy is initiated, virologic evaluation is necessary only if patients develop reactivated disease while on ganciclovir. In these situations, viral isolates should be evaluated for ganciclovir resistance, particularly when obtained from patients who fail to respond to reinduction with ganciclovir.

ACKNOWLEDGMENTS

This work was supported in part by Public Health Service grants AI-27563, AI-27670, and AI-28270 from the National Institutes of Health.

REFERENCES

1. Stinski MF. Cytomegalovirus and its replication. In Fields BN, Knipe DM (Eds), Fields Virology, Raven Press, New York, 1990, pp 1959-1980.

2. Costa J, Rabons AS. Viral diseases. In Kissane JM (Ed), Anderson's Pathology, CV Mosby, St Louis, 1990, pp 362-390.

3. Goldstein LC, McDougall J, Hackman R, Meyers JD, Thomas ED, Nowinski RC. Monoclonal antibodies to cytomegalovirus: rapid identification of clinical isolates and preliminary use in diagnosis of cytomegalovirus pneumonia. Infect Immunol 1982; 38:273-281.

4. Hackman RC, Myerson D, Meyers JD, Shulman HM, Sale GE, Goldstein LC, Rastetter M, Flournoy N, Thomas ED. Rapid diagnosis of cytomegaloviral pneumonia by tissue immunofluorescence with a murine monoclonal antibody. J Infect Dis 1985; 151:325-329.

5. Stirk PR, Griffiths PD. Use of monoclonal antibodies for the diagnosis of cytomegalovirus infection by the detection of early antigen fluorescent foci (DEAFF) in cell culture. J Med Virol 1987; 21:329-337.

6. Myerson D, Hackman RC, Nelson JA, Ward DC, McDougall JK. Widespread presence of histologically occult cytomegalovirus. Hum Pathol 1984; 15:430-439.

7. Myerson D, Hackman RC, Meyers JD. Diagnosis of cytomegaloviral pneumonia by *in situ* hybridization. J Infect Dis 1984; 150:272-277.

8. Spector SA, Spector DH. The use of DNA probes in studies of human cytomegalovirus. Clin Chem 1985; 31:1514-1520.

9. Spector SA, Hsia K, Denaro F, Spector DH. Use of molecular probes to detect human cytomegalovirus and human immunodeficiency virus. Clin Chem 1989; 35:1581-1587.

10. Toorkey CB, Carrigan DR. Immunohistochemical detection of an immediate early antigen of human cytomegalovirus in normal tissues. J Infect Dis 1989; 160:741-751.

11. Starr SE, Friedman HM. Human cytomegalovirus. In Lennette EH, Balows A, Hausler WJ, Shadomy HJ (Eds), Manual of Clinical Microbiology, 4th ed, ASM, 1985, pp 711-719.

12. Gleaves CA, Smith TF, Schuster EA, Pearson GR. Comparison of standard tube and shell vial culture techniques for the detection of cytomegalovirus in clinical specimens. J Clin Microbiol 1985; 21:217-221.

13. Gleaves CA, Smith TF, Schuster EA, Pearson GR. Rapid detection of cytomegalovirus in MRC-5 cells inoculated with urine specimens by low-speed centrifugation and monoclonal antibody to an early antigen. J Clin Microbiol 1984; 19:917-919.

14. Griffiths PD, Panjwani DD, Stirk PR, Ball MG, Ganczakowski M, Blacklock HA, Prentice HG. Rapid diagnosis of cytomegalovirus infection in immunocompromised patients by detection of early antigen fluorescent foci. Lancet 1984; 2:1242-1244.

15. Martin WJ, Smith TF. Rapid detection of cytomegalovirus in bronchoalveolar lavage specimens by a monoclonal antibody method. J Clin Microbiol 1986; 23:1006-1008.

16. Swenson PD, Kaplin MA. Rapid detection of cytomegalovirus in cell culture by indirect immunoperoxidase staining with monoclonal antibody to an early nuclear antigen. J Clin Microbiol 1985; 21:669-673.

17. Shuster EA, Beneke JS, Tegtmeier GE, Pearson GR, Gleaves CA, Wold AD, Smith TF. Monoclonal antibody for rapid laboratory detection of cytomegalovirus infections: Characterization and diagnostic application. Mayo Clin Proc 1985; 60:577-585.

18. Spector SA. Diagnosis of cytomegalovirus infection. Sem Hematol 1990; 27:11-16.

19. Hanshaw JB. Cytomegalovirus complement fixing antibody in microencephaly. N Engl J Med 1966; 275:476-479.

20. Kettering JD, Schmidt NJ, Lennette EH. Improved glycine-extracted complement-fixing antigen for human cytomegalovirus. J Clin Microbiol 1977; 6:647-649.

21. Kettering JD, Schmidt NJ, Gallo D, Lennette EH. Anti-complement immunofluorescence test for antibodies to human cytomegalovirus. J Clin Microbiol 1977; 6:627-632.

22. Rao N, Waruszewski DT, Armstrong JA, Atchison RW, Ho M. Evaluation of anti-complementary immunofluorescence test in cytomegalovirus infection. J Clin Microbiol 1977; 6:633-638.

23. Betts RF, George SD, Rundell BR. Comparative activity of immunofluorescent antibody and complement-fixing antibody in cytomegalovirus infection. J Clin Microbiol 1976; 4:151-156.

24. Dienstag JL, Cline WL, Purcell RH. Detection of cytomegalovirus antibody by immune adherence hemagglutination. Proc Soc Exp Biol Med 1976; 153:543-548.

25. Lennette EH, Lennette DA. Immuno adherence hemagglutination: alternative to complement fixation serology. J Clin Microbiol 1978; 7:282-285.

26. Yeager AS. Improved indirect hemagglutination test for cytomegalovirus using human O erythrocytes in lysine. J Clin Microbiol 1979; 10:64-68.

27. Plummer G, Benyesh-Melnick MA. A plaque reduction neutralization test for human cytomegalovirus. Proc Soc Exp Biol Med 1964; 117:145-150.

28. Chou S, Scott KM. Rapid quantitation of cytomegalovirus and assay of neutralizing antibody by using monoclonal antibody to the major immediate-early viral protein. J Clin Microbiol 1988; 26:504-507.

29. Hunt AF, Allen DL, Brown RL, Robb BA, Puckett AY, Entwistle CC. Comparative trial of six methods for the detection of CMV antibody in blood donors. J Clin Pathol 1984; 37:95-97.

30. Adler SP, McVoy M, Biro VG, Britt WJ, Hider P, Marshall D. Detection of cytomegalovirus antibody with latex agglutination. J Clin Microbiol 1985; 22:68-70.

31. Chou S, Scott KM. Latex agglutination and enzyme-linked immunosorbent assays for cytomegalovirus serologic screening of transplant donors and recipients. J Clin Microbiol 1988; 26:2116-2119.

32. Cappel R, de Cuyper F, de Braekeleer J. Rapid detection of IgG and IgM antibodies for cytomegalovirus by the enzyme-linked immunosorbent assay (ELISA). Arch Virol 1978; 58:253-258.

33. Sarov I, Andersen P, Andersen HK. Enzyme-linked immunosorbent assay (ELISA) for determination of IgG antibodies to human cytomegalovirus. Acta Pathol Microbiol Scand 1980; 88:1-9.

34. Kiefer DJ, Phelps DA, Halbert SP. Normalized enzyme-linked immunosorbent assay for determining immunoglobulin G antibodies to cytomegalovirus. J Clin Microbiol 1983; 18:33-39.
35. Dylewski JS, Rasmussen L, Mills J, Merigan TC. Large-scale serological screening for cytomegalovirus antibodies in homosexual males by enzyme-linked immunosorbent assay. J Clin Microbiol 1984; 19:200-203.
36. Nielsen SL, Ronholm E, Sorensen I, Andersen HK. Detection of immunoglobulin G antibodies to cytomegalovirus antigen by antibody capture enzyme-linked immunosorbent assay. J Clin Microbiol 1986; 24:998-1003.
37. Friedman HM, Tustin NB, Hitchings MM, Plotkin SA. Comparison of complement fixation and fluorescent immunoassay (FIAX) for measuring antibodies to cytomegalovirus and herpes simplex virus. Am J Clin Pathol 1981; 76:305-307.
38. Brandt JA, Kettering JD, Lewis JE. Immunity to human cytomegalovirus measured and compared by complement fixation, indirect fluorescent-antibody, indirect hemagglutination, and enzyme-linked immunosorbent assays. J Clin Microbiol 1984; 19:147-152.
39. Booth JC, Hannington G, Bakir TM, Stern H, Kangro H, Griffiths PD, Heath RB. Comparison of enzyme-linked immunosorbent assay, radioimmunoassay, complement fixation, anticomplement immunofluorescence and passive haemagglutination techniques for detecting cytomegalovirus IgG antibody. J Clin Pathol 1982; 35:1345-1348.
40. Phipps PH, Gregoire L, Rossier E, Perry E. Comparison of five methods of cytomegalovirus antibody screening of blood donors. J Clin Microbiol 1983; 18:1296-1300.
41. Beckworth DG, Halstead DC, Alpaugh K, Schweder A, Blount-Fronefield DA, Toth K. Comparison of a latex agglutination test with five other methods for determining the presence of antibody against cytomegalovirus. J Clin Microbiol 1985; 21:328-331.
42. Tardy JC, Pouteil-Noble C, Touraine JL, Aymard M. Prognostic value of anti-cytomegalovirus IgM in kidney graft recipients. Transplant Proc 1987; 19:4066-4067.
43. Demmler GJ, Six HR, Hurst SM, Yow MD. Enzyme-linked immunosorbent assay for the detection of IgM-class antibodies to cytomegalovirus. J Infect Dis 1986; 153:1152-1155.
44. Joassin L, Reginster M. Elimination of nonspecific cytomegalovirus immunoglobulin M activities in the enzyme-linked immunosorbent assay by using anti-human immunoglobulin G. J Clin Microbiol 1986; 23:576-581.
45. Chou S, Kim Dy, Scott KM, Sewell DL. Immunoglobulin M antibody to cytomegalovirus in primary and reactivation infections in renal transplant recipients. J Clin Microbiol 1987; 25:52-55.
46. Gray JJ, Alvey B, Smith DJ, Wreghitt TG. Evaluation of a commercial latex agglutination test for detecting antibodies to cytomegalovirus in organ donors and transplant recipients. J Virol Methods 1987; 16:13-19.
47. Spector SA, Rua JA, Spector DH, McMillan R. Detection of human cytomegalovirus in clinical specimens by DNA-DNA hybridization. J Infect Dis 1984; 150:121-126.

48. Chou S, Merigan TC. Rapid detection and quantitation of human cytomegalovirus in urine through DNA hybridization. N Engl J Med 1983; 308:921-925.
49. Buffone GJ, Schimbor CM, Demmler GJ, Wilson DR, Darlington GJ. Detection of cytomegalovirus in urine by nonisotopic DNA hybridization. J Infect Dis 1986; 154:163-166.
50. Schuster V, Matz B, Wiegand H, Traub B, Kampa D, Neumann-Haefelin D. Detection of human cytomegalovirus in urine by DNA-DNA and RNA-DNA hybridization. J Infect Dis 1986; 154:309-314.
51. Spector SA, Spector DH. The use of DNA probes in studies of human cytomegalovirus. Clin Chem 1985; 31:1514-1520.
52. Saltzman RL, Quirk MR, Jordan MC. Disseminated cytomegalovirus infection. Molecular analysis of virus and leukocyte interactions in viremia. J Clin Invest 1988; 81:75-81.
53. Shibata D, Klatt EC. Analysis of human immunodeficiency virus and cytomegalovirus infection by polymerase chain reaction in the acquired immunodeficiency syndrome. An autopsy study. Archives Path Lab Med 1989; 113:1239-1244.
54. Hsia K, Spector DH, Lawrie J, Spector SA. Enzymatic amplification of human cytomegalovirus sequences by polymerase chain reaction. J Clin Microbiol 1989; 27:1802-1809.
55. Jiwa NM, Van Gemert GW, Raap AK, Van de Rijke FM, Mulder A, Lens PF, Salimans MM, Zwaan FE, Van Dorp W, Van der Ploeg M. Rapid detection of human cytomegalovirus DNA in peripheral blood leukocytes of viremic transplant recipients by the polymerase chain reaction. Transplantation 1989; 48:72-76.
56. Demmler GJ, Buffone GJ, Schimbor CM, May RA. Detection of cytomegalovirus in urine from newborns by using polymerase chain reaction DNA amplifications. J Infect Dis 1988; 158:1177-1184.
57. Olive DM, Simsek M, Al-Mufti S. Polymerase chain reaction assay for detection of human cytomegalovirus. J Clin Microbiol 1989; 27:1238-1242.
58. Spector SA, Michelotti V. Diagnosis of Epstein-Barr virus and cytomegalovirus. Diagnosis 1985; 7:65-79.
59. Griffiths PD, Kangro HO. A user's guide to the indirect solid-phase radioimmunoassay for the detection of cytomegalovirus specific IgM antibodies. J Virol Methods 1984; 8:271-282.
60. Griffiths PD, Stagno S, Pass RF, Smith RJ, Alford CA. Congenital cytomegalovirus infection: diagnostic and prognostic significance of the detection of specific immunoglobulin M antibodies in cord serum. Pediatrics 1982; 69:544-549.
61. Stagno S, Tinker MK, Elrod C, Fuccillo CA, Cloud G, O'Beirne AJ. Immunoglobulin M antibodies detected by enzyme-linked immunosorbent assay and radioimmunoassay in the diagnosis of cytomegalovirus infections in pregnant women and newborn infants. J Clin Microbiol 1985; 21:930-935.
62. Dieterich DT, Dugan M, Blank K, Chachoua A. Ganciclovir (DHPG) treatment of cytomegalovirus infections in 183 AIDS patients. IV International Conference on AIDS, Stockholm, 1988, abstract 7193.
63. Rene E, Verdon R, Roze C, Vallot T, Matheron S, Leport C, Marche C, Ruszniewski P. Intestinal infections during AIDS: Who should be investigated? Gastroenterology 1990; 98:A471.

64. Neiman P, Wasserman PB, Wentworth BB, Kao GF, Lerner KG, Storb R, Buckner CD, Clift RA, Fefer A, Fass L, Glucksberg H, Thomas ED. Interstitial pneumonia and cytomegalovirus infection as complications of human marrow transplantation. Transplantation 1973; 15:478-485.

65. Meyers JD, Harrison CS, Watts JC, Gregg MB, Stewart JA, Troupin RH, Thomas ED. Cytomegalovirus pneumonia after human marrow transplantation. Ann Intern Med 1975; 82:181-188.

66. Atkinson K, Storb R, Prentice RL, Weiden PL, Witherspoon RP, Sullivan K, Noel D, Thomas ED. Analysis of late infections in 89 long-term survivors of bone marrow transplantation. Blood 1979; 53:720-731.

67. Peterson PK, Balfour HH, Marker SC, Fryd DS, Howard RJ, Simmons RL. Cytomegalovirus disease in renal allograft recipients: A prospective study of the clinical features, risk factors and impact on renal transplantation. Medicine 1980; 59:283-300.

68. Glenn J. Cytomegalovirus infections following renal transplant. Rev Infect Dis 1981; 3:1151-1178.

69. Betts RF. Cytomegalovirus infection in transplant patients. Prog Med Vir 1982; 28:44-64.

70. Trachtman H, Weiss R, Spigland I, Greifer I. Clinical manifestations of herpesvirus infections in pediatric renal transplant recipients. Ped Infect Dis 1985; 4:480-486.

71. Gorensek MJ, Stewart RW, Keys TF, McHenry MC, Goormastic M. A multivariate analysis of the risk of cytomegalovirus infection in heart transplant recipients. J Infect Dis 1988; 157:515-522.

72. Jacobsen MA, Mills J. Serious cytomegalovirus disease in the acquired immunodeficiency syndrome (AIDS). Ann Intern Med 1988; 108:585-594.

73. Bower M, Barton SE, Nelson MR, Bobby J, Smith D, Youle M, Gazzard BG. The significance of the detection of cytomegalovirus in the bronchoalveolar lavage fluid in AIDS patients with pneumonia. AIDS 1990; 4:317-320.

74. Emanuel D, Peppard J, Stover D, Gold J, Armstrong D, Hammerlung U. Rapid immunodiagnosis of cytomegalovirus pneumonia by bronchoalveolar lavage using human and murine monoclonal antibodies. Ann Intern Med 1986; 104:476-481.

75. Gleaves CA, Myerson D, Bowden RA, Hackman RC, Meyers JD. Direct detection of cytomegalovirus from bronchoalveolar lavage samples by using a rapid *in situ* hybridization assay. J Clin Microbiol 1989; 27:2429-2432.

76. Ruutu P, Ruutu T, Volin L, Tukiainen P, Ukkonen P, Hovi T. Cytomegalovirus is frequently isolated in bronchoalveolar lavage fluid of bone marrow transplant recipients without pneumonia. Ann Intern Med 1990; 112:913-916.

77. Gleaves CA, Meyers JD. Rapid detection of cytomegalovirus in bronchoalveolar lavage specimens from marrow transplant patients: evaluation of a direct fluorescein-conjugated monoclonal antibody reagent. J Virol Meth 1989; 26:345-349.

78. Woods GL, Thompson AB, Rennard SL, Linder J. Detection of cytomegalovirus in bronchoalveolar lavage specimens—spin amplification and staining with

a monoclonal antibody to the early nuclear antigen for diagnosis of cytomegalovirus pneumonia. Chest 1990; 98:568-575.

79. Zaia JA. Epidemiology and pathogenesis of cytomegalovirus disease. Sem Hem 1990; 275:5-10.

80. So YT, Holtzman DM, Abrams DI, Olney RK. Peripheral neuropathy associated with acquired immunodeficiency syndrome: Prevalence and clinical features from a population based survey. Arch Neurol 1988; 45:945-948.

81. Miller RG. Distal symmetric polyneuropathy and lumbosacral polyradiculopathy. AAEM Course B 1990; pp 21-25.

82. Miller RG, Story JR, Greco CM. Ganciclovir in the treatment of progressive AIDS-related polyradiculopathy. Neuro 1990; 40:569-574.

83. Fuller GN, Gill SK, Guiloff RJ, Kapoor R, Lucas SB, Sinclair E, Scaravilli F, Miller RF. Ganciclovir for lumbosacral polyradiculopathy in AIDS. Lancet 1990; 335:48-49.

Index

Absorption of drug, 73-74
ACIF (anticomplement immunofluor-
    escence), 219
Acquired immunodeficiency syn-
    drome (AIDS), 5, 15, 145
  animal models of, 17
  asymptomatic infections in, 176
  drug resistance and, 151, 185, 188,
    189, 191, 192, 193
  drug safety and, 35-49, 53, 54, 57,
    58, 59, 60, 61, 62-63
  GI disease and, 24, 38, 129-140,
    166, 224, 226 (*see also* Gastro-
    intestinal disease)
  heterogeneity of disease in, 156
  pathogenesis of disease in, 158
  peripheral nervous system dysfunc-
    tion in, 225
  pharmacokinetics and, 71, 73-74,
    75, 76, 77, 78

[Acquired immunodeficiency syn-
    drome]
  pneumonia and, 224
  retinitis and, 6, 24, 37-38, 40, 42,
    45, 47-48, 49, 63, 73-74, 75,
    83-89, 94, 105-113, 115-127,
    151, 188, 189, 193, 198-211
    (*see also* Retinitis)
  serological diagnosis of, 220
  virologic monitoring in, 226
Acute leukemia, 171
ACV (*see* Acyclovir)
Acyclovir (ACV), 1, 2, 3, 5, 31, 105,
    145, 160, 165, 167, 187, 198
  in animal models, 16, 18, 20, 22,
    25, 26
  interactions with other drugs, 58,
    79
  pharmacokinetics of, 71, 72, 73,
    75, 79

[Acyclovir]
prophylaxis with, 175-176
resistance to, 191, 192
Acyclovir-monophosphate, 3
Acyclovir-triphosphate, 3
AD169 strain, 2, 4, 5, 19, 186, 190
Adenine arabinoside (Vidarabine),
1, 145, 165, 167, 191
Adenosine arabinoside, 198
Adrenal gland disorders, 18, 24, 158,
159
Alkaline phosphatase, 48, 136
Amebiasis, 129-130
Amphotericin, 58
Anemia, 40-41, 44, 87
Animal models, 5, 15-27
in vitro assessment and, 17, 18-19
of latent infections, 19, 24
of lethal infections, 19-21, 24
replication in (*see* Replication)
in safety studies, 32-35
testing methods in, 17-18
Anophthalmia, 34
Anticomplement immunofluorescence
(ACIF), 219
Antigens, 60, 175, 193
human leukocyte, 162
IE, 218, 224
MHC, 26, 175
p24, 203, 208-211
Antimetabolites, 59
Antithymocyte globulin (ATG), 21,
24
Aphidocolin, 186
Aplasia:
erythroid, 52-53
marrow, 150
pancreatic, 34
renal, 34
Ara-A (vidarabine), 1, 145, 165, 167,
191
Aspermatogenesis, 59, 60, 62
Asymptomatic infections, 158, 176-
177, 215 (*see also* Latent in-
fections)
ATG (antithymocyte globulin), 21, 24

Autologous bone marrow transplants
(BMT), 35, 164, 166
Azidothymidine (AZT) (*see* Zidovu-
dine)
Azoospermia, 87
AZT (*see* Zidovudine)

Bacteremia, 45, 87
Barium swallow, 134
β-actin mRNA, 162
Biliary tree, 133, 135-136
Bilirubin, 47
BIOLF-62, 2
Biopsies, 133, 135, 136, 137, 138,
215-216, 221
Biotin-avidin, 217
Blepharitis, 110
Blindness, 86, 94, 101, 113, 125, 198
transient cortical, 174
Blood-brain barrier, 74
Blood donors, 175
Blood urea nitrogen (BUN), 33, 45-
46, 55
BMT (*see* Bone marrow transplants)
Bone marrow aplasia, 150
Bone marrow transplants (BMT),
2, 26, 218
autologous, 35, 164, 166
disease prevention following, 175-
177
drug distribution and, 74
drug resistance and, 151, 192, 193
drug safety and, 50-53, 54, 55, 59,
63-64
GI disease and, 51-52, 166
GM-CSF and, 53
heterogeneity of disease in, 156-157
IP and, 155, 156, 158, 159-160,
161, 163-165, 167-175, 176-177
(*see also* Interstitial pneumonia)
pathogenesis of disease in, 157-163
pneumonia and, 26, 27, 50, 52, 63-
64, 148, 151-152, 159, 220,
224-225 (*see also* Pneumonia)

[Bone marrow transplants]
  prophylaxis in, 151
  renal dysfunction and, 54-55, 172, 174
  solid-organ transplants compared with, 155-156, 163
  syndromes following, 163-166
Brachygnathia, 34
Breakthrough retinitis, 100, 120
Breakthrough viremia, 193, 207
Breast milk, 75
Bronchoalveolar lavage (BAL), 165, 170, 172-173, 176, 177, 216, 224, 225
BUN (blood urea nitrogen), 33, 45-46, 55

Candida esophagitis, 134
Carcinogenicity, 34, 57
Catheter-associated infections, 87, 106
CAVHD (continuous ateriovenous hemodialysis), 76, 77
CD4 cells, 40, 92, 204, 205
Cellular kinases, 2, 72
Cellular polymerases, 32
Central nervous system complications, 87, 150, 156, 157, 159, 167
CF (complement fixation), 219
Chemotherapy, 86, 165
Chlamydia, 165
Cholangitis, 135
Cholecystitis, 135
Cholestatic liver, 135
Chorioretinitis, 193, 221
Choroiditis, 125
Chromosomal damage, 34
Chronic administration, 77-78, 87
Chronic lymphocytic leukemia, 171, 174, 188, 189
Chronic toxicity studies, 33
Clearance of drug, 75-76
Cleft palate, 34

Clinical safety (*see* Drug safety)
Clotrimazole, 134
Cocaine, 110
Colitis, 1, 129-130, 136, 139, 193
  drug resistance and, 188
  drug safety and, 38, 41-42, 43, 46, 47, 48, 59
Colon diseases, 133, 136-137, 224 (*see also* specific types)
Colonoscopy, 133, 136, 139
Coma, 150
Complement fixation (CF), 219
Congenital abnormalities, 15
Congenital cytomegalic inclusion disease, 221, 223
Conjunctivitis, 110
Continuous arteriovenous hemodialysis (CAVHD), 76, 77
Cortisone, 21, 23-24, 25
Cotton-wool spots, 94, 118, 122, 127
Creatinine, 45-46, 50, 55, 56, 58, 61, 62, 63, 76, 205
Cryptosporidiosis, 135
CSG strain, 19
Cyclogyl, 126
Cyclophosphamide, 25, 26
Cyclosporine, 55, 63
Cytokines, 6, 161 (*see also* specific types)
Cytology, 224
Cytopenia, 36, 58
Cytosine arabinsoide, 1
Cytostaticity, 59, 62
Cytotoxicity, 32, 59
Cytotoxic lymphocytes, 160

Davis strain, 19
ddI (2′,3′-dideoxyinosine), 58
2′-Deoxyguanosine, 2, 31
Deoxyguanosine kinase, 72
dGTP, 72
Diagnosis, 215-226
  of congenital cytomegalic disease, 221, 223

[Diagnosis]
  of GI disease, 131-133, 221-224
  of pneumonia, 224-225
  of polyradiculopathy, 225-226
  of retinitis, 93-94, 221
  techniques in, 215-221 (*see also*
    specific techniques)
Diarrhea, 130, 133, 135, 136, 139,
  140, 166
Dideoxycytidine, 5
2′,3′-Dideoxyinosine (ddI), 58
Distribution of drug, 74-75
DNA, 158, 191
DNA amplification, 220-221
DNA elongation, 3, 8, 72
DNA hybridization, 6-7, 8, 9-10, 17,
  217, 224
DNA polymerase, 2, 3, 4, 16, 32
  drug resistance and, 186, 190, 191,
    192
DNA probes, 6, 138, 217
DNA synthesis, 3, 6-7, 17, 61, 72
Dosage, 32-33, 56-57, 61-62, 77-79,
  87
Drug absorption, 73-74
Drug clearance, 75-76
Drug distribution, 74-75
Drug elimination, 75-76, 77, 79
Drug excretion, 75
Drug interactions, 58-59, 79
Drug metabolism, 75
Drug resistance (*see* Resistance)
Drug safety, 31-64
  for AIDS patients, 35-49, 53, 54,
    57, 58, 59, 60, 61, 62-63
  animal studies of, 32-35
  cellular level studies of, 31-32
  dosing adjustments and, 61-62
  drug interactions and, 58-59
  for geriatric patients, 58
  gonadal function and, 59-60
  immunosuppressive effects and,
    60-61
  in intravitreal therapy, 35, 60
  long-term, 56-57
  for pediatric patients, 57-58, 63

[Drug safety]
  for transplant patients, 49-56, 59-
    60, 63-64
Drug toxicity (*see* Toxicity)
Dysphagia, 134, 166

EIA (enzyme immunoassays), 219
Elimination of drug, 75-76, 77, 79
ELISA (enzyme-linked immunosor-
  bent assay), 73
Embryolethality, 33, 34
Encephalitis, 159
Endophthalmitis, 109, 112
Endoscopy, 132, 133, 134, 136-137
Enteritis, 135, 156, 157, 159-160,
  166
Enzyme immunoassays (EIA), 219
Enzyme-linked immunosorbent assay
  (ELISA), 73
Eosinophilia, 206, 207-208, 211
Epithelial cells, 138
Erythrocytes, 33, 40, 52
Erythroid aplasia, 52-53
Esophageal disease, 133, 134, 135,
    138, 140, 166, 193, 224 (*see
    also* specific types)
Excretion of drug, 75

Fertility, 33, 34
Fetal infections, 34, 158
Fever, 48, 63, 150, 156, 157, 159,
    163, 166, 207
FIAC (2′-fluoro-5-iodoarabinosyl-
    cytosine), 191
FIAU (2′-fluoro-5-iodoarabinosyl-
    uridine), 191
Fibroblasts, 186, 218
Fibronectin, 162
FIC (fractional inhibitory concentra-
    tion) method, 88
Fluconazole, 134
Fluorescein angiography, 125

2′-Fluoro-5-iodoarabinosylcytosine (FIAC), 191
2′-Fluoro-5-iodoarabinosyluridine (FIAU), 191
Folate inhibitors, 59
Follicle-stimulating hormone (FSH), 59
Foscarnet, 1, 2, 3, 4-5
  for GI disease, 139, 140
  for IP, 165, 167, 173, 176
  prophylaxis with, 176
  resistance to, 186, 191, 194
  for retinitis, 1, 88, 106, 110, 112, 167
Fractional inhibitory concentration (FIC) method, 88
Frosted-branch angiitis, 119
FSH (follicle-stimulating hormone), 59
Fulminant retinitis, 118-119

Ganciclovir diphosphate, 72
Ganciclovir monophosphate (GCV-MP), 2, 31
Ganciclovir triphosphate (GCV-TP), 2, 3, 32, 72, 186
Gastritis, 134, 135, 193
Gastroenteritis, 71, 139
Gastrointestinal (GI) disease, 38, 129-140, 224, 226 (*see also* specific types)
  AIDS and (*see* Acquired immuno-deficiency syndrome)
  animal models of, 24, 33
  BMT and, 51-52, 166
  diagnosis of, 132-133, 221-224
  incidence of, 130-132
  manifestations and sites of, 133-137
  pathology of, 137-138
  surgery for, 135, 137
  transplants and, 131-132, 133, 136, 139 (*see also* specific types)
  treatment for, 138-139

GCV-MP (ganciclovir monophosphate), 2, 31
GCV-TP (ganciclovir triphosphate), 2, 3, 32, 72, 186
Gentamicin, 110
GGT (glutamyl transpeptidase), 47, 48
GGTP, 136
GI disease (*see* Gastrointestinal disease)
Glomerulofiltration, 79
Glutamate-pyruvate transaminase (SGPT), 33, 47, 48
Glutamic-oxaloacetic transaminase (SGOT), 33, 47, 48
Glutamyl transpeptidase (GGT), 47, 48
GM-CSF (*see* Granulocyte-macrophage colony stimulating factor)
GMP (guanosine monophosphate) kinase, 3
Gonadal function, 59-60, 87
GPCMV (guinea pig cytomegalovirus), 16, 18-19
Graft failure, 166, 174
Graft vs. host reaction (GVHR), 26, 157, 159, 160, 164, 166, 174, 175
Granular retinitis, 119
Granulocyte-macrophage colony stimulating factor (GM-CSF), 6, 45, 53, 62
  for GI disease, 140
  interactions with other drugs, 58
  for retinitis, 45, 88, 100, 112, 198-211, 226
    pharmacokinetics of, 202, 205-211
Granulocytopenia, 86, 99-100, 106 (*see also* Leukopenia)
Granulomas, 48
Guanosine kinases, 32 (*see also* specific types)
Guanosine monophosphate (GMP) kinase, 3

Guinea pig cytomegalovirus (GPCMV), 16, 18-19
GVHR (*see* Graft vs. host reaction)

Hallucinations, 150
Heart-lung transplants, 53, 147, 156
Heart transplants, 147, 151, 156
  drug safety and, 53, 55, 56, 63, 64
Hematological complications, 5, 6
  in AIDS patients, 35-45, 53, 54, 62, 63
  in transplant patients, 50-54
Hematopoietic function, 33
Hematopoietic growth factors, 200
Hematoxylin, 216
Hemodialysis, 76, 77, 151
Hemofiltration, 151
Hemolysis, 150
Hemorrhage, 40, 166
  retinal (*see* Retinal hemorrhage)
Hepatic dysfunction, 24, 63, 77, 133
    (*see also* specific diseases)
  AIDS and, 47-48, 135-136
  solid-organ transplants and, 150
Hepatic transplants, 53, 148, 149, 156
Hepatitis, 19, 193
  AIDS and, 132, 136
  BMT and, 156, 157, 159, 166
  incidence of, 132
  solid-organ transplants and, 148, 149, 156
  transplants and, 132, 133, 136 (*see also* specific types)
Hepatomegaly, 221
Herpes simplex virus (HSV), 2, 3, 160
    (*see also* specific types)
  animal models of, 16
  resistant strains of, 191-192
  retinitis and, 94
  ulcers and, 133, 134
Herpes simplex virus-1 (HSV-1), 3, 7, 72
Herpes simplex virus-2 (HSV-2), 4, 7, 72

H&E staining, 138
High-performance liquid chromatography (HPLC), 72-73
Histopathology, 216-217, 224
HLA (human leukocyte antigen) system, 162
Homosexuals, 130, 204
Host vs. graft reaction (HVGR), 157, 159
HPLC (high-performance liquid chromatography), 72-73
HPMPA [(s)-9-(3-hydroxy-2-phosphonyl-methoxypropyl)adenine], 191, 194
HPMPC, 186, 191, 194
HSV (*see* Herpes simplex virus)
Human immunodeficiency virus (*see* Acquired immunodeficiency syndrome)
Human leukocyte antigen (HLA) system, 162 (*see also* Major histocompatibility complex antigens)
HVGR (host vs. graft reaction), 157, 159
Hydrocephaly, 34
8-Hydroxy-gancilovir, 75
(s)-9-(3-Hydroxy-2-phosphonyl-methoxypropyl)adenine (HPMPA), 191
Hypocalcemia, 88
Hypospermatogenesis, 33, 59, 62

IE antigens, 218, 224
IFA (indirect immunofluorescence), 219, 224
IFN (*see* Interferon)
Ig (*see* Immunoglobulin)
IHA (indirect hemagglutination), 219
IL (interleukin), 61, 160
Imipenem-cilastatin, 59
Immune adherence hemagglutination assay, 219
Immunocytochemistry, 217

Immunoglobulin (Ig), 27, 52, 151-152,
165, 168-172, 174-175, 188
(*see also* specific types)
prophylaxis with, 176
Immunoglobulin G (IgG), 219-220,
222
Immunoglobulin M (IgM), 221, 223
Immunohistochemistry, 224
Immunoperoxidase staining, 138
Immunosuppression, 60-61
Indirect hemagglutination (IHA), 219
Indirect immunofluorescence (IFA), 219
Indirect ophthalmoscopy, 110, 115,
122-123, 127
Inflammatory bowel disease, 129
Interactions of drugs, 58-59, 79
Interferon (IFN), 1, 145, 165, 167
(*see also* specific types)
α-Interferon (IFN), 198
β-Interferon (IFN), 4, 42, 43, 44, 46
γ-Interferon (IFN), 61, 163
Interleukin-1 (IL-1), 160
Interleukin-2 (IL-2), 61, 160
Interstitial pneumonia (IP), 155, 156,
158, 159-160, 161, 163-165
animal models of, 24, 25
asymptomatic, 176-177
diagnosis of, 165
prevention of, 176
treatment of, 167-175
Intravenous drug users, 130, 204
Intravitreal therapy, 35, 60, 74, 75,
88, 105-113
administration technique in, 110-
111
complications of, 111-112
indications for, 109-110
pharmacokinetics of, 107, 108-109
toxicity of, 108-109
In vitro inhibition, 1-10
in animal models, 17, 18-19
mechanism of action in, 2-4
pharmacokinetics of, 72
sensitivity testing in, 6-8
In vivo inhibition, 4-5, 17-18, 84
IUDR, 1

Kaposi's sarcoma, 135
Ketoconazole, 134

Latent infections, 19, 24, 215, 217
(*see also* Asymptomatic infections)
Latex agglutination, 219
Legionella pneumophila, 165
Lethal infections, 18, 19-21, 24
Leukemia, 165, 171, 174, 188, 189
Leukocyte interferon (IFN), 145, 167
Leukocytes, 33, 36, 52, 166, 172, 220
drug resistance and, 193
GM-CSF and, 206, 207
in polyradiculopathy, 226
in virologic monitoring, 226
Leukopenia, 193 (*see also* Granulo-
cytopenia)
in AIDS patients, 36-39, 41-42, 48,
199
in BMT patients, 50, 53, 156
drug interactions and, 58
long-term dosing and, 57
LH (luteinizing hormone), 59
Long-term dosing, 56-57
Luteinizing hormone (LH), 59
Lymphoblast interferon (IFN), 167
Lymphocytes, 34, 60-61, 100, 160
(*see also* T cells)
Lymphoma, 135, 188

Macrophages, 160, 200, 208
Major histocompatibility complex
(MHC) antigens, 26, 175
MCMV (*see* Murine cytomegalovirus)
Meningitis, 95
Mesenchymal cells, 138
Metabolism of drug, 75
Methylprednisolone, 168
MHC (major histocompatibility com-
plex) antigens, 26, 175
Microcephaly, 221

Microphthalmia, 34
Monoclonal antibodies, 25, 224
Monocytes, 200, 201, 208
Mononucleosis, 156, 157, 159
Mortality
    in animal models, 17, 18, 19-21,
        24, 32-33
    GI disease and, 138, 140
    IP and, 164, 167, 174
mRNA, 162
Murine cytomegalovirus (MCMV),
        16-17, 18, 19, 20, 21, 22-24,
        25-27, 169
Mutations, 34, 57, 62, 186, 187
Mycobacterium avium intracellulare, 48
Mycobacterium tuberculosis, 165
Mycoplasmas, 165
Myelosuppression, 83-84, 86, 87, 88,
        106, 166, 199
Myelotoxicity, 33, 46, 62, 78, 168

Nausea, 87, 166
Neonates, 75, 77, 156, 221
Neo-Synephrine, 126
Nephrotoxicity, 88, 106
Neutralization, 219
Neutropenia, 4, 106, 227
    in AIDS patients, 36-39, 41-42, 44,
        45, 46, 48, 49, 54, 62, 63, 78,
        87, 88, 140, 199, 200, 201, 202,
        203, 204, 205, 207, 208, 211
    in BMT patients, 50-51, 52, 53, 63,
        157, 163
    drug interactions and, 58
    GM-CSF and, 53, 62, 88, 200, 201,
        202, 203, 204, 205, 207, 208,
        211
    intravitreal therapy and, 106, 108
    renal function relation to, 46
    in solid-organ transplant patients,
        53, 63, 150
    in transplant patients, 78-79 (*see also*
        specific types)
    ZDV and, 44, 45, 54

Neutrophils (*see* Granulocytopenia;
        Neutropenia)
Normal-angle cameras, 123-124
Nucleic acid detection, 220-221

Ocular fundus photography, 115,
        123-127
Odynophagia, 134
OKT3, 151
Ophthalmoscopy, 110, 115, 122-123,
        127
Oral administration, 88
Organ transplants, 34, 130, 220 (*see
        also* Bone marrow transplants;
        Solid-organ transplants)
    drug resistance and, 185, 187, 192
    drug safety and, 49-56, 59-60, 63-
        64
    GI disease and, 131-132, 133, 136,
        139
    pharmacokinetics and, 77, 78-79
    pneumonia and, 54
    retinitis and, 91
    virologic monitoring in, 226
Oropharyngeal disorders, 133-134
Overdosage, 61-62

PAA (phosphonoacetic acid), 186,
        190
Pancolitis, 137
Pancreatic disorders, 133
Pancytopenia, 87
p24 antigens, 203, 208-211
PCR (polymerase chain reaction),
        220-221, 224
Pediatric patients, 57-58, 63, 75, 77,
        156, 221
Pentamidine, 58
Peptide vaccines, 176
Peripheral nervous system dysfunc-
        tion, 225
Petechiae, 221

PFA (phosphonoformic acid) (*see* Foscarnet)
Pharmacokinetics, 71-79
 absorption in, 73-74
 assays in, 72-73
 distribution in, 74-75
 dosage in, 77-79
 drug interactions in, 79
 elimination in, 75-76, 77, 79
 of GM-CSF, 202, 205-211
 of intravitreal therapy, 107, 108-109
 in vitro, 72
 renal dysfunction and (*see* Renal dysfunction)
Phorbol ester, 160
Phosphokinase-C, 162
Phosphonoacetic acid (PAA), 186
Phosphonoformic acid (PFA) (*see* Foscarnet)
Phosphorylation, 2, 3-4, 31-32, 84, 94-95
 drug interactions and, 59
 drug resistance and, 186, 189-190
Plaque-reduction assays, 4, 6, 8-9, 18
Platelets (*see* Thrombocytopenia)
Pneumocystis carinii, 95, 125, 165
Pneumonia, 71, 193
 AIDS and, 224
 BMT and, 26, 148, 159, 220
 diagnosis of, 224-225
 drug safety and, 50, 52, 63-64
 Ig for, 27, 151-152
 drug resistance and, 188
 interstitial (*see* Interstitial pneumonia)
 MCMV-associated, 25-27
 solid-organ transplants and, 64, 145, 146-148, 156
 transplants and, 54 (*see also* specific types)
Polymerase chain reaction (PCR), 220-221, 224
Polyradiculopathy, 225-226
Probenecid, 79
Proparacaine, 110
Prophylaxis, 151, 164, 165, 175-176

Radiation, 165
Radioimmunoassay (RIA), 73
Rash, 48, 63, 87, 150, 174
Reactivation of virus, 155-156, 175
Rectal disorders, 136-137
Relapse:
 drug resistance and, 192, 193-194
 in GI disease, 140, 226
 in hepatitis, 148
 in pneumonia, 147-148
 in retinitis, 95, 99, 100-101, 102, 150
Remission:
 of GI disease, 138
 of leukemia, 171
 of retinitis, 84, 96-97, 100
Renal aplasia, 34
Renal dysfunction (*see also* specific diseases):
 AIDS and, 45-46, 58
 animal studies of, 33
 BMT and, 54-55, 172, 174
 dose adjustments and, 61
 Ig and, 168
 neutropenia relation to, 46
 pharmacokinetics in, 75, 76, 76-77, 79
 solid-organ transplants and, 63, 150, 151
Renal transplants, 2, 156
 drug resistance and, 187
 drug safety and, 53, 59-60
 hepatitis and, 149
 pneumonia and, 145, 148
 prophylaxis and, 176
Replication, 109, 215
 in animal models, 16, 17, 18, 19, 21-24, 25, 26
 BMT and, 160, 162, 175
 diagnosis and, 217
 foscarnet and, 88
 in retinitis, 94-95
Reproductive toxicity, 33 (*see also* specific disorders)
Resistance, 6, 7-8, 226, 227
 in AIDS patients, 151, 185, 188, 189, 191, 192, 193

[Resistance]
in BMT patients, 151, 192, 193
fatal disease due to, 186-189
frequency of, 189
implications for treatment, 192-194
mechanisms involved in, 189-192
in mutants, 186, 187
in retinitis, 84, 100, 151, 188, 189, 192, 193
in transplant patients, 185, 187, 192 (*see also* specific types)
Reticulocytes, 33
Retinal detachment, 49, 63, 86-87, 94, 101, 118, 125, 188
intravitreal therapy and, 109, 112
Retinal hemorrhage, 40, 93, 118-119, 121
ocular fundus photography of, 125, 127
ophthalmoscopy of, 122
Retinitis, 6, 49, 71, 83-89, 91-102, 115-127
AIDS-associated (*see* Acquired immunodeficiency syndrome)
animal models of, 18, 24
BMT and, 159, 224
breakthrough, 100, 120
diagnosis of, 93-94, 221
drug absorption and, 73-74
drug distribution and, 75
drug resistance and, 84, 100, 151, 188, 189, 192, 193
drug safety and, 37-38, 40, 42, 47-48, 60, 63
epidemiology of, 91-93
fluorescein angiography of, 125
foscarnet for, 1, 88, 106, 110, 112, 167
fulminant, 118-119
GM-CSF for, 45, 88, 100, 112, 198-211, 226 (*see also* Granulocyte-macrophage colony stimulating factor)
granular, 119
healed, 119-120, 121
HSV-associated, 94

[Retinitis]
improvement in, 127
intravitreal therapy for (*see* Intravitreal therapy)
leukemia-related, 188
natural history of, 93-94
ocular fundus photography of, 115, 123-127
ophthalmoscopic appearance of, 116-119
ophthalmoscopy of, 110, 115, 122-123, 127
reactivation of, 105, 106, 120-121
retinal detachment in (*see* Retinal detachment)
solid-organ transplants and, 149-150
stabilization in, 127
transplants and, 91 (*see also* specific types)
treatment for, 138 (*see also* specific agents)
efficacy of, 84-87, 94-99
failure of, 127
long-term outcome of, 100-101
new strategies in, 88-89
side effects of, 87, 99-100
varicella zoster-associated, 94
Retinopathy, 63, 94, 200 (*see also* specific disorders)
Retrovir (*see* Zidovudine)
RIA (radioimmunoassay), 73
Ribavirin, 5
RNA, 162, 220
RNA probes, 217
Rubella, 15

Salivary glands, 22, 24, 25
Scotoma, 86, 93
Seizures, 59, 150
Sepsis, 37, 38-39, 56, 106, 174
Serological diagnosis, 219-220
SGOT (glutamic-oxaloacetic transaminase), 33, 47, 48

SGPT (glutamate-pyruvate trans-
      aminase), 33, 47, 48
Shell-vial culture, 224
Sigmoidoscopy, 136, 139
Single doses, 32-33, 77-78
Slot/dot blot hybridization, 220, 224
Small bowel diseases, 135, 166 (*see
      also* specific types)
Solid-organ transplants, 145-152 (*see
      also* specific types)
   adverse treatment effects and, 150-
      151
   BMT compared with, 155-156, 163
   drug dosage and, 151
   drug resistance and, 192
   drug safety and, 53-54, 55, 63
   graft rejection in, 166
   hepatitis and, 148, 149, 156
   pneumonia and, 64, 145, 146-148,
      156
   renal function and, 55
   retinitis and, 149-150
Spermatogenesis, 59, 87
Splenomegaly, 221
Spontaneous remission, 84
Staphylococcus epidermidis, 109
Steroids, 134, 165
Stomach diseases, 134-135, 166 (*see
      also* specific types)
Sulfa congeners, 86
Sulfadoxine-pyrimethamine, 48
Surgery, 135, 137

T-cell immune therapy, 176
T cells, 25, 26, 136, 162, 175
Tenesmus, 136
Teratogenicity, 34, 62
Testicular atrophy, 33
Testicular hypoplasia, 59
Testosterone, 59
Thrombocytopenia, 4, 99, 100, 193,
      227
   in AIDS patients, 39-40, 42-43, 45,
      58, 62, 87, 199, 206

[Thrombocytopenia]
   in BMT patients, 52, 156, 157,
      163, 166
   drug interactions and, 58
   GM-CSF and, 206
   intravitreal therapy and, 110
   long-term dosing and, 57
   in solid-organ transplant patients,
      53, 150, 156
   ZDV and, 45
Thrush, 134
Thymic involution, 33
Thymidine kinase (TK), 2, 3, 16, 72
   drug resistance and, 190-191, 192
Tissue culture diagnosis, 217-218, 224
Tissue specimens, 215-216
TK (*see* Thymidine kinase)
TNF-α (tumor necrosis factor-α), 160,
      163
Torulopsis globrata, 133
Toxicity, 33, 78, 99-100, 108-109 (*see
      also* specific types)
Toxoplasma gondii, 95, 118
Transfusion recipients, 204
Transient cortical blindness, 174
Trifluorothymidine, 1
Trimethoprime-sulfamethoxizole, 58
Triphosphorylation, 94-95
Tumor necrosis factor-α (TNF-α),
      160, 163

Ulcers, 133
   colon, 137, 166
   esophageal, 134, 138, 166
   oropharyngeal, 133-134
   small bowel, 166
   stomach, 135, 166
Ultrawide-angle cameras, 124

Vaccines, 176
Varicella zoster, 94, 191, 192
Vidarabine (ara-A), 1, 145, 165, 167,
      191

Vinblastine, 84
Vinca alkyloids, 59
Viral shedding, 158, 199, 215
   drug resistance and, 189, 192-
      193
   monitoring of, 226
Viremia, 188, 193, 199, 207,
      220
Virlologic monitoring, 226-227
Viruria, 199, 207
Virus reactivation, 155-156, 175
Virus replication (*see* Replica-
      tion)
Vitrectomy, 112
Vomiting, 166

Wasting syndrome, 135
Wide-angle photography, 124, 126, 127
Wright-Giemsa, 216

ZDV (*see* Zidovudine)
Zidovudine (ZDV), 5, 189
   for GI disease, 134
   hematological effects of, 37, 40,
      41, 42, 43, 44-45, 54, 62
   interactions with other drugs, 58, 79
   myelosuppression by, 84, 86, 87
   for retinitis, 94, 100, 106
      GM-CSF and, 201, 202, 207-208,
      209

About the Editor

STEPHEN A. SPECTOR is Chief, Division of Pediatric Infectious Diseases and Professor of Pediatrics, Department of Pediatrics, University of California, San Diego. Additionally, he is a Member of the Center for Molecular Genetics at the University of California, San Diego, an Attending Physician at Mercy Hospital, San Diego, and a Senior Consultant at Children's Hospital and Health Center, San Diego. He is Co-Principal Investigator of the National Institutes of Health–sponsored AIDS Clinical Trials Unit at the University of California, San Diego, Principal Investigator of the Pediatric AIDS Clinical Trials Unit, and Director of the Children's and Women's HIV Program. Dr. Spector is the author or coauthor of more than 100 peer-reviewed articles, book chapters, and reviews; a Fellow of the Infectious Diseases Society of America and Pediatric Infectious Diseases Society; and a member of the Society for Pediatric Research, among other societies. He received the B.A. degree (1971) from the State University of New York at Buffalo and M.D. degree (1975) from Tufts University School of Medicine, Boston, Massachusetts.